DO NOT REMOVE

Nursing History and Humanities

This series provides an outlet for the publication of rigorous academic texts in the two closely related disciplines of Nursing History and Nursing Humanities, drawing upon both the intellectual rigour of the humanities and the practice-based, real-world emphasis of clinical and professional nursing.

At the intersection of Medical History, Women's History and Social History, Nursing History remains a thriving and dynamic area of study with its own claims to disciplinary distinction. The broader discipline of Medical Humanities is of rapidly growing significance within academia globally, and this series aims to encourage strong scholarship in the burgeoning area of Nursing Humanities more generally.

Such developments are timely, as the nursing profession expands and generates a stronger disciplinary axis. The MUP Nursing History and Humanities series provides a forum within which practitioners and humanists may offer new findings and insights. The international scope of the series is broad, embracing all historical periods and including both detailed empirical studies and wider perspectives on the cultures of nursing.

'Curing queers'

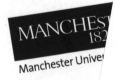

MANCHESTER
182

Manchester Univer

'CURING QUEERS'

Mental nurses and their patients, 1935–74

TOMMY DICKINSON

Manchester University Press

Published by Manchester University Press
Altrincham Street, Manchester M1 7JA
www.manchesteruniversitypress.co.uk

British Library Cataloguing-in-Publication Data
A catalogue record for this book is available from the British Library

Library of Congress Cataloging-in-Publication Data applied for

ISBN   978 0 7190 9588 7   hardback

First published 2014

Typeset by Servis Filmsetting Ltd, Stockport, Cheshire
Printed in Great Britain by TJ International Ltd, Padstow

To Mum, for all that you are
and
In memory of Mrs Lyle, a truly inspirational teacher

I can no other answer make but thanks,
And thanks, and ever thanks.
(William Shakespeare, *Twelfth Night*)

Contents

Figures

Front cover: Patient receiving electrical aversion therapy at Nerthern Hospital, UK. (Photograph reproduced by kind permission of *Times* Newspapers Ltd/NewsSyndication.com)

The inclusion of places or people who appear in the photographs in this book does not imply anything about their sexual orientation or their involvement with treatments for sexual deviations, either now or then. Every effort has been made to trace copyright owners of the images used in this book and anyone claiming copyright should get in touch with the author.

Note on terminology

Homosexuality

At this stage, in books on queer life at least, it is customary to offer a note about terminology, as finding appropriate language with which to discuss the historical organisation of male sexual practices and identities is particularly challenging. Matt Houlbrook argues that the terms 'gay'/'homosexual' and 'straight'/'heterosexual' are modern terms, and position such practices within a specific interpretive framework that cannot be applied easily to the past. Indeed, prior to the early 1970s, many men who had sex with other men did not consider themselves to be gay. The word only came into popular usage in the United Kingdom with the advent of Gay Liberation during the 1970s. Different labels were given to these men in the eighteenth, nineteenth and twentieth centuries, and included 'mollies', 'sodomites', 'inverts', 'maryannes', 'homosexuals', 'queens', 'queans', 'trade', 'gays', 'artistic', 'so', 'queers', and 'TBH' – 'to be had'. However, these labels were not necessarily synonymous, with each representing a different understanding of identity and desire. Therefore, I have used the term 'queer' in the title of this book to reflect queer in its broadest sense – not to collapse people together but to mean those considered queer in whatever (gendered or sexualised) ways.

However, for many men who suffered stigma in the last century – not least those whom I examine here, the term 'queer' may have pejorative meanings. It would seem ironic – and for the subjects themselves, inappropriate – to re-use that term within the book, albeit with a difference in meaning. I therefore use the labels of 'gay' and 'homosexual' (as appropriate in context) interchangeably throughout the book to describe men who self-identified as mainly being sexually and romantically attracted to other men. However, I acknowledge that some of these men would not have used these words to describe themselves during the time they were receiving treatments for their sexual deviations, even though they apply it to themselves retrospectively.

Transvestism

The term 'transvestite' was first coined by Magnus Hirschfeld in 1910. Hirschfeld invented the word from Latin *trans*, 'across, over' and *vestitus*, 'dressed' to refer to the sexual interest in cross-dressing. The definition of transvestite has always been contentious – not least for the two individuals interviewed for this book who received treatments for transvestism. The two participants never identified themselves as homosexual and stated that they did not get any sexual gratification from cross-dressing. They expressed an obsessive desire to assume the genitals and body of the opposite sex. Indeed, both the participants subsequently underwent gender reassignment surgery (GRS) and are now living as females. However, the first GRS was not undertaken in the UK until the 1940s, when Dr Harold Delf Gillies carried out GRS on Laurence Michael Dillon (born Laura Maud Dillon). Consequently, most men who sought or were referred for medical help relating to cross-dressing were labelled as transvestites even though the majority of them would never have identified themselves with this label. Therefore, in keeping with the terminology used during the period being discussed, I use the term 'transvestite' (as appropriate in context) to describe men who cross-dressed in the opposite sex's clothes. However, I acknowledge that both the participants in this book and many other men may not have used this word to describe themselves at the time when they were receiving treatments.

Mental health nursing

Mental health nurses have also been known by different names in the past. For the majority of the period being explored in this book, the most commonly used term was 'mental nurse'. This term is used throughout the book for consistency. For the same reason, the term 'patient' is used. However, I recognise that many people today would use contemporary terms such as 'service user', 'client' or 'survivor'. Furthermore, I acknowledge that the terms 'mental' 'lunatic' and 'mental hospital' that I also use in this book can have derogatory connotations for individuals today. Nevertheless, using contemporary terminology would impose current categories on the past. Therefore, the language of the past has been used to preserve clarity.

Acknowledgements

Like all histories, this book is a collaboration between its author and a vast number of historians, librarians, lecturers and archivists. My interest in history was first aroused by the reminiscences of my late nana, Mary Dickinson (nee Lambert), and grandfather, Joseph Murro. As a child, I would listen attentively to their fascinating anecdotes of living through World War II, especially my grandfather's experiences as an evacuee; they would have been delighted to see me complete this book. I miss them.

I am really excited that this book is appearing in the Manchester University Press (MUP) series, *Nursing History and Humanities*. The team at MUP have been a pleasure to work with. I am particularly grateful to the anonymous reviewers who took the time out of their schedules to read the manuscript for MUP; I have acted on much of their good advice.

My colleagues in the School of Health at the University of Central Lancashire, the Faculty of Health and Social Care at the University of Chester; and most recently at the School of Nursing, Midwifery and Social Work at the University of Manchester have been great. I have benefited remarkably from the open exchange of ideas with Geoff Speight, Susan Ramsdale, Professor Joy Duxbury, Dr Mick McKeown, Emma Walker, Marie Mather, Heather Turner, Sharon Pagett, Dr Bernard Gibbon, Professor Elizabeth Mason-Whitehead, Caroline Gibbon and Ian Denoual. Meanwhile Kim Greening offered some incisive comments and advice on several chapters. At Manchester, I have found a fresh energy from colleagues and students alike, which provided me with an exciting intellectual environment to complete the project. My thanks go to Professor Christine Hallett, Dr Jane Brooks,

Dr Sarah Kendal, Dr John Baker, Professor John Keady, Professor Karina Lovell, Professor Chris Todd and Dr Valerie Harrington. I would also like to thank Dr Matt Cook at Birkbeck, University of London, Professor John Playle at the University of Huddersfield, Dr Claire Chatterton at the Open University and Emeritus Professor of Staffordshire University, Peter Nolan. Their comments on various bits of this book, from sentences to entire chapters, have made me reconsider my work and think harder about my arguments. All encouraged me to clarify my prose and revisit ideas I had taken for granted. I hope they can find traces of their ideas which have helped guide this book. It is much better as a result of their input – thank you.

Researching my curiosities has been immensely enjoyable, and has been made all the more so by staff at the following institutions: the Lesbian and Gay News Media Archive (LAGNA), London; the British Library, London; the 'Opening Doors London' Project, Age Concern, Camden; the Glenside Hospital Museum, Bristol; Gay's the Word bookshop, London; the National Archives, Kew; the Bookshop Darlinghurst, Sydney; the National Archives of Scotland, Edinburgh; the Hall Carpenter Archives, London; the Royal College of Nursing Archives, Edinburgh; the 'Out in the City' Project, Age Concern, Manchester; and the former Oscar Wilde Bookshop, New York City. I'd also like to thank those who took the time to talk to me or respond to my emails (Professor Chris Waters, Professor Michael King, Dr Helen Sweet and Professor Janet Hargreaves).

I want to express my gratitude and thanks to Dr Anne Hickley at Penguin Office Services for her technological support, particularly when I was ready to throw my computer out of the window! The following for their permission to use illustrative material reproduced in this book: The Glenside Hospital Museum; *Times* Newspapers Ltd/NewsSyndication.com; *Nursing Times*; Trinity Mirror Group; and The Seattle Post-Intelligencer Collection, Museum of History & Industry, Seattle, Washington, USA. Also, the writer Alastair Jessiman for granting me permission to use his poem in the prologue.

Amazingly, organisations have funded this study. Therefore, my sincere gratitude goes to the University of Manchester: Mona Grey prize; The Royal College of Nursing: Monica Baly Award; The Royal Historical Society; and the Wellcome Trust.

Acknowledgements

I am lucky enough to have an amazing set of friends and family who have always been there when I needed them; they mean the world to me. They have humoured me, tolerated me, given their opinion on various cover pictures and generally coped with my obsession with 'Curing Queers'. For what it's worth, I offer my thanks to Donna Taylor, Sam Byers, Paul Tiebout, Leanne Ballantyne, Craig Joyce, Simon Hagley, Mark Faulkner, Bruce Heath, Jon Davies and Georgina Stubbs. To Will Osmond and Nicci Yarnold for carefully and scrupulously reading the whole manuscript and offering some intellectually savvy comments; and last but by no means least, Darren-Luke Mawdsley, for reminding me how much fun it is to be gay and for the careless nights out in London. It's been a joy being able to discuss the links between my study and theatre.

Most heartfelt thanks are reserved for my parents, Henry and Sheila. Their kindness and support has been unfailing.

Finally, my deepest gratitude goes to the twenty-five men and women whom I have interviewed for this book. Without them 'Curing Queers' would not have been possible. Thank you for inviting me into your homes and sharing your experiences. Some of the testimonies, especially those of former patients, were quite difficult to hear, and I admire your bravery in retelling me your stories. Your voices are finally being heard and I am forever in your debt.

Abbreviations

AIDS	Acquired Immunodeficiency Syndrome
APA	American Psychiatric Association
COHSE	Confederation of Health Service Employees
CMN	Chief Male Nurse
DHEW	Department of Health, Education and Welfare
DSM	Diagnostic Statistical Manual
ECT	electroconvulsive therapy
FANY	First Aid Nursing Yeomanry
GAA	Gay Activist Alliance
GLBTIQ	gay, lesbian, bisexual, transgendered, intersex, and queer/questioning
GLF	Gay Liberation Front
GNC	General Nursing Council
GP	general practitioner
GRID	gay-related immune deficiency
GRS	gender reassignment surgery
HCA	Hall Carpenter Archives
HMC	Hospital Management Committee
ICD	International Classification of Diseases
MPA	Medico-Psychological Association
NA	National Archives
NHS	National Health Service
PoW	prisoner of war
RAF	Royal Air Force
RCN	Royal College of Nursing
RHB	Regional Hospital Board
RMN	Registered Mental Nurse

RMPA	Royal Medico-Psychological Association
RN	registered nurse
SEAN	state enrolled assistant nurse
SEN	state enrolled nurse
SOE	Special Operations Executive
SRN	state registered nurse
SS	Schutzastaffel (Defence Detachment)
USPHS	United States Public Health Service
USSR	Union of Soviet Socialist Republics
WHO	World Health Organization

Prologue

A cautionary tale of Tom,
who denied his own nature and became a vegetable.

On a dark and fateful day in May,
Tom told his parents he was gay.
His mother shrieked; his father scolded.
(His granddad's pacemaker exploded.)
'Oh God!' roared dad, 'Our son's a pansy!
A fag! A fruit! A queer! A Nancy!'

Oh tell me, God, what have we done
To merit such cruelty from our son?
'My lad', said he, 'you've quite appalled
Your granddad, me, and most-of-all –
Your mother, who most painfully bore you.
Tom, for our sakes, I implore you
Go and see a doctor, *please*;
He'll cure you of this vile disease.'

So next day they took Tom to see
Doctor Tuffnell Williams MBE,
A man renowned through all the lands
For treating sexual deviants.
'Doc', said Dad, 'our son's a bender:
He fancies those of his own gender.
So make him normal, if you can,
And we'll make you a wealthy man.'
So Dr Williams set about

Trying to get Tom straightened out.
At first he started to cure Tom's ills
By filling him full of hormone pills –
To no avail. So then he jabbed him,
Poked him, pricked him, pierced him, stabbed him.
Tom didn't respond; he got much worse;
He'd fallen for a cute male nurse
Called Kenny, who had lovely dimples.
And a dial entirely free from pimples.
Ken loved Tom too. What bliss! What joy!
True love requited: Boy loves Boy!
So one night Ken and Tom eloped,
using their bed-sheets for a rope . . .

They fled by boat across the sea
And set up house quite near Portree
In a little cottage. Oh, what bliss!
There they'd cuddle, smooch and kiss,
And do the things that can't be done
Under the age of 21.
Those happy days continued, still
Down from the farm and over the hill
Came the farmer's son, one Dhonald Maclay,
And stole the heart of Ken away!
Oh fickle youth: Tom's love Ken spurned –
And all for a smile, and a large milk-churn!

Not caring whether he lived or died,
Tom forever left the shores of Skye,
And on the mainland went to see
Doctor Tuffnell, William, MBE,
And sadly said, 'Now listen, Tuff,
Make me normal – I've had enough.'
So, after a course of sixteen talks
On *The Joys of Marriage*, and electric shocks,
And little tablets for his genes,
And pornographic magazines –
Tom was cured. (So Tufnell said.)

And two years later, Tom was wed.
His parents were both overjoyed
That he's married a girl instead of a boy:
'And Mabel's such a lovely wife:
She'll see to him – she'll change his life.'
And they were right, for very soon her
Fruitful womb bore Tuffnell Junior.

But Tom ignored his little boy;
His heart was closed to any joy.
He rarely smiled – just watched the telly,
Ate KP nuts, and saw his belly
Grow and grow, till very soon
It had grown to the size of a barrage balloon.
Now and then, on a Saturday night,
He'd wander the streets, and perhaps he might
Visit a cottage (alas; not in Skye)
And find, perhaps, a lonely guy
Like him. But Mabel stopped all that,
And Tom grew silent, moped and sat
Chewing his nuts, grew fatter still,
Ate, moped, and grew, until
With a loud report TOM's BELLY BURST,
Filling the house with a cold, grey dust
'He never had time to say 'Beg your pardon',
Wept Mabel as they buried him in the garden.

And in that garden every year
Carrots, beans and sprouts appear
Where Tom was buried. There you'll find
Vegetables of every kind.

Moral

My poem's done. The ending's sad.
But can't we be both gay *and* glad?
It can be so (it's up to you),
If to yourself you remain true.
(Alastair Jessiman, 1982)

Introduction

On a winter evening in 1966, Percival Thatcher visited a public toilet on his way home from work in his family's butcher's shop in east London.[1] Percival did not need to use the facilities in the public toilet; he was 'looking for love'.[2] Here an 'exceptionally good looking young man'[3] approached Percival and made a sexual advance towards him. When Percival responded to his advance, he was arrested – the young man was an undercover police officer. Percival was charged and subsequently convicted of importuning and conspiring to incite the police officer to 'commit unnatural offences'.[4] He was given the option of imprisonment or to be remanded provided he was willing to undergo psychological treatment to 'cure' his 'condition'. In the belief that the psychological treatment would be a 'better option'[5] than imprisonment, he chose to receive the treatment.

Percival was transferred to a local National Health Service (NHS) psychiatric hospital and was subjected to what he described as 'a barbaric torture scene by the Gestapo in Nazi Germany trying to extract information from me'[6] and he thought he 'was going to die'.[7] What Percival had agreed to was to undergo aversion therapy in a bid to cure him of his homosexuality. The behaviour of the police officer was not unusual and entrapment by undercover police officers during the 1950s and 1960s was common practice.[8] Nurses were frequently involved in administering aversion therapies to cure such individuals of what were seen as their 'sexual deviations'.[9]

The heart of this book is primarily focused on such characters and narratives, which will be used as a way of interrogating questions of experience, motivation, feeling and perception in relation to the use of aversion therapy to 'cure' homosexuality and transvestism.

In this way, it seeks to offer fresh insight into both patients' and nurses' perspectives on these treatments. It uses testimonies of patients and nurses to explore the subject in ways that have not been attempted before, and to texture more broadly focused histories of these treatments and this period. This echoes recent moves towards micro-histories particularly when looking at sexuality and nursing, as a way of framing and answering questions about everyday life, experience and thought in relation to discourse and the bigger narratives and cultural assumptions we make about sexuality and nursing.[10]

This introductory chapter outlines the time scale and the geographical location of the research upon which this book is based, and goes on to debate the concept of 'deviance' and 'sexual deviance'. It provides an overview of the book, considers personal testimony as a historical source, and discusses key moments in the history of sexuality and mental health nursing (1533–1929), which are relevant to this book.

Anecdotal evidence of the testimonies of patients who received treatments for sexual deviations and medical attitudes towards them are scattered in the written and recorded accounts of gay, lesbian, bisexual, transgendered, intersex and queer/questioning (GLBTIQ) people.[11] However, with the notable exception of the joint work of Glenn Smith, Michael King and Annie Bartlett,[12] there is a paucity of academic literature exploring the experiences of individuals who were subjected to these treatments. In 2004, Smith and his colleagues conducted oral history interviews with twenty-nine people who received treatments to change their sexual orientation in the UK. The study concluded that the definition of same-sex attraction as an illness and the development of treatments to eradicate such attractions have had a negative long-term impact on the individuals who received them.[13]

The same year, King and his colleagues also conducted a study exploring the experiences of thirty health care practitioners caring for these individuals. They concluded that 'social and political assumptions sometimes lie at the heart of what we regard as mental pathology and serve as a warning for future practice'.[14] However, their study mainly focused on the testimonies of doctors and psychologists and only included one nurse. The role of the nurse in regard to nursing individuals receiving treatments for sexual deviations is a hitherto neglected aspect of nursing history. In addition, no study has specifically explored the testimony of men who received treatments for transvestism. Therefore, this book seeks to rectify these omissions by adopting oral history as the prime research tool to examine the experiences of and meanings that nurses and patients attached to certain 'treatments' to change sexual deviation in the UK. Furthermore, it seeks to explore why men received such treatments, how they experienced them, how they affected their lives, and their aftermath, to obtain a better understanding of the topic in question.

There is little written or published material that explores the perceptions of former patients' views in the history of nursing. Roy Porter warned that if patients' views are ignored in the history of health care, there is the potential for gross distortion. He argues that the omission of the patient perspective may lead to the continued silencing of 'those who travel in silence' through the mental health system.[15] Therefore, by using the experiences of former patients, as told through their own accounts, the researcher can obtain a better understanding of the topic in question and claim a 'history from below' which allows historians to see past practice from a new perspective.[16]

The period this book examines is 1935 to 1974. This period began with the publication of the first official report on aversion therapy being used to treat homosexuality. The report was by Louis Max, a psychiatrist, who required a homosexual patient to fantasise about an attractive same-sex sexual stimulus in conjunction with receiving an electric shock.[17] The book ends in 1974 with the seventh printing of the American Psychiatric Association (APA) *Diagnostic Statistical Manual* (DSM) version II, which removed homosexuality as a category of psychiatric disorder. Although published in the USA, this manual was widely utilised in the UK to aid healthcare practitioners to diagnose mental illness.[18]

This book is specifically about the treatments developed for sexual deviations in the UK. The treatments were administered elsewhere – not least in the USA and South Africa during apartheid.[19] However, given the dearth of literature specifically discussing these treatments in the UK, I decided to focus the book on this geographical area. Nevertheless, the APA is based in the USA and this is where the majority of the rhetoric regarding the eventual removal of homosexuality from the DSM took place. Therefore, Chapter 5 explores this literature and the implications it had for the UK.

Deviance

Given that the notions of what is considered appropriate and inappropriate result from complex interaction of institutionalised norms and laws, it is pertinent that the notion of 'deviance' is explored. My main concern, within this book, is with its shifting definition predominantly in relation to views of homosexuality, and the consequences of these changes. I am particularly interested in how nurses came to see the treatments they were administering for sexual deviation as appropriate and then inappropriate as the ideas of deviance shifted throughout the period covered by this book.

There are many ways to study what sociologists call deviance. Peter Conrad and Joseph Schneider note that there are two general orientations to consider in sociology that lead in distinctive directions and produce altered, sometimes conflicting conclusions about what deviance is and how sociologists and others should conceptualise it.[20] These are the positivist and the interactionist approaches. Conrad and Schneider state that the positivist approach accepts that deviance is real, that it occurs in the objective knowledge of the individuals who engage in deviant acts and those who respond to them. Essentially, this view rests on a second important notion – 'that deviance is definable in a basic manner as behaviour not within permissible conformity to social norms'.[21] The focus of positivists' study of deviance has mainly been on searching for its causes. From a sociological point of view, such causes have been attributed to terms such as social and/or cultural environment and one's socialisation. However, Conrad and Schneider suggest that positivists outside sociology typically search for causes in physiology and/or the psyche.[22] Therefore, the medical model of deviance is essentially a positivist one.[23]

Peter Aggleton suggests that the interactionist orientation to deviance perceives that the morality of society is 'socially constructed and relative to actors, context and historical time'.[24] Of fundamental importance to this view is the assumption that moral codes do not just happen; rather they are socially constructed and since they are

4

socially constructed, there must be constructors. Therefore, morality, and hence definitions of deviance, are arguably the product of certain people making claims based on their own vested interests, values, beliefs and views of the world. People who command comparatively more power within society are characteristically better able to impose their rules and sanctions on the less powerful.[25] Deviance, therefore, becomes the conditions that are defined as inappropriate to or in violation of certain powerful groups' ideals and moral codes. The interactionist view assumes that the behaviours defined as deviant are mainly voluntary and that people exercise some degree of 'free will' in their lives.[26] Arguably, deviance is socially defined, and research should focus on how such definitions are constructed, how these labels are attached to particular behaviours and people and what the consequences are, both for those labelled as deviant and for the authors of such attributions. It is pertinent at this juncture to note, however, that it does not mean that positivist and interactionist approaches are never combined in research; according to Conrad and Schneider, some of the best studies have adopted elements of both.[27] However, as discussed above, given that the notions of what is deemed appropriate and inappropriate result from complex interaction of institutionalised norms and laws, shared and internalised norms or mores, the main approach taken within this book is decidedly interactionist. My main concern is with the shifting of definitions of deviance, the explanations of such shifts, and the implications of these changes.

Sexual deviance

The definition of what is considered deviant sexual behaviour has slowly transformed within British society. This has not been a change in behaviour so much as a change in how behaviour is defined. Those deviant behaviours once defined as immoral, sinful or criminal were later interpreted as medical conditions, hence requiring treatment as opposed to punishment. Rehabilitation eventually replaced punishment. However, Michael King and Annie Bartlett suggest that medical treatments became a new form of punishment and social control.[28] These changes have not ensued by themselves; nor have they been the consequence of a 'natural' development of society or the inevitable advancement of medicine. The roots of these changes lie deep within our social and cultural heritage.[29] This book presents an analysis of the historical transformation of the definitions of sexual deviance from a 'crime' to 'sickness' and finally on to 'acceptance' and discusses the significances of these changes and the implications in terms of treatments administered for sexual deviance.

As awareness of the variability and multifariousness of sexual behaviour increased throughout the period examined in this book, the boundaries between normal and deviant sexual behaviour became more blurred. However, certain forms of sexual behaviour were generally held to be deviant. Paul Scott adumbrated the features that characterised such behaviour as follows:

> The elements of a comprehensive definition of sexual perversion should include sexual activity or fantasy directed towards orgasm other than genital intercourse with a willing partner of the opposite sex and of similar maturity, persistently recurrent, not merely a substitute for preferred behaviour made difficult by the immediate environment and contrary to the generally accepted norm of sexual behaviour in the community.[30]

This definition, which is taken from the 1960s, which is towards the latter part of the period covered by this book, emphasises that it is the continued and habitual substitution of some other act for heterosexual genital intercourse which primarily characterised behaviours called sexual deviation. Sexual deviations were separated into categories according to the predominant or outstanding sexual behaviour. These categories included homosexuality, prostitution, sexual activity with immature partners of either sex (paedophilia), transvestism and sex with dead people (necrophilia), animals (bestiality) or inanimate objects (fetishism). Also included were sado-masochism, sexual violence, rape, incest, exhibitionism, voyeurism and transsexualism.[31]

Treatments were developed for all of these categories of sexual deviations.[32] However, homosexuality was the category which predominately received treatments and where we can see clear shifts in attitudes towards individuals.[33] Six participants in this book received treatments for homosexuality. Transvestism was also treated fairly widely; however, not to the same extent as homosexuality, and only two participants in this book received treatments for this.[34] It is important to consider transvestism alongside homosexuality, as I discuss below how an arraignment in the late nineteenth century cast doubts over the distinctions between 'cross dressers' and 'sodomites'.

Moreover, transvestism currently remains classifiable as a mental disorder.[35] Nevertheless, while this book discusses the treatments developed for transvestism and the testimonies of the individuals who received treatment for this, it predominantly explores the cultural and medical attitudinal shifts towards homosexuality, which initially led to treatments being developed for this 'disorder', and subsequently on to the eventual removal of homosexuality from psychiatric diagnostic manuals.

This book is mainly about the treatments for sexual deviations in men. That is not to say that women were not subjected to psychiatric evaluation or advised to undergo these treatments – they were.[36] However, of all reported cases in the medical literature, only one published study discussed aversion therapy being administered to women.[37] Furthermore, no women came forward as research participants for this book. It is important to note that while female sexual deviation – predominantly prostitution – was inscribed within forms of investigation that mirrored the regulation of male sexualities, lesbianism remained invisible in the law.[38] When we consider that one of the main ways in which men were referred for these treatments was through a court order,[39] this could offer a context to explain the limited response from females to the study upon which this book is based and their limited presence in the literature. Moreover, the experience of homosexual women in relation to these treatments is likely to have been qualitatively different from that of men, and therefore out of the scope of this study.

Personal testimony as a historical source

The main source of primary data within this book is oral history testimonies. Oral history can be defined as:

> A systematic collection, arrangement, preservation and publication ... of recorded verbatim accounts and opinions of people who were witnesses to or participants in events.[40]

Ken Plummer argues that there are merits to this particular research method when scholars wish to explore hidden or taboo subjects.[41] Subsequently, John D'Emilio suggests that oral history 'has the power to enrich, deepen and expand enormously' the history of sexuality.[42]

Advantages of oral evidence to the history of nursing are that it can reveal the voices of women, ethnic and other minority groups, working people and sections of the middle classes who did not write autobiographies and who have been essentially hidden from history.[43] Further, official written records rarely cover the private yet crucial areas of family relationships, influences in childhood and episodes that prompted career decisions. This is pertinent to nursing, as so much nursing practice has been transmitted through the oral tradition, and it supplements the domains that have existing written and official material. Indeed, Kirby has argued:

> The conversations in the corridors on the way to meetings, or the chance remark when the committee had closed its business, add to the composite picture of negotiations around significant nursing legislation and policy making.[44]

Until recently the sources for gay history have been largely based on the writings of experts, writers and celebrities, with the 'ordinary' world of lesbians and gay men essentially hidden.[45] Oral histories, therefore, give a voice to those who have been marginalised so far. They can go further than complementing other available information sources: oral histories can also allow individuals varied interpretations of accounts from eyewitnesses that can stand alone. The benefit is that subjects do not have a wide-ranging agenda that have the potential to influence generations to come. Instead, they can relate events as they saw them and thus provide historians with the ability to use them in the way they see fit.[46]

Twenty-five participants were interviewed for this book: seventeen former nurses and eight former patients. Five participants were recruited from flyers posted on noticeboards of various gay bars, and seven participants were recruited from an article I wrote in a mental health nursing journal.[47] Two participants were recruited following an interview I conducted on the radio regarding the study. Another participant was recruited from a short presentation I made at a social group for older GLBTIQ individuals. The remaining participants were recruited by means of snowball sampling: the initial participants put me in contact with other individuals who had similar stories to tell.[48] I used face-to-face semi-structured interviews, which lasted a maximum of two hours, as any longer tends to overtire the

8

interviewee.[49] The interviews took place in the participant's home so as to be as informal as possible. These were audio-taped and transcribed.

Of the seventeen mental nurses interviewed, there were eight men and nine women. At the time of their interviews, their ages ranged from 63 years to 98 years. Two commenced nursing in the 1930s, five in the 1950s and eight in the 1960s. All the nurses had worked in NHS hospitals. All of the nurses identified themselves as having Caucasian ethnicity. One was originally from France and three were originally from the Republic of Ireland; the rest were from the UK, Jersey and the Isle of Man. The eight patients were male at the time they received treatments for their sexual deviations; however, two later underwent gender reassignment surgery and are now living as females. At the time of their interviews they ranged from 65 years to 97 years. Seven of the former patients identified themselves as Caucasian and one as having African Caribbean ethnicity. One was originally from Jamaica; the remaining former patients were from the UK and the Isle of Man (see Appendix for brief biographical details of the participants). Cook highlights the lack of research in the history of sexuality in the UK beyond the metropolis.[50] It was, therefore, a deliberate feature of the research for this book that participants were recruited from throughout the UK, the Channel Islands and the Isle of Man, thus offering a broader history of sexuality.

Intersubjectivity and composure

The intersubjectivity between the interviewer and interviewee and how this may have affected the 'composure' of the individuals in the book is a pertinent factor and needs exploration. However, to discuss the nature of intersubjectivity in oral history, one must initially be aware of the nature of the subjective and the objective within history and also of the concept of composure. Penny Summerfield argues that the 'concept of composure refers to the process by which subjectivities are constructed in life-story telling'. It occurs when an interviewee composes a story about themselves. It also refers to the way in which the interviewee seeks a sense of 'composure' from establishing themselves as the subject of their story.[51] Further, concerning intersubjectivity in psychoanalysis, Stolorow and Atwood suggest that:

The perspective of intersubjectivity is, in its essence, a sweeping methodological and epistemological stance calling for a radical revision of all aspects of psychoanalytic thought. An intersubjective field exists at a higher level of generality and this can encompass dimensions of experience – such as trauma, conflict, defence, and resistance – other than the self-object dimension.[52]

Therefore, using this definition of intersubjectivity, we can begin to understand that subjectivity from the interviewee's perspective involves a deeper analysis of the story being told than can be seen from a purely objective standpoint. Once intersubjectivity is brought into play, which involves the subjective nature of both interviewee and interviewer, it is a narrative told which involves the lives of both parties.

The recollections of sensitive experiences were often disclosed as a result of the confiding relationship of trust that was often built up with the participants.[53] The fact that I am gay may have helped to put the former patient interviewees at ease in terms of their confidence in telling their own personal stories. This concurs with the writings of James Sears.[54] Further, it aided in the ability of the individuals to compose their narrative, in that I was able to identify and empathise with elements of their story. Conversely, it could also have been counterproductive in some cases, particularly when interviewing the nurses, as they may not have wanted to tell me the whole truth about the treatments for fear that it might offend me.

However, as I am also a mental health nurse, I was also in some respects an 'insider' in relation to the mental nurses I interviewed.[55] Kate Prebble also believed she was an 'insider' to the mental nurses she interviewed. I would concur with her in that this status created a level of trust with the interviewees. She argues that this was mainly due to many mental nurses often experiencing the effect of stigma by association with mental illness and feeling misunderstood by other nurses and by the general public.[56] Nevertheless, my sexuality meant that I was in other respects an 'outsider' who had to demonstrate trustworthiness as a researcher. In spite of having an understanding of the practice, concepts and language of mental health nursing, I had to be aware that in relation to my interviewees' lived experience of providing these treatments I was indeed an outsider.[57]

Debates between the subjective and objective nature of various components of the telling of history are not new, and this is certainly the case in terms of oral history. In recent years, in a variety of disciplines, there has been a shift towards recognising and accepting the subjective nature of oral history, in so far as 'what the informant believes is indeed a fact (that is, the fact that he or she believes it) just as much as what "really" happened'.[58] A pertinent aspect of this subjectivity, therefore, is the role of the interviewer, who is facilitating the interviewee in their interpretation of their oral history, which has been described as the 'self-conscious analysis of the intersubjectivity of the interview'.[59] Michelle Palmer and her colleagues place this analysis within modern ethnographic theory, by which intersubjectivity is acknowledged rather than ignored, and as a result of which, through other people's stories, we become aware of our own story. Moreover, Grele argues that a purely objective view is 'a view from nowhere'.[60]

The rise of interest in intersubjectivity in oral history (and in many other disciplines) can therefore be seen as a consequence to a challenge to the reality of a supposedly objective viewpoint, which has also been influenced by a noticeable shift from quantitative to qualitative methods of information-gathering in history.[61] This move away from a putatively objective and quantitative standpoint to a more subjective and qualitative standpoint, allied with an appreciation of the challenge of the interviewer to be fully objective, has augmented the validity of intersubjectivity in oral history.

This has particularly been the case in terms of oral histories from a queer perspective. In *Edwin and John: A Personal History of the American South*, Sears appreciates not only the story of Edwin and John but also readily identifies with his own homosexuality as he enters the world of their story.[62] There is, therefore, an interaction of intersubjectivity taking place within the testimony of John, as he tells his story, and Sears as he relates to the story and as it brings his own story into stark relief.

Memory and subjectivity

The debate over the 'reliability' of memory has generated a great deal of contention in the historical literature. Alessandro Portelli argues that memory 'functions as an incessant work of interpretation and re-interpretation, and organisation of meaning.[63] Geertje Boschma and her colleagues argue that memories are very rarely a precise account of what happened, but are always a reconstruction of events and experiences. These change over time and through the process of selection, recollection and connection with other memories.[64]

Indeed, some participants' memories of dates and details of events did not always concur with written historical records. Nevertheless, over the years oral historians have come to view this 'unreliability' of memory as a resource rather than a flaw, which can provide vital clues to the meaning people attach to certain events.[65] As I analysed and interpreted the participants' testimonies, it became apparent that there were times when their memories were more important as an indication of personal meaning than as a source of empirical data.

Barrington Crowther-Lobley, for example, when recalling his time in hospital receiving aversion therapy, stated that, 'it was a miserable chapter of my life . . . the weather was always dark, cold and gloomy when I was in there too.'[66] Arguably his particular experience of the weather was coloured by his unhappy memories of his time in hospital. As I scanned for the incidence of internal and external discrepancies and incongruities, I was able to gain an understanding of the subjective experience and the numerous constructed identities, especially in relation to the meanings that nurses placed on aversion therapies. Indeed, Elizabeth Kenny argues that to supplement the authenticity of the data, one must learn from the subjective nature of oral history interviews.[67]

Arguably, in examining intersubjectivity, we can see a shift from the modern to the post-modern: a change from a modernist perspective, where there are accounts that can be observed and interpreted from an objective perspective, to a series of narratives where the subject, and therefore the intersubjective, are much more important, with objectivity less important than (as Sears suggests) authenticity.[68] Moreover, instead of seeing subjectivity as a limitation, I agree that it should be viewed as a positive, in so far as this allows the historian to see the authenticity of the data as complementary to 'empirical' insights. Indeed, these rich, subjective stories, in feminist historians Gluck and Patai's words, 'turn up the muted channel'.[69]

Of course, there is a danger with this type of history, which pays close attention to individuals' attitudes and values regarding a sensitive issue that the interviewees, particularly the former nurses, could give me what they think I want to hear. For example, interviewees may express their objections towards aversion therapy to 'cure' gay men and transvestites in today's *expected* language of abhorrence – having ironed out their doubts and hesitations in the intervening years. Indeed Harry Cocks argues that personal testimonies can be 'strategic and performative articulations'.[70] There is the potential that a book such as this could overlook continuity and overemphasise change, by measuring progress from a presentist perspective. On this point Jeffrey Weeks argues that it is challenging not to give a 'Whig interpretation of sexual history [. . .] who in their right senses would not prefer living today rather than fifty years ago?'[71]

Therefore, presenting evidence through the eyes of those interviewed, I do not intend to dwell on the benefit of historical hindsight or rely on progress narratives. Instead, I aim to adopt a similar approach to that utilised in Simon Szreter and Kate Fisher's book, which provides a nuanced and empirically based portrait of sexuality and intimacy within marriages, 1918–1963.[72] Szreter and Fisher do not dismiss the issues of 'selection, omission, distortion and retrospection' identified by the critics of the oral history methodology.[73] They recognise that the narratives of the participants in their book are influenced with layers of 'cultural consciousness [. . .] communal conventions, idealisation and nostalgia'.[74] Nevertheless, they go on to argue that dialogue with the present should be seen as productive rather than distorting.[75]

There is no denying that the present had an influence on the participants in this book. However, many participants were aware of the ways their own views had been challenged and transformed in the intervening years. Many of the former nurses now hold different (usually more liberal) views on homosexuality and transvestism and reflected constructively and informatively on their attitudinal shifts. Meanwhile, many of the former patients interviewed now felt aggrieved regarding the medical treatments they received, yet at the time they actually *chose* aversion therapy to avoid prison, as we have seen in the case of Percival Thatcher, or to free themselves of their own same-sex desires. My aim, therefore, is to explore these contentions and offer some interpretations for why nurses and patients came to see the treatments they were administering or receiving for sexual deviation as appropriate and then inappropriate, as ideas of deviance shifted throughout the period covered by this book.

Equality between researcher and participant

I was greeted into all the participants' homes and the majority welcomed the opportunity to reminisce about their lives. It was also apparent that they were aware that they were delivering their testimonies into the public domain, and despite sometimes finding the subject matter difficult, many sought to be helpful. Some participants had made active preparations for my visit by finding old photographs, hospital badges and nursing certificates to show me during the interview. There was evidence that most participants were keen to give a positive impression of themselves. Many of the interviewees had tidied and cleaned the house, dressed very smartly, and had prepared refreshments, as if for a special occasion. Indeed one of my most memorable interviews was with Una Drinkwater,[76] which was conducted over a pre-prepared afternoon tea consisting of smoked Scottish salmon and cream cheese sandwiches; freshly baked scones with strawberry jam and clotted cream; and a selection of handmade miniature cakes – all served on her best bone china. Nevertheless, despite these attempts to welcome me into their homes and put me at ease, Judith Stacey has gone so far as to state that the ideal of equality between academic researchers and their subjects is impossible to achieve.[77]

This possible power imbalance may have affected the composure in Albert Holliday. When describing his upbringing, he was able to articulate a very detailed picture of growing up in a working-class mining town where money was scarce, with his parents having six other brothers and sisters to feed. However, he commented:

> Although, I suppose your upbringing was very different and you didn't have to worry about such things. I imagine you are from a very middle class background.[78]

This comment clearly displays that the participant did not perceive me to be someone 'level' with himself in terms of social class, education and occupational identity. It is difficult to determine the extent to which this complex interplay between the interviewer and interviewee affected the 'composure' in the interviewee. However, it arguably affected the readiness of the interviewee to develop a relationship with me, as he may have believed that the perceived class difference made it difficult to relate to me; this would in turn impinge on the interviewee's ability to compose a story. On reflection, though, I was dressed very smartly, as I had given a paper at a conference earlier that day, and I introduced myself as a university lecturer. It was only at the end of the interview, when the recorder had been turned off and we were both chatting about where I grew up and my 'working-class' and nursing background, that I felt some equilibrium in the 'level' at which he perceived me. Therefore, for subsequent interviews, I found it beneficial to give a brief synopsis of myself and my background at the start of the interview.

Anonymity

Some feminist oral historians recommend that interviewers should encourage openness in their respondents by guaranteeing their anonymity.[79] Maintaining the participants' anonymity is done to protect respondents from public recognition, but this contradicts one of the aims of homosexual history, which is to allow a platform for gay people to embrace and share their pasts that have often been hidden from history.[80] However, in the process of engaging, interpreting and analysing their testimony, I decided to offer all participants anonymity, owing to my own role in writing about their past. My reason for this concurs with that of Paul Baker and Jo Stanley, who changed all participants' names in their study for their protection.[81]

Summerfield also gave all participants in her study pseudonyms, as she wanted to screen them from the public embarrassment, 'which [her] arbitration between their words and "the public" might cause'.[82] Summerfield goes on to argue that anonymity protects interviewees from the ultimate manifestation of the power inequity in the oral history relationship: 'the historian's interpretation and reconstruction in the public form of print of intimate aspects of their lives'.[83] In light of these arguments, pseudonyms are used throughout the book.

The medicalisation of sex

Sodomy was initially outlawed as a capital crime in England by the 1533 Buggery Act, under Henry VIII.[84] It was also the settled practice of the common law to treat any attempt to commit a crime as an offence in itself. Therefore, any homosexual act was regarded in the law as an attempt to commit sodomy, and, therefore, fell under the jurisdiction of this Act.[85] Harry Cocks argues that during the eighteenth century the common law had also made it possible to prosecute a number of fairly new offences, which fell under the auspices of 'unnatural crimes'. This term included sodomy, bestiality and any homosexual act or invitation to the act, usually described as indecent assault or 'assault with intent to commit sodomy'.[86] Until around the 1830s, men convicted of these crimes were often exposed in the 'pillory', which sometimes resulted in their being permanently injured or mutilated by the angry crowds.[87]

Starting in around 1780 and lasting throughout the nineteenth century, there was a sustained increase in the number of men who were being prosecuted for homosexual offences.[88] These crimes were considered to be some of the most loathsome and serious. However, the trial process was affected by the necessity of silence. Many judges and legal officials believed that the reports of these trials threatened to spread moral corruption and even encourage such offences – allowing even the notion of sodomy to enter the public's conscience was deemed to be dangerous within itself.[89]

However, given the rising tide of prosecutions, public discourse could not be prevented and the homosexual (and transvestite) were rarely out of the public eye during the course of the late nineteenth century, as headlines regarding these individuals were ever present in the press.[90] The influential press made it more obvious than ever that the sexual deviant was a matter of national and imperial interest, as they were seen to threaten the strength of the Empire.[91] This is important to note, as the media had a similar influence on the minds of unsuspecting observers in relation to sexual deviation and its medicalisation in the 1950s and 1960s, which is explored in Chapter 1.

The second half of the nineteenth century saw significant changes in the press.[92] Technological advances meant that newspapers could be produced more quickly than before, while the earlier abolition of advertisement, stamp and paper duties – in 1853, 1855 and 1862 respectively – and improved national and local transport infrastructures meant that more newspapers were on the market and were more widely available.[93] Cook argues that there was also a change in style within the press during the late 1800s, and the articles published were more direct and headlines and sub-headings became more descriptive, delivering mini-narratives at a glance. The new style press often took on a crusading mantle; they did not merely report on parliamentary, court and police action but also highlighted inaction and corruption.[94]

This could be said for a series of articles entitled *A Night in a Workhouse*, written by James Greenwood but reprinted under the pseudonym 'The Amateur Casual', which appeared in the *Pall Mall Gazette* in 1866.[95] Within these articles, Greenwood masqueraded as one of the poor to experience first-hand what it meant to be an inmate in a workhouse for indigent wayfarers, tramps and other homeless people.[96] Greenwood's writing had a sodomitical subtext, and suggested that sodomy was so contagious within the wards of these workhouses that it threatened to corrupt even innocent bystanders compelled by circumstances to witness it. This in turn fuelled its Victorian readers because it both helped to create and drew upon widely held fantasies and anxieties about poor men and their sexuality.[97] The publication of *A Night in a Workhouse* made visible the complex intersection of sexual and social politics in Britain at the time. These articles are important, as they demonstrate how the media began to reinforce the perception that homosexuals were a contagious risk who essentially polluted society. This notion prevailed until the 1970s and appeared to re-emerge with the AIDS crisis in the 1980s (discussed in Chapters 1 and 5, and within the epilogue).

Conversely, men had crossed-dressed for the English stage for centuries, and as a result of this, cross-dressing was more accepted by society. Rictor Norton argues that cross-dressing men and their associates have formed and retained their own set of customs and institutions since the early eighteenth century.[98] These men developed an identity among themselves in the eighteenth century as 'mollies' or 'mary-annes', and they established an intricate system of safe spaces and supportive relationships that enabled their connection with similar men to satisfy their sexual and emotional needs. These men were intermittently 'discovered' and prosecuted throughout the eighteenth and nineteenth centuries for same-sex sexual activity, as were those men who took advantage of casual opportunities for sex with other men in toilets and well-known cruising[99] areas, primarily in cities. However, Charles Upchurch argues that the state lacked either the means or the predisposition to mount a continued and pervasive campaign against them.[100]

Nevertheless, an arraignment in 1870 would bring two crossdressing men into intimate contact with the law, media and medicine. This indictment was the case of the *Queen* vs. *Boulton and Others*, which involved the arrest and trial of Boulton and Park for 'a misdemeanour related to their public cross-dressing'.[101] Ernest Boulton and Fredrick Park – known popularly as 'Stella' and 'Fanny' respectively – were arrested outside the Strand Theatre on 28 April 1870. They were dressed completely in women's clothes, and it was in this attire that they were brought before the Bow Street magistrates for 'conspiracy to commit a felony'.[102]

The prosecution in this case included the testimony of doctors who, having subjected the two men to an invasive physical examination, claimed to have 'medical proof' that the defendants had engaged in recurrent acts of anal intercourse.[103] This medical evidence cast doubts over the distinctions between 'cross-dresser' and 'sodomite', and Upchurch argues that this medical testimony essentially 'collapsed these two categories of individuals into each other'.[104] Peter Ackroyd argues that the cross-dressing of Boulton and Park had no malice and was not fetishistic, but 'outrageous and exhibitionistic', yet their behaviour merited public condemnation and the threat of vengeance. He goes on to argue that the reasons for this were that their appearance explicitly defied the fundamental ethos of their society; by refusing to adopt the 'phallic and utilitarian model' of male clothing, and by asserting instead the primacy of 'pleasure and ornamentation, they inverted the codes of a society, which had created its sexual and social images in the name of economic progress and material acquisition'.[105]

This arraignment was heavily publicised by the British press, with *The Times* referring to the proceedings as 'the most extraordinary case we can remember to have occurred in our time'.[106] Meanwhile the *Pall Mall Gazette* warned of the serious threat that the Boulton and Park case posed to the Empire's reputation, and advocated that fathers might feel obligated to keep their newspapers under lock and key for the duration of the arraignment.[107] The media were keen to express that there was a threat to British morality and manhood if sodomites such as Boulton and Park were living in central London. Upchurch argues that the mainstream press from the 1820s onwards heavily influenced societal perceptions of sexual deviations. He proposes that newspapers did not simply provide information about sex acts and offences but also offered readers normative judgements about appropriate and inappropriate male social identities and same-sex behaviour.[108] The media were instrumental in shaping images of deviance and therefore controlling and regulating it.[109] This arraignment is significant because it not only demonstrates the way that pathology starts to be written into accounts of sexual deviation, but also displays the influence that the media had in regard to shaping public perceptions of transvestism and homosexuality. In essence, the media were making the concept of effeminacy and cross-dressing more broadly threatening.

With each of these publicised sensations, Britons came closer to developing a vocabulary and an intellectual framework within which to place their understanding of the relationship between same-sex desires and behaviours on the one hand and homosexual identity on the other. It was within this highly charged atmosphere that Liberal MP Henry Labouchère changed the law regarding sodomy in an attempt to augment public morals. On 6 August 1885, the Labouchère Amendment to the Criminal Law Amendment Act was passed, which brought all practices of homosexuality between men under the auspices of the criminal law, and these were made illegal, whether conducted in private or in public.[110]

The late nineteenth century also witnessed a variety of scientific investigations into sexual pathology.[111] These investigations began on the continent in the 1860s, when, the German writer Karl-Heinrich Ulrichs began to describe the different types of homosexuality, or 'Uranism' as he called it, as a way of arguing for its social acceptance. Ulrichs identified three major categories: lesbians ('urninds'), homosexual men ('urnings'), and bisexuals ('uranodionings'). His ideas focused on the notion of the homosexual as a particular type of person that had characteristics, which were determined by their physiology, desire and psychology.[112] In 1886, Richard von Krafft-Ebing, a professor of psychiatry at the University of Vienna, published his seminal *Psychopathia Sexualis, mit besonderer Berucksichtigung der contraren Sexualempfindung* (Psychopathia Sexualis, with Especial Reference to Antipathic Sexual Instinct).[113] This publication offered a clinical analysis and formal classification of most major 'sexual perversions'. Krafft-Ebing's work is pertinent, as it transformed the approach to the perceived problem of sexual deviation from stringent legal containment and great social taboo to one of genuine and sympathetic medical concern.[114]

Early attempts to 'cure' homosexuality initially used hypnotic suggestion therapy, and in 1888, Krafft-Ebing began treating homosexuals using this approach.[115] However, Albert von Schrenck-Notzing of Munich was arguably the most noteworthy advocate of this therapy to treat homosexuality. Schrenck-Notzing first announced that he could cure homosexuality by hypnotism and suggestion theory in August 1889 at the First International Congress of Hypnotism, held in Paris. He reported that his homosexual patient had required forty-five hypnotic sessions over four months in order to reverse his homosexual desires. Three years later, Schrenck-Notzing published his monograph on suggestion therapy and sexual sense, which reported on seventy similar cases where homosexual and other 'perverse inclinations' had been either completely cured or significantly reduced through hypnotic theory. (In addition to hypnotic suggestion, Schrenck-Notzing's treatment included trips to local brothels in order to bolster these therapeutic suggestions!)[116]

In 1896, Havelock Ellis and John Addington Symonds published their masterwork on 'contrary sexual feeling' *Das konträre Geschlechtsgefühl* three years after Symonds' death.[117] The Symonds family later strove to have their name removed from the publication, which has subsequently been ascribed simply to Havelock Ellis. Ellis and Symonds were sexologists based in the UK; however, they initially published their work in German, as British publishers were frightened to print any works dealing with homosexuality in the aftermath of Oscar Wilde's well-publicised trial and conviction for gross indecency in 1895. Nevertheless, their work was published in English in 1897 entitled *Sexual Inversion*.[118] In using the umbrella term 'sexual inversion', Ellis and Symonds shifted away from the more detailed classificatory system presented in Krafft-Ebing's *Psychopathia Sexualis*.

20

Furthermore, Cocks argues that *Sexual Inversion* was the first British attempt to synthesise biological, anthropological and psychological knowledge on the subject of sexuality.[119]

Sexology was born as the study and classification of sexual behaviours, identities and relations. Lucy Bland and Laura Doan argue that the aim of sexologists was positive in that they wanted to stop discrimination and show that differences in sexual behaviour and desires were biologically and psychologically based rather than an unnatural perversion.[120] Ellis and Symonds employed the methods of sexology in order to show that 'perversity' of all kinds was merely one aspect of human sexuality and should be judged accordingly. They and other sexologists, such as Magnus Hirschfeld in Germany, opposed attempts to criminalise homosexuality. They advocated that sexual behaviour, and hence homosexuality, was inherent to the personality, as something inborn and congenital, either physiologically or psychologically. They argued, therefore, that it did not require treatment or punishment.[121] Sexology is important, as it was the first attempt to mark out a specialism and a unique discourse in relation to the medicalisation of sexual deviation, and it remained in vogue as the main method of classifying sexual behaviours, identities and relations from the late nineteenth century until the early twentieth century.[122]

In 1898, with virtually no debate, Parliament passed an amendment to the 1824 Vagrancy Act. The main impetus of the 1898 amendment was to expand the state's capacity to imprison bullies or pimps who lived on the earnings of female prostitution; however, it soon also became the Victorian state's draconian regulation of all forms of sex between men.[123] According to the Act, 'every male person who in any public place persistently solicits or importunes for immoral purposes shall be deemed a rogue and a vagabond and may be dealt with accordingly'.[124] Seth Koven posits that, in practice, the law was applied only to men who 'importuned' or 'solicited' other men for sex.[125] However, Cook argues that the 1898 provision of the Vagrancy Act heightened the significance of behaviour that was not explicitly sexual (such as the use of cosmetics and the way a man walked). The police did not simply arrest because homosexual acts had actually been committed, but also on the basis of a judgement they had made about the predilection of an individual to commit such acts.[126]

Michel Foucault has suggested that the period between 1870 and 1900 was significant in relation to the medicalisation of sexual behaviour, as this is where the sexological categories and lived social identities of both the 'homosexual' and the 'heterosexual' first came into being.[127] Koven concurs and argues that the period between the 1860s and 1890s irrefutably constituted a watershed in the histories of sexualities and the medicalisation of sexually deviant behaviour in Great Britain.[128]

In 1905, Freud's *Three Essays on the Theory of Sexuality* were published in German. This was a seminal work where he first described his psychoanalytical 'theories on the development, aberrations, and transformations of the sexual instinct from its earliest beginnings in childhood'.[129] Freud's new psychoanalytical paradigm on human behaviour combined two major casual tiers (one for *current* causes and one for *childhood* factors), along with a series of universal psychical mechanisms such as displacement and repression. With his new insights on human behaviour, Freud became a fundamental part of the burgeoning science of sexology. Freud's approach allowed him to adopt the best of the psychological and biological ideas advanced in sexology at the time. Moreover, Frank Sulloway argues that it was this dual construction to his theorising as a sexologist, which made Freud's thinking as a psychoanalyst so enduring.[130]

Following translation, Freud's work began to have a pioneering influence in the treatment and understanding of sexual deviation in Britain.[131] Freud believed that 'homosexual and heterosexual object choices were simply two outcomes of each person's unique development, a process that began in a shared, polymorphous, infant bisexuality'.[132] Freud purported that 'every male had to pass through a phase of homosexuality as a way of delivering himself from the Oedipus complex'.[133] Freudian arguments of homosexuality in Britain had made considerable headway by the 1930s:

> Homosexuality is nothing to be ashamed of, no vice, no degradation; it cannot be classified as an illness; we consider it to be a variation of the sexual function, produced by certain arrest of sexual development.[134]

In the 1930s, Chris Waters suggests that optimism regarding psychiatric treatment of the homosexual offender, and other psychiatric conditions was widespread and this is explored in Chapter 2. Though in that decade few of the suggestions pertaining to treatment of the former were implemented, doctors, magistrates and barristers began calling for institutions where homosexuals could be isolated and treated, as psychological explanations for sexual behaviour were more frequently cited in court cases.[135] Such ideas were indebted to Freud in so far as they developed from the idea that, as one medical officer put it, homosexuality was a mental disorder that arose 'from repressive influences in infancy and childhood which retard or distort the normal development of the sex instinct' – a state of arrested development that required therapeutic intervention.[136] However, one Dorset doctor had a more antipathetic view of how to manage these individuals, advocating that special gas chambers should be attached to courts for the immediate execution of such 'sex perverts' post-prosecution.[137]

Nevertheless, with the outbreak of World War II, there appeared to be a relaxing of attitudes towards homosexuality; this is discussed further in Chapter 1. A cultural shift in the immediate post-war years, however, urged the nation to return to pre-war values, and during the 1950s and 1960s treatments for sexual deviations really came to the fore. The narrative of the ways in which homosexuals and transvestites have been regarded and treated by British society is taken further in Chapter 1 where the introduction of aversion therapies for 'sexual deviance' are considered.

History of mental nursing

Not only were there changes and developments in the ways that homosexuals and transvestites were viewed by society and the treatment they received: the profession of mental nursing has also seen considerable changes and developments over the years. Since this book is exploring the role nurses played in the treatment of sexual deviants, and given the nature of newness of this book in relation to the history of nursing, it is pertinent that the wider history of the profession is also explored.

Prebble shows that histories of mental nursing have proliferated since the 1980s. She goes on to posit that in the first instance, they were add-on aspects of broader nineteenth-century asylum studies, but they later shifted to consider the workers themselves.[138] Historians such as Michael Arton, Diane Carpenter, Patricia D'Antonio, Anne

Digby, John Hopton, Nancy Tomes, Ellen Dwyer, Olga Church, Peter Nolan, Geertje Boschma, Veryl Tripisk, John Adams, Angela Martin, Kate Prebble, Claire Chatterton and Philip Maude have produced noteworthy accounts of the life and work of attendants and nurses.[139] As a leading scholar in the field, Peter Nolan argues that the history of mental nursing has at best been considered an appendage either to general nursing or to medicine and, at worst, an insignificance meriting minimal or no credit in the history of care.[140] He goes on to explain: 'having a history confirms the legitimacy of the services one provides'.[141]

Initially, staff who worked within the early asylums in the UK were referred to as 'keepers', a title that applied to both male and female staff and dated back to medieval times.[142] Following the 1845 Lunacy Act the term 'attendant' became the norm. This also reflected a cultural shift within the asylums, as attendants were now expected to 'attend' to the patients and the institution rather than simply 'keep' them confined.[143] The asylums were expected to be self-financing and self-sufficient; this meant that labour costs had to be kept to a minimum. Therefore, staff and patients were expected to undertake a wide variety of duties, which included maintaining the buildings and farming duties.[144] The large majority of the workforce was made up of male attendants who occupied the middle ground between doctors and the patients. Their status was considered very much inferior to that of the medical staff. However, their closeness to the patients made them extremely pertinent in the patients' lives.[145] The majority of asylums, like general hospitals, referred to the female attendants as 'nurses'.[146] Nolan argues, however, that these attendants and nurses were all pioneers and laid down the foundations of contemporary mental health nursing. They represented cheap labour, and in the majority of asylums during the 1850s and 1860s, they received no training; nor was there any career structure for them.[147]

Initially, the attendants' role was not clearly defined; this largely depended on the way the medical superintendent of the asylum saw it. Some viewed the attendants as obedient servants of the institution to keep and enforce rules; others saw them as principally servants to the patients; others again saw their role as that of spiritual guides. There was also the view that the attendants were simply intermediaries between doctors and patients.[148] Moreover, these individuals did not have a body of knowledge upon which to base a coherent system of care and treatment.

It was not until 1884 that the Medico-Psychological Association (MPA), which was run by doctors, finally accepted that there was some advantage in training attendants, and Drs Campbell Clark, McIvor Campbell, Turnball and Urquart were commissioned to prepare a handbook which would help attendants 'to a due understanding of their work in which they were engaged'.[149] In 1885, they completed their task and *The Handbook for the Instruction of Attendants on the Insane* was published.[150]

Nolan has argued that this handbook was a milestone in the history of training mental health nurses, as it gave the attendants a semblance of scientific credibility and the beginning of a literature base. Nurses who wanted to advance had to be able to read and quote from it.[151] By 1889, the MPA had decided that a national training scheme was required for attendants. Therefore, the decision was made that attendants would undergo a two-year training course, following a three-month probation period. At the end of this, the attendants would sit an exam, with successful completion leading to a Certificate in Nursing the Insane and registration with the MPA. Once attendants' names were entered on the Association Register, their Superintendents were held responsible for their conduct and anyone found guilty of misconduct was to be reported to the Registrar, who could remove his/her name from the Register and advise dismissal.[152] Nevertheless, despite a new education system, nursing was still based on '"common sense" assumptions and concern with neatness rather than on research-based theory'.[153] This ideological structure has important implications for this book, and is explored further in Chapters 2, 3 and 4.

In 1890, the Lunacy Act came into force, and confirmed that the practice of psychiatry was firmly established within the confines of mental institutions.[154] There were very few developments in mental nursing between 1890 and 1918. However, the World War I was a critical period in the history of psychiatry. The mental hospitals were depleted of able-bodied staff called up for military service, while the patient population of certain hospitals increased immensely, as patients were transferred from other hospitals that had been commissioned to treat wounded soldiers.[155]

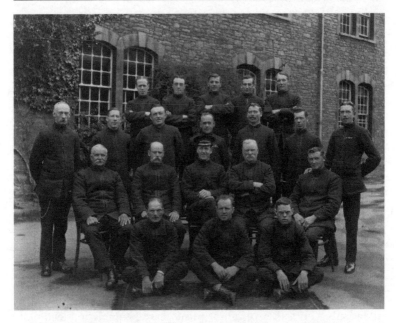

1 Male attendants at Bristol Lunatic Asylum, circa 1910s

At the end of 1919, the Nurses' Registration Act for England, Scotland, Wales and Ireland received royal assent. This established a register for general nurses with supplementary sections for other groups, including 'mental nurses',[156] and at the end of 1919, nursing registration became enshrined in law.[157] Then, in 1920, the General Nursing Council (GNC) agreed to accept holders of the MPA's Certificate in Nursing the Insane, as eligible for admission to the supplementary register for a 'period of grace'.[158] In the early 1920s, the GNC also set up their own alternative qualification, and the first cohort of mental nurse trainees sat the GNC's examination in 1922.[159]

New honours, however, could not disguise the confusion which was widespread among doctors, nurses and boards of governors as to the role of mental hospitals. The staffing levels were reducing yet patient numbers were increasing, and the country was in an economic depression which deprived health services of resources.[160] A similar incident happened after World War II, and the effects of this are discussed in Chapter 2, as it contributed and influenced the work of mental nurses caring for patients receiving treatments for their sexual deviations.

In response to these pressures, in the 1920s, psychiatry began to look to community care as a way of relieving the pressure on hospitals. The very early moves towards community care were consolidated in the Mental Treatment Act 1930, and with this new Act, asylums formally became hospitals.[161] Although asylum doctors had long been talking about 'patients' with 'mental illness', and had constantly sought closer contact with general medicine, it was not until the passing of the Act that the concept of mental disorder as illness was cautiously accepted.[162] This was the first major revision of mental health policy since the 1890 Lunacy Act and brought to the fore new and innovative ideas such as observation wards, outpatient clinics and aftercare facilities. It also provided for the voluntary admission of patients to mental hospitals and placed a new emphasis on a model of treatment. The implications of the introduction of this new Act of 1930 are explored in Chapter 2.

The structure ahead

This book shuttles between two levels of discussion throughout. The first part of the book – here in the introduction and in Chapter 1 – sketches out and discusses some broader histories and approaches which couch the detailed oral history work that follows. The main chapters (2–4) deliberately focus on the oral history interviews conducted as part of this book. However, I fully recognise the significance of the documentary, printed and published sources. Indeed, a number of the 'published sources' in the bibliography are, in fact, primary sources, which demonstrates the wealth of primary sources upon which this book is based. The oppression and suppression of the sexual deviant are examined in Chapter 1. The narrative of the ways in which homosexuals and transvestites have been regarded and treated by British society are explored and the introduction of aversion therapies for sexual deviance considered. The mixed and muddled messages nurses were receiving about these individuals are also discussed.

During the 1930s–1950s, mental health care witnessed a spirit of 'therapeutic optimism' as new somatic treatments and therapies were introduced in mental hospitals. Chapter 2 examines the impact these had on the role of mental nurses and explores how such treatments may have essentially normalised nurses to implement painful and distressing 'therapeutic' interventions to patients in their care. Attention is also given to investigating the effect of hospital conditions, as despite these new therapeutic approaches the nurses were still working within asylum type conditions. Overcrowding, lack of resources and understaffing all contributed and influenced the work of mental nurses. Finally, the chapter reveals a hitherto undiscovered history of gay life among homosexual male nurses in mental hospitals.

Some nurses in this book appeared to have behaved in a subservient, unenquiring and unquestioning manner that resulted in, or at least contributed to, their behaviour and participation in what could now be perceived as professionally incongruent activities. Chapter 3 deconstructs and offers some possible interpretations for why these nurses may have behaved in this way.

Some nurses in this book, albeit very few, conscientiously objected to the medical treatments for sexual deviations. These nurses engaged in some fascinating subversive behaviours in order to avoid participating in this aspect of clinical practice. Chapter 4 examines and interprets the testimonies of these 'subversive nurses'.

By the 1970s, individuals were beginning to question the definition of 'difference'. Gay men and women were starting to unite and promote sexual and subcultural difference as positive and life-enhancing as gay liberation emerged – individuals were actively and vocally refuting the sickness label and the treatment that had come to accompany it. This eventually led the APA to remove the term 'homosexuality' from its DSM. Chapter 5 considers these issues and also explores the inception of 'nurse therapists' and discusses their role in administering aversion therapy. This chapter deliberates the implications of these changes and examines how nurses began to view medical treatments for sexual deviation as inappropriate as ideas of deviance shifted.

'Curing Queers' draws to a close by offering some concluding remarks regarding the research upon which it is based. Ideas are drawn together in order to cast light on the possible meanings that nurses attached to the treatments for sexual deviations. The final section serves as an epilogue. In spite of the fact that these treatments appeared to peter out in the mid- to late 1970s, following the decision by the APA to remove homosexuality as a diagnosis and a growing gay liberation movement, it was not until 1992 that the World Health Organization (WHO) removed 'homosexuality' from its diagnostic manual. Therefore, the period 1974–1992 is explored to offer a context to help interpret why the WHO did not follow the example of the APA and remove 'homosexuality' from its diagnostic manual until 1992.

Notes

1 Percival Thatcher (pseudonym), interviewed 29 April 2010. All participants have been given pseudonyms. For a detailed discussion regarding anonymity of the participants, please see above; biographical details of all participants in the book can be found in the appendix.

2 Percival Thatcher, interviewed 29 April 2010.

3 Percival Thatcher, interviewed 29 April 2010.

4 Percival Thatcher, interviewed 29 April 2010.

5 Percival Thatcher, interviewed 29 April 2010.

6 Percival Thatcher, interviewed 29 April 2010.

7 Percival Thatcher, interviewed 29 April 2010.

8 For an exploration of the police regulation of homosexuality: see, e.g., Matt Houlbrook, *Queer London: Perils and Pleasures in the Sexual Metropolis, 1918–1957* (Chicago, 2005), pp. 19–43; Patrick Higgins, *Heterosexual Dictatorship: Male Homosexuality in Postwar Britain* (London, 1996); Stephen Jeffery-Poulter, *Peers, Queers & Commons. The Struggle for Gay Law Reform from 1950 to the Present* (London, 1991), pp. 169–172.

9 See, e.g., 'A Nursing Sister's Advice to Homosexuals', *Johannesburg Star* (25 November 1968).

10 See, e.g., Carlo Ginzburg, John Tedeschi and Anne C. Tedeschi, 'Microhistory: Two or Three Things That I Know about It', *Critical Inquiry* 20 (1993), pp. 10–35; Matt Cook, 'Gay Times': Identity, Locality, Memory, and the Brixton Squats in 1970s London', *Twentieth Century History* 9 (2011), pp. 1–26; Diana Gittins, *Madness in its Place: Narratives of Severalls Hospital, 1913–1997* (London, 1997); John Adams, 'Challenge and Change in a Cinderella Service: A History of Fulbourn Hospital, Cambridgeshire, 1953–1995' (PhD thesis, The Open University, 2009).

11 See, e.g., Duncan Fallowell and April Ashley, *April Ashley's Odyssey* (London, 1982), pp. 30–32; Pete Price, '*Namesdropper*' (Liverpool, 2007), pp. 85–90; Chris Brickell, *Mates & Lovers: A History of Gay New Zealand* (Auckland, 2008) pp. 272–273; Alkarim Jivani, *It's Not Unusual: A History of Lesbian*

and *Gay Britain in the Twentieth Century* (London, 1997), pp. 122–128; Roger Davidson, *And Thus Will I Freely Sing: An Analogy of Gay and Lesbian Writings from Scotland* (Edinburgh, 1989), pp. 154–159; Bob Cant, *Footsteps and Witnesses: Lesbian and Gay Life Stories from Scotland* (Edinburgh, 1993), p. 49.

12 Glenn Smith, Michael King and Annie Bartlett, 'Treatments of Homosexuality in Britain since the 1950s – An Oral History: The Experience of Patients', *British Medical Journal* 1136 (2004), pp. 1–4.

13 Smith, King and Bartlett, 'Treatments of Homosexuality in Britain since the 1950s', p. 2.

14 Smith, King and Bartlett, 'Treatments of Homosexuality in Britain since the 1950s', pp. 187–201.

15 Kerry Davies, 'Silent and Censured Travellers? Narratives and Patients Voices: Perspectives on the History of Mental Health since 1948', *Social History of Medicine* 14 (2) (2001), p. 271.

16 Roy Porter, 'The Patient's View: Doing History from Below', *Theory and Society* 14 (2) (1985), pp. 175–198.

17 Louis W. M. Max, 'Breaking up a Homosexual Fixation by the Conditional Reaction Technique: A Case Study', *Psychological Bulletin* 32 (1935), p. 734.

18 American Psychiatric Association, *Seventh Printing Diagnostic Statistical Manual Version II* (Arlington, 1974). It is important to note that the World Health Organization only decided to drop the term 'homosexuality' as a diagnosis in 1990. It was eventually removed from their diagnostic manual in 1992, with the introduction of the *International Classification of Diseases edition 10 Classification of Mental and Behavioural Disorders* (ICD-10). Nevertheless, there is a paucity of literature describing treatments for homosexuality after 1974, and the literature (explored in Chapter 5), describes how the publication of the seventh printing of the DSM II, combined with a fresh gay liberation movement in the 1970s, was seminal in the curtailment of these treatments. Additionally, no participants in this book reported receiving treatments after this date. Therefore, the decision was made to end the book in 1974. However, the period, 1974–1992 is discussed in the epilogue.

19 See, e.g., Ronald Bayer, *Homosexuality and American Psychiatry: The Politics of Power* (Princeton, 1987); Jack Drescher and Joseph P. Merlino, *American Psychiatry and Homosexuality: An Oral History* (New York, 2007); 'A Neurosis Is Just A Bad Habit', *New York Times* (4 June 1967); Robert M. Kaplan, 'Treatment of Homosexuality During Apartheid', *British Medical Journal* 329 (2004), p. 1415.

20 Peter Conrad and Joseph W. Schneider, *Deviance and Medicalization: From Badness to Sickness* (Philadelphia, 1980), p. 1.

21 Conrad and Schneider, *Deviance and Medicalization*, p. 2.

22 Conrad and Schneider, *Deviance and Medicalization*, p. 2.
23 Peter Aggleton, *Deviance* (London, 1987), p. 17; Conrad and Schneider, *Deviance and Medicalization*, p. 2.
24 Aggleton, *Deviance*, p. 17.
25 Conrad and Schneider, *Deviance and Medicalization*, p. 2.
26 Conrad and Schneider, *Deviance and Medicalization*, p. 2.
27 Conrad and Schneider, *Deviance and Medicalization*, p. 2.
28 Michael King and Annie Bartlett, 'British Psychiatry and Homosexuality', *British Journal of Psychiatry* 175 (1999), pp. 106–113.
29 Conrad and Schneider, *Deviance and Medicalization*, p. 1.
30 Paul D. Scott, *Definition, Classification, Prognosis and Treatment of Sexual Deviation* (London, 1964), p. 34.
31 Ismond Rosen, *Sexual Deviation* (Oxford, 1979), p. 3.
32 See, e.g., John Bancroft, *Deviant Sexual Behaviour: Modification and Assessment* (Oxford, 1974); Rosen, *Sexual Deviation*.
33 Rosen, *Sexual Deviation*, p. 5.
34 Bancroft, *Deviant Sexual Behaviour*, p. 29.
35 The current versions of the Diagnostic Statistical Manual and the International Classification of Diseases both classify transvestism as a mental disorder: 'Transvestic Fetishism' (DSM: 302.3) American Psychiatric Association, *Diagnostic Statistical Manual Version IV* (Washington, 1994); 'Transvestism' (ICD: F64.1) World Health Organization, *The International Classification of Diseases version 10 Classification of Mental and Behavioural Disorders* (Geneva, 1992).
36 See, e.g., Jennifer Terry, 'Lesbians under the Medical Gaze: Scientists Search for Remarkable Differences', *The Journal of Sex Research* 27 (1990), pp. 317–339; Jivani, *It's Not Unusual*, p. 127; Henry L. Minton, 'Community Empowerment and the Medicalization of Homosexuality: Constructing Sexual Identities in the 1930s', *Journal of the History of Sexuality* 6 (1996), pp. 435–458.
37 Michael J. McCulloch and Michael P. Feldman, 'Aversion Therapy in the Management of 43 Homosexuals', *British Medical Journal* 4 (1967), p. 595.
38 See, e.g., Judith Walkowitz, Prostitution and Victorian Society: Women, Class and the State (Cambridge, 1980), pp. 7–8; Houlbrook, *Queer London*, p. 10; Lillian Faderman, *Surpassing the Love of Man: Romantic Friendship and Love Between Women from Renaissance to the Present* (London, 1985).
39 John Bancroft, 'Aversion Therapy of Homosexuality: A Pilot Study of 10 Cases', *The British Journal of Psychiatry* 115 (1969), p. 1418.
40 Winnifred W. Moss, *Oral History Programme Manual* (New York, 1974), p. 7; see, also, Paul Thompson, *The Voice of the Past: Oral History* (Oxford, 2000), p. 2.

41 Ken Plummer, *Telling Sexual Stories: Power, Change and Social World* (London, 1995), p. 35.

42 John D'Emilio, 'Afterword: "If I knew then . . .", in Nan A. Boyd and Horacio N. Roque Ramirez (eds), *Bodies of Evidence The Practice of Queer Oral History* (Oxford, 2012), p. 269.

43 Gina Safier, 'What is Nursing History? What are the Advantages and Disadvantages of Oral History? How can it be Used in Nursing History?', *Nurse Researcher* 25 (5) (1976), p. 384; Moss, *Oral History Programme Manual*, p. 35.

44 Stephanie Kirby, 'The Resurgence of Oral History and the New Issues it Raises', *Nurse Researcher* 5 (1997), p. 47.

45 Jeffrey Weeks and Kevin Porter, *Between the Acts: Lives of Homosexual Men 1885–1967* (London, 1998), p. viii.

46 Joan W. Scott, 'The Evidence of Experience', *Critical Inquiry* 17 (4) (1991), p. 776.

47 Tommy Dickinson, 'Nursing History: Aversion Therapy', *Mental Health Practice* 13 (5) (2010), p. 13.

48 Kirby, 'The Resurgence of Oral History and the New Issues it Raises', p. 48.

49 P. Abbott and R. Sapsford, *Research Methods for Nursing and the Caring Professions* (London, 2007), p. 267.

50 Matt Cook, Personal Communication.

51 Penny Summerfield, 'Culture and Composure: Creating Narratives of the Gendered Self in Oral History Interviews', *Cultural and Social History* 1 (2004), p. 69.

52 Robert D. Stolorow and George E. Atwood, *Context of Being: The Intersubjective Foundations of Psychological Life* (Hillsdale, 1992), pp. 18–42.

53 Simon Szreter and Kate Fisher, *Sex Before the Sexual Revolution: Intimate Life in England, 1918–1963* (Cambridge, 2010), p. 6.

54 James T. Sears, *Edwin and John: A Personal History of the American South* (New York, 2009).

55 Perks and Thomson, *The Oral History Reader*, p. 67.

56 Prebble, 'Ordinary Men and Uncommon Women', p. 23.

57 Prebble, 'Ordinary Men and Uncommon Women', p. 23.

58 Perks and Thomson, *The Oral History Reader*, p. 178.

59 Michelle Palmer, Marianne Esolen, Susan Rose, Andrea Fishman and Jill Bartoli, 'I Haven't Anything to Say': Reflections of Self and Community in Collecting Oral Histories, in Ronald K Grele (ed.), *International Annual of Oral History, 1990: Subjectivity and Multiculturalism in Oral History* (New York, 1992), pp. 9–42.

60 Grele, *International Annual of Oral History*, 1990, p. 2.

61 Donald A. Ritchie, *Doing Oral History: A Practical Guide* (New York, 2003), pp. 103–104.

62 Sears, *Edwin and John: A Personal History of the American South*, p. xv.

63 Alessandro Portelli, 'What Makes Oral History Different?', in Robert Perks and Alistair Thompson (eds), *The Oral History Reader*, 2nd edn (London, 1998), p. 33.

64 Geertje Boschma, Margaret Scaia, Nerrisa Bonifacio and Erica Roberts, 'Oral History Research', in Sandra B. Lewenson & Eleanor K. Herrman (eds.) *Capturing Nursing History: A Guide to Historical Methods in Research* (New York, 2007), p. 84; on this point, see also Cook, *Brixton Squats in 1970s London*; Paul Connerton, *How Societies Remember* (Cambridge, 1989); Mary Evans, *Missing Persons: The Impossibility of Auto/Biography* (London, 1998).

65 Alistair Thomson, 'Fifty Years On: An International Perspective on Oral History', *The Journal of American History* (September 1998), pp. 584–588.

66 Barrington Crowther-Lobley, interviewed 28 April 2010.

67 Elizabeth Lapovsky Kennedy, 'Telling Tales: Oral History and the Construction of Pre-Stonewall Lesbian History', Robert Perks and Alistair Thomson (eds), *The Oral History Reader*, 2nd edn (New York, 2006), p. 281.

68 Sears, *Edwin and John: A Personal History of the American South*, p. xvi.

69 Sherna Gluck and Daphne Patai, *Women's Words* (New York, 1991), p. 11.

70 Harry Cocks, 'Review: The Growing Pains of the History of Sexuality', *Journal of Contemporary History* 39 (4), p. 665.

71 Jeffrey Weeks, *The World We Have Won: The Remaking of Erotic and Intimate Life* (London, 2007), p. 4.

72 Szreter and Fisher, *Sex Before the Sexual Revolution*.

73 Szreter and Fisher, *Sex Before the Sexual Revolution*, p. 51.

74 Szreter and Fisher, *Sex Before the Sexual Revolution*, p. 51.

75 Szreter and Fisher, *Sex Before the Sexual Revolution*, p. 11.

76 Una Drinkwater, interviewed 29 December 2009.

77 Judith Stacey, 'Can There Be a Feminist Ethnography?', in Gluck and Patai (eds), *Women's Words*, pp. 111–119.

78 Albert Holliday, interviewed 27 June 2010.

79 Gluck, 'What's So Special About Women?', p. 5.

80 Plummer, 'Telling Sexual Stories Power', p. 43.

81 Baker and Stanley, *Hello Sailor!*, p. 16.

82 Penny Summerfield, *Reconstructing Women's Wartime Lives* (Manchester, 1998), p. 26.

83 Summerfield, *Reconstructing Women's Wartime Lives*, p. 32.

84 Morris B. Kaplan, *Sodom and the Thames. Sex, Love and Scandal in Wilde Times* (New York, 2005), p. 23; Harry Cocks, *Nameless Offences: Homosexual Desire in the 19th Century* (London, 2010), p. 17; Randolph Trumbach, 'Renaissance Sodomy, 1500–1700', in Matt Cook (ed.), *A Gay History of Britain: Love and Sex Between Men Since the Middle Ages* (Oxford, 2007), pp. 49–50.

85 Cocks, *Nameless Offences*, p. 17.

86 Cocks, *Nameless Offences*, pp. 17–18.

87 Louis Crompton, *Byron and Greek Love: Homophobia in Nineteenth-Century England* (Berkeley, 1985), pp. 158–171.

88 Cocks, *Nameless Offences*, pp. 7–8.

89 Kaplan, *Sodom and the Thames*, p. 24. Charles Upchurch argues, however, that the reporting of sex between men was used to check state power and abuses of class privilege during the 1820s, which ultimately led to publicity winning over silence: Charles Uphurch, 'Politics and the Reporting of Sex Between Men in the 1820s', in Brian Lewis (ed.), *British Queer History: New Approaches and Perspectives* (Manchester, 2013), pp. 17–38.

90 See, e.g., Matt Cook, *London and the Culture of Homosexuality, 1885–1914* (Cambridge, 2003), pp. 42–55.

91 Harry Cocks, 'Secrets, Crimes and Diseases, 1800–1914', in Matt Cook (ed.), *A Gay History of Britain: Love and Sex Between Men Since the Middle Ages* (Oxford, 2007), p. 110.

92 Cook, *London and the Culture of Homosexuality*, p. 49.

93 Matt Cook, '"A New City of Friends": London and Homosexuality in the 1890s', *History Workshop Journal* 56 (2003), pp. 33–58; Cook, *London and the Culture of Homosexuality*, p. 49.

94 Cook, *London and the Culture of Homosexuality*, p. 49.

95 'A Night in a Workhouse', *Pall Mall Gazette* (4 January 1866).

96 Seth Koven, *Slumming, Sexual and Social Politics in Victorian London* (Princetown, 2004), p. 26.

97 Koven, *Slumming*, p. 57.

98 Rictor Norton, *Mother Clap's Molly House: The Gay Subculture in England, 1700–1830* (London, 1992), p. 35.

99 Cruising areas are public places where gay men search for a sexual partner and sometimes engage in sexual acts.

100 Charles Upchurch, 'Forgetting the Unthinkable: Cross-Dressers and British Society in the Case of the Queen vs. Boulton and Others', *Gender and History* 12 (2000), p. 127. See also Randolph Trumbach, 'London's Sodomites: Homosexual Behaviour and Western Culture in the Eighteenth Century', *Journal of Social History* 11 (1977), pp. 4–5.

101 Upchurch, 'Forgetting the Unthinkable', p. 127. For a detailed discussion regarding Ernest Boulton and Fredrick Park, see Neil McKenna, *Fanny and Stella: The Young Men Who Shocked Victorian England* (London, 2013).

102 Ackroyd, *Dressing Up*, p. 83.

103 Kaplan, *Sodom and the Thames*, p. 23; Norton, *Mother Clap's Molly House*, p. 47; Upchurch, 'Forgetting the Unthinkable', p. 140.

104 Upchurch, 'Forgetting the Unthinkable', p. 140.

105 Ackroyd, *Dressing Up*, p. 85.

106 *The Times* (31 May 1870).

107 *Pall Mall Gazette* (8 June 1870).

108 Upchurch, 'Forgetting the Unthinkable', p. 137.

109 Cook, *London and the Culture of Homosexuality*, p. 50.

110 Jeffrey Weeks, *Coming Out: Homosexual Politics in Britain from the Nineteenth Century to Present* (London, 1990), p. 35.

111 Frank J. Sulloway, *Freud Biologist of the Mind* (London, 1979), p. 297. See, also, Ivan Crozier, 'Philosophy in the English Boudoir: Havelock Ellis, Love and Pain, and Sexological Discourses on Algophilia', *Journal of the History of Sexuality* 13 (2004), pp. 275–305; Cocks, 'Secrets, Crimes and Diseases, 1800–1914', pp. 134–135.

112 Cocks, 'Secrets, Crimes and Diseases, 1800–1914', p. 135.

113 Richard von Kraft-Ebing, *Psychopathia Sexualis, mit besonderer Berucksichtigung der contraren Sexualempfindung* (Vienna, 1886). This was translated into English in 1892: Richard von Kraft-Ebing, *Psychopathia Sexualis* (Philadelphia, 1892).

114 Sulloway, *Freud Biologist of the Mind*, p. 279.

115 Robert Nye, *Sexuality* (Oxford, 2000), p. 57.

116 Sulloway, *Freud Biologist of the Mind*, p. 287.

117 'Sexual inversion' was one of the many terms developed by sexologists to refer to same-sex desire: Cocks, 'Secrets, Crimes and Diseases, 1800–1914', p. 110.

118 Havelock Ellis and John Addington Symonds, *Studies in the Psychology of Sex, Vol. 1: Sexual Inversion* (London, 1897).

119 Cocks, 'Secrets, Crimes and Diseases, 1800–1914', pp. 134–135.

120 Lucy Bland and Laura Doan, *Sexology Uncensored: The Documents of Sexual Science* (Cambridge, 1998), p. 1; Despite fundamental differences in their approach to the subject and their attitudes towards sexology as a science, Symonds and Ellis both sought to use their study to challenge the 1885 Labouchère amendment, which had made sexual contact between men subject to harsh criminal punishment. Their study drew heavily on case histories written by 'inverts' who attempted to make sense of their own sexual histories. See also Faderman, *Surpassing the Love of Man*, p. 67.

121 Crozier, 'Philosophy in the English Boudoir', p. 300; Cocks, 'Secrets, Crimes and Diseases, 1800–1914', p. 135; Sulloway, *Freud Biologist of the Mind*, p. 257.

122 See, e.g., Crozier, 'Philosophy in the English Boudoir, pp. 275–305; Bland and Doan, *Sexology Uncensored The Documents of Sexual Science*.

123 Koven, *Slumming*, p. 73; see also Angus McLaren, *The Trials of Masculinity: Policing Sexual Boundaries, 1870–1930* (Chicago, 1997), p. 16.

124 Cocks, 'Secrets, Crimes and Diseases, 1800–1914', p. 110.

125 Koven, *Slumming*, p. 73.

126 Cook, *London and the Culture of Homosexuality*, p. 57.

127 Michel Foucault, *The History of Sexuality, Vol. 1: An Introduction* (Oxford, 1990), pp. 57–68.

128 Koven, *Slumming*, p. 74.

129 Sigmund Freud, *Three Essays On The Theory Of Sexuality* (Vienna, 1905).

130 Sulloway, *Freud Biologist of the Mind*, p. 279.

131 In 1924, the Hogarth Press became the publisher for the papers of the International Psycho-Analytical Institute. In doing so, it became the official publisher for Sigmund Freud in England and was the first publisher to make psychoanalytic theory available in English. See, also, Chris Waters, 'Havelock Ellis, Sigmund Freud and the State: Discourses of Homosexual Identity in Interwar Britain', in Lucy Bland and Laura Doan (eds), *Sexology in Culture Labelling Bodies and Desires* (Cambridge, 1998).

132 Doan and Waters, 'Homosexuality', in Lucy Bland and Laura Doan (eds), *Sexology Uncensored*, p. 43.

133 Sigmund Freud, 'Some Neurotic Mechanisms in Jealously, Paranoia, and Homosexuality', *The International Journal of Psycho-analysis* 4 (1923), p. 1; Doan and Waters, 'Homosexuality', p. 43.

134 Sigmund Freud, Anonymous (letter to an American Mother) reprinted in *The Letters of Sigmund Freud* (New York, 1935).

135 Chris Waters, 'Havelock Ellis, Sigmund Freud and the State', pp. 173–174; for psychological explanations in court cases, see e.g., 'Porter's Punishment', *News of the World* (30 October 1932).

136 Chris Waters, 'Havelock Ellis, Sigmund Freud and the State', pp. 173–174.

137 'If Guilty They Would be Gassed While in Court', *Reynold's News* (18 December 1938).

138 Kate Prebble, 'Ordinary Men and Uncommon Women: A History of Psychiatric Nursing in New Zealand Public Mental Hospitals' (unpublished PhD thesis, University of Auckland, 2007), p. 2. For a broader history of mental health services in the UK, see, e.g., Roy Porter, *Madness: A Brief History* (Oxford, 2002).

139 Michael Arton, 'The Professionalization of Mental Nursing in Great Britain' (unpublished PhD thesis, University College London, 1998); Diane Carpenter, 'Above All a Patient Should Never Be Terrified: An Examination of Mental Health Care and Treatment in Hampshire' (unpublished PhD thesis, University of Portsmouth, 2010); Patricia D'Antonio, 'Negotiated Care: A Case Study of the Friends Asylum, 1800–1850' (unpublished PhD thesis, University of Pennsylvania, 1992); Anne Digby, *Madness, Morality and Medicine: A study of the York Retreat, 1796–1914* (Cambridge, 1985); John Hopton, 'Prestwich Hospital in the Twentieth Century: A Case Study of Slow and Uneven Progress in the Development of Psychiatric Care', *History of Psychiatry* (1999), p. 351; Nancy Tomes, *A Generous Confidence: Thomas Story Kirkbride and the Art of Asylum-Keeping, 1840–1883* (Cambridge, 1984); Ellen Dwyer, *Homes for the Mad: Life Inside Two*

Nineteenth-century Asylums (New Brunswick, 1987); Olga Church, 'That Nobel Reform: The emergence of psychiatric nursing in the United States, 1882–1963' (unpublished PhD thesis, University of Illinois, 1982); Peter Nolan, 'Psychiatric Nursing Past and Present: The Nurses' Viewpoint' (unpublished PhD thesis, University of Bath, 1989); Peter Nolan, *A History of Mental Health Nursing* (London, 1993); Geertje Boschma, *The Rise of Mental Health Nursing: A History of Psychiatric Care in Dutch Asylums, 1890–1929* (Amsterdam, 2003); Veryl Tipliski, 'Parting in the Crossroads: The Development of Education in Psychiatric Nursing in Three Canadian Providences, 1909–1955' (unpublished PhD thesis, University of Manitoba, 2003); Adams, *Challenge and Change in a Cinderella Service*; Angela Martin, 'Determinants of Destiny: The Professional Development of Psychiatric Nurses in Saskatchewan' (unpublished MA thesis, University of Regina, 2003); Prebble, 'Ordinary Men and Uncommon Women'; Claire S. Chatterton, '"The Weakest Link in the Chain of Nursing?" Recruitment and Retention in Mental Health Nursing, 1948–1968' (unpublished PhD thesis, University of Salford (Salford, 2007); Philip Maude, 'The Development of the Community Mental Health Nursing Services in Western Australia: A History (1950 to 1995) and Population Profile' (unpublished Master of Nursing thesis, Edith Cowan University, 1996).

140 Nolan, *A History of Mental Health Nursing*, p. 22.
141 Nolan, *A History of Mental Health Nursing*, p. 1.
142 Arton, 'The Professionalization of Mental Nursing in Great Britain, 1850–1950', p. 14; Chatterton, 'The Weakest Link in the Chain of Nursing?', p. 5.
143 Peter Nolan, *A History of Mental Health Nursing* (London, 1993), p. 6.
144 Walk, 'The History of Mental Nursing', p. 12.
145 Nolan, *A History of Mental Health Nursing*, p. 47.
146 Carpenter, Above All a Patient Should Never Be Terrified, p. 57; Nolan, *A History of Mental Health Nursing*, p. 47.
147 Nolan, *Psychiatric Nursing Past and Present*, p. 67; Nolan, *A History of Mental Health Nursing*, p. 47; Walk, 'The History of Mental Nursing', p. 12.
148 Peter Nolan, 'A History of the Training of Asylum Nurses', *Journal of Advanced Nursing* 18 (1993), p. 1197; Nolan, *A History of Mental Health Nursing*, p. 53.
149 Henry R. Rollin, 'The Red Handbook: An Historic Centenary', *Bulletin of the Royal College of Psychiatrists* 10 (1986), p. 279; Nolan, 'A History of the Training of Asylum Nurses', p. 1197.
150 Medico-Psychological Association, The Handbook for the Instruction of Attendants on the Insane (London, 1885).
151 Carpenter, 'Above All a Patient Should Never Be Terrified', p. 61; Nolan, *A History of Mental Health Nursing*, p. 64.

152 Walk, 'The History of Mental Nursing', p. 17; Nolan, 'A History of the Training of Asylum Nurses', p. 1199; Nolan, *A History of Mental Health Nursing*, p. 67.

153 Hopton, 'Prestwich Hospital in the Twentieth Century', p. 360.

154 Nolan, *A History of Mental Nursing*, p. 8.

155 Psychiatry's contribution to the war effort was acknowledged in 1926 when the Medico-Psychological Association was awarded a Royal Charter and became the Royal Medico-Psychological Association (RMPA). See also Peter Nolan, 'Mental Health Nursing – Origins and Developments', in Monica E. Baly (ed.), *Nursing & Social Change* (New York, 1995), p. 254.

156 The title of 'mental nurse' endured until the 1960s, when it was replaced by the term 'psychiatric nurse'. This had no statutory basis, however, and registered nurses were officially known as registered mental nurses (RMNs) from the 1920s until the inception of Project 2000 in the late 1980s and early 1990s, when the term 'mental health nurse' was embraced: Chatterton, 'The Weakest Link in the Chain of Nursing?', p. 6.

157 Claire Chatterton, '"Caught in the Middle"? Mental Nurse Training in England 1919–51', *Journal of Psychiatric and Mental Health Nursing* 11 (2004), p. 32.

158 Chatterton, '"Caught in the Middle"?', p. 32.

159 The number of mental nurses registering with the GNC rose steadily until 1930, and thereafter, approximately 5000 nurses registered annually. Each year the number of female mental nurses increased, resulting in there being far more qualified female nurses than males: Nolan, *A History of Mental Health Nursing*, p. 81. See also Valerie Harrington, 'Voices Beyond the Asylum: A Post War History of Mental Health Services in Manchester and Salford' (unpublished MPhil/PhD transfer report, University of Manchester, 2005). See, also Chapter 2 for a fuller exploration of mental health nurse education.

160 Nolan, 'Mental Health Nursing – Origins and Developments', p. 254.

161 Harrington, 'Voices Beyond the Asylum', p. 4; Nolan, 'Mental Health Nursing – Origins and Developments', p. 254.

162 Karen Jones, 'The Culture of the Mental Hospital', in German E. Berrios and Hugh Freeman (eds), *150 Years of British Psychiatry 1841–1991* (London, 1991), p. 121.

1

Oppression and suppression of the sexual deviant, 1939–1967

I would sometimes question the treatments we were giving. [. . .] Then I would get home and turn on the television [. . .] and all over it was either 'homosexuals should be accepted', or 'homosexuality is illegal, it is wrong, these people are irredeemable'. And thank goodness; 'psychiatry is trying to do something about it.' [. . .] I just didn't know who was right and what was wrong, it left me very perplexed.[1]

Introduction

Nurses caring for patients receiving treatments for sexual deviations received mixed and muddled messages regarding their patients' place in society. Public debate surrounding sexual deviations refocused on to issues of aetiology rather than punishment, in a highly charged discourse which centred on finding a cure.[2] This chapter draws upon publications within the medical press and news media, along with literary, film, legal and sociological depictions of homosexuality to explore the complex social and cultural climate in which the homosexuals, transvestites and mental nurses were living from the 1930s to the 1960s. In doing so, it offers a context to explain why treatments for sexual deviations came to be developed and implemented.

World War II

The start of World War II and mobilisation meant that men who had never been away from home suddenly found themselves on the move. They were mixing with other people of their own age and were responsible only to themselves – it is not surprising to find that the war created new sexual experiences and shaped more liberal attitudes towards variations in sexual desires.[3] During the first year of the war many male nurses were called up for military service and assigned to the Royal Army Medical Corps.[4] When the war ended many returned to the mental hospitals and numerous ex-service personnel who had not previously worked in mental health were noted to join the profession owing to limited employment opportunities.[5] Nolan argues that one of the main attractions of mental nursing to demobilised soldiers was the military-style atmosphere of the hospitals and their excellent sporting facilities.[6] Julian Wills was called up for military service during the war, and after demobilisation went on to train as a mental nurse. He recalls working with a fellow soldier during the war who was homosexual:

> I remember one young chap who I served with in the 1940 Campaign in France. He was overtly camp and didn't really hide it. He was a good source of entertainment for us; he could always be relied upon to lighten the mood. I had never met an overtly gay person before, but if he 'had my back' then I had his I suppose. It opened my mind and I was less prejudiced against it. That is why I really struggled once I was expected to administer aversion therapies to the poor chaps later on.[7]

On the home front in World War II, the blackout in major cities provided cover for erotic encounters, with Quentin Crisp noting: 'When the blackout came, London became a vast double bed.'[8] Bert Sutcliffe a Canadian soldier stationed in England for six months in 1942 was overwhelmed by the sexual possibilities offered in wartime London: 'I suddenly found out that Leicester Square, Piccadilly Circus were just hotbeds of gay bars. Just jam-packed with them. In London you could have almost had sex twenty-four hours a day.'[9] Indeed, despite its prime target for the Luftwaffe, London managed to sustain its leading position as the metropolis of queer sociability.[10] Meanwhile, 'Roy' recalled Edinburgh being 'full of sailors' who were 'quite easy; quite quite easy. The place was as if the world had gone mad because it was so easy.'[11] Many of the testimonies of gay men who lived during the war pertain to a sense of living for the moment – death may have been imminent for each of them, and this necessarily changed the way they and many others responded to sexual possibility: moral codes, old inhibitions, class divisions and customs were compromised in certain places and at certain times.

Herbert Bliss, who received aversion therapy in the 1960s, recalled his wartime experiences. He joined the Royal Air Force (RAF) in 1939 at the age of 19, but was captured by the Japanese during the fall of Singapore and spent the rest of the war in prisoner of war (PoW) camps; he recalls such transcending of class divisions and the tolerance of his colleagues:

> We all just got on with it, we had a common goal, which was to beat Hitler and the Japanese, and that was it, really. I had had what you might call a fairly privileged background, but I was working alongside the 'salt of the Earth' type people and it didn't bother me or them – class didn't come into war. In the PoW camp I met a young chap from Liverpool. He had been a builder's labourer before the war and we became lovers. The other lads in the camp knew and just turned a blind eye to it really. After a while, he was sent to another camp, though. I tracked him down after the war and we met up again; but it wasn't the same. He had decided that he wanted to get married and have kids, and that it was the segregation from females that had developed his homosexual feelings. I was upset, but I understood. We still remained friends, though. In fact I'm godfather to his daughter.[12]

As we have seen from the testimony of Julian Wills above, overtly camp[13] gay men could find themselves relatively accepted in the services. Jo Denith recalls a homosexual colleague under his command. Denith notes that immediately before they disembarked from the landing craft during the D-Day landings his colleague began to daub his lips with lipstick and, when asked to explain his actions, said, 'I must look pretty for the Germans.' Denith recalled that everybody on board erupted in laughter.[14] Meanwhile, John Beardmore, an officer in the Navy, recalls Freddy, who was a coder on his ship. He had the job of relaying messages from the captain to the rest of the ship:

> During moments of high drama he sometimes diffused the tension by camping it up. So when the captain issued orders to open fire, he simply repeated 'open fire dear', which would crack up the troops. He ... was immensely popular on the ship – everybody loved him and he loved everybody else.[15]

Freddy and the colleague described by Denith provided light relief for the troops. It is interesting to note that John, who related the story about Freddy, also identified himself as homosexual. However, he clearly saw himself as being in a different category to Freddy, which could be due to the fact he was an officer, and men in higher ranks had to be especially cautious.[16] This highlights the hidden and complex impact of class within homosexual culture.[17] There appear to be some similarities between this wartime pattern and the dynamic between the more effeminate homosexual lower-ranking nurses and their senior administrators, who were also homosexual, in mental hospitals during the study period. This will be explored in Chapter 2.

Cook argues that such 'campery' could be tolerated and enjoyed in the forces.[18] Nevertheless, while sexual contact between people of the same sex appears to have been fairly common in the forces, and some had a more liberal attitude towards this, it still remained furtive and secret. Being caught would mean a certain court martial and subsequent disgrace, not only for having committed a 'crime' but, furthermore, because the ejection from the post meant that the individual was not 'doing his bit'.[19] Indeed, courts martial for sex between men increased during the war years – rising from 48 in 1939 to 324 in 1944/45.[20] Moreover, pathological, psychological and psychoanalytical interpretations and analysis of homosexuality can be seen to be appearing on both sides of the Atlantic during World War II.

Psychiatrists within the US army were promoting the concept that homosexuality was a pathology and making a concerted effort to eradicate homosexuals from their ranks.[21] Psychiatrists tried to detect homosexual men at induction stations either by their 'effeminate looks or behaviour or by repeating certain "homonyms" (words from the homosexual vocabulary) and watching for signs of recognition'.[22] These arbitrary homonyms were: 'blow', 'fairy', 'French', 'fruit', 'queer', 'rear', 'suck', 'pansy' and 'Greek'.[23] However, a problem arose when men who did not want to fight faked homosexuality in order to be discharged. Therefore, diagnostic tests were devised, including one by Nicolai Giosca, which was published after the war. Giosca came to the scientifically dubious notion that homosexual men did not display a gag reflex when a tongue depressor was put in their throat.[24] A. C. Cornsweet, a commander in the US Naval Reserve, and Dr Hayes, an army physician, conducted a survey among 200 homosexual men. They concluded that they had discovered a specific reaction common to all those 'confirmed to the practice of sexual oralism'. This constituted a localisation of pleasure which could only be described by a true homosexual.[25]

There were also studies describing the characteristics of homosexuals. George Henry studied thirty-three homosexual mental patients. He concluded that the homosexual male is characterised by a feminine carrying angle of the arm, long legs, narrow hips, large muscles, deficient hair on the face, chest and back, feminine distribution of pubic hair, a high-pitched voice and a small penis and testicles.[26] Alkarim Jivani suggests that an indication of how futile these studies were came at the end of the war when *Newsweek* ran an article on the US Army's own figures on homosexuality that had just been tabulated. During the course of World War II, between 3,000 and 4,000 men were discharged for this 'abnormality' and an unspecified number were released as 'neuropsychiatric cases'.[27]

An indication of the British Army's policy on homosexuality is given by a War Office document made public in 1950, entitled 'The Second World War: Army Discipline', which stated: 'confirmed homosexuals whose rehabilitation is unlikely should be removed from the Army by the appropriate means'.[28] The regulation only refers to 'confirmed' homosexuals, which could suggest that repeated offences were necessary and even then expulsion from the army was only considered appropriate for those confirmed homosexuals who could not be rehabilitated.[29] Dudley Cave recalls being discharged from the army and being referred to an army psychiatrist who told him: 'Well, my advice to you is to find someone of like mind and settle down with him and stop bothering.'[30] However, when Quentin Crisp went for his physical examination for the army, he was asked if he was homosexual. He replied, 'Yes.' Nevertheless, he was still examined, which caused great consternation among the medics: 'All the doctors were in a terrible state when they saw me. They were terribly flustered, rushed about and talked to each other in whispers.'[31] Following his examination, he was given his exemption papers, which stated that he suffered from 'sexual perversion'.[32] Emma Vickers argues, however, that Quentin Crisp appears to have been the exception rather than the rule, as given the desperate need for manpower, the British armed forces did not have the luxury of being able to exclude those that were judged to desire members of their own sex.[33]

Nevertheless, John Costello argues that the British military authorities did take homosexuality seriously, and reports were commissioned on the behaviour of homosexual soldiers. A report by a medical officer highlighted a threat to the navy and nation from the 'dry rot' of 'homosexualists' bent on 'racial suicide'.[34] Additionally, a study by Charles Anderson on sexual offenders in the British Army accentuated that homosexuals 'achieved gratification from those of their comrades who turned towards them as substitutes for women'; they were also known 'to dominate the group, obtain love, respect, and acknowledgement of prowess. He must lead, cannot be led, and finds it intolerable to be in a passive position of obeying.' More than a third of the cases examined 'had Fascist leanings and were facile exponents of power politics'. The report concluded that homosexuals 'form a foreign body in the social macrocosm' and vindicated the wartime policy of offenders being 'quietly invalided out of service, with appropriate advice about medical treatments, unless they had to be brought up before a court martial'.[35]

Joanna Bourke suggests that psychiatrists never tired of implying that men who collapsed under the strain of war were 'feminine' or 'latent homosexuals'. She proposes that a respected psychiatrist, Philip S. Wagner, used judgemental comments such as, 'socially and emotionally immature soldiers' who 'shrunk from combat with almost feminine despair and indignation' to describe homosexual soldiers in the military.[36] Worried that such 'socially and emotionally stunted' individuals were being rewarded by being excused from combat, he recommended that they be immediately forced back to the battlefields and threatened with disciplinary actions should their symptoms reappear.[37] These reports highlight that the homosexual was considered a case for psychological interpretation. In some cases, such interpretations were used to underscore familiar stereotypes of homosexual treachery and to draw an implicit analogy between a passive position in the forces and homosexual sex.[38]

While there is some evidence of the pathologising of homosexuality by the Allies during the war, across Europe, it was on the Nazi side that homosexuals were to become subject to unprecedented persecution, torture and medicalisation in the 1930s and 1940s. While it could be argued that the majority of nurses practising in the UK during the 1950s and 1960s would not have known about the treatment of homosexuals in Germany during Nazi rule, because the testimonies of homosexual men who lived through this period were not in the wider public domain until the late 1970s following the gay liberation movement,[39] an exploration of this period is pertinent to this book, and is used for comparison purposes in Chapters 3 and 4.

The Nazi campaign to rid Germany of its homosexuals began in 1933, with the rise of the Nazi Party in Germany. The initial target was Hirschfeld's Institute of Sexual Research, condemned by the Nazis as 'the international centre of the white-slave trade' and 'an unparalleled breeding ground of dirt and filth'.[40] A mob of around one hundred young extremists descended upon the institute, smashing everything they could lay their hands on. Then in 1935, Nazi lawyer Hans Frank warned that the 'epidemic of homosexuality' was threatening the new Reich.[41] This sparked the re-wording of the original Paragraph 175 (1871), which was a provision of the German Criminal Code that made homosexual acts between males a crime.

On 28 June 1935, Paragraph 175 was revised to extend the concept of 'criminally indecent activities between men'.[42] It permitted the authorities to arrest any male on the most trivial charges, such as furtive glances at other men. The specialists in the Ministry of Justice were not content until anything that could remotely be perceived as sex between males was labelled a transgression.[43] As with British law, lesbians were not regarded as a threat to Nazi racial policies and were not generally targeted for persecution. This vicious campaign against Germany's homosexuals was led by the head of the Schutzastaffel (SS, defence detachment), Reichsfuhrer (leader) Heinrich Himmler.[44]

The Nazi persecution of homosexuals was staunchly informed by the influential eugenics movement. Eugenics strongly advocated white, middle-class fertility and discouraged childbirth among the poor and the mentally 'unfit'.[45] Himmler's obsession with eugenics led him to name homosexuals 'contragenics'.[46] He saw them as unlikely to produce children and increase the German birth rate and, therefore, believed they deserved to be systematically exterminated before they spread the 'poison of racial suicide'.[47] He was particularly eager to ensure that such behaviour was not practised in his military ranks. Himmler announced in 1940:

When a man in the Security Service, in the SS, or in the government has homosexual tendencies, then he abandons the normal order of things for the perverted world of the homosexual. Such a man drags ten others after him, otherwise he can't survive. We can't permit such a danger to the country: the homosexual must be entirely eliminated.[48]

After toying with the idea of drowning homosexuals in swamps, Himmler persuaded Hitler to issue a directive in 1941 warning that:

Any member of the SS or Gestapo who engages in indecent behaviour with another man or permits himself to be abused by him for indecent purposes will, regardless of age, be condemned to death and executed. In less grave cases, a term of not less than six years' penal servitude or imprisonment may be imposed.[49]

The period between 1937 and 1939 saw the peak of the Nazi persecution of homosexual men, and it is estimated that between 5,000 and 15,000 were interned in concentration camps.[50] These prisoners were marked with a pink triangle to signify their homosexuality and according to many survivor accounts, homosexuals were among the most abused in the camps.[51] The Nazis believed that homosexuality was a sickness that could be cured. Therefore, they designed policies to cure homosexuals of their disease through humiliation and hard work.[52] Guards often derided and beat homosexual internees upon arrival, regularly separating them from other inmates; they were also subjected to medical experiments to cure them of their disease.[53] Moreover, nurses played a role in assisting with the medical experiments undertaken within concentration camps in Nazi Germany and other occupied countries; this will be explored in Chapter 3.[54]

The influx of foreign troops and a 'live for the moment' attitude expressed by many exposed the British to different and more liberal sexual attitudes during the war. The majority of homosexual men were just as enthusiastic to fight as their compatriots. Some provided comedic relief in highly stressful situations. In doing so they were arguably displaying exactly the emotional self-control and courage valued by the military. Nevertheless, they were fighting for a country that did not recognise their right to be who they were without fear. Additionally, the notion that homosexuality was a pathology can be seen to be appearing during World War II. This was mainly driven by army psychiatrists. Jivani claims, however, that gay men in the UK had what could be called a 'good' war.[55] World War II had chipped away some of the old taboos. Servicemen living in close proximity to each other were made aware that men who chose a sexual relationship with other men were not suffering from a deadly disease, nor were they cowards or effeminates. Indeed, Costello argues that the very act of bringing so many homosexuals together, may have contributed to the evolution of the future Gay Liberation movement.[56] Set against the war years, in the backlash that followed, complained Crisp, 'the horrors of peace were many'.[57]

Rebuilding the Empire, 1945–1951

After World War II, fears surrounding homosexuality acquired a particularly powerful resonance, and narratives of sexual danger as corruption predominated in public discourse.[58] For many observers, the rapid social changes unleashed by the war seemed to have rendered Britain's stability problematic. In the immediate post-war years, Harry Hopkins argues that the country had the atmosphere of one 'huge transit camp'.[59] Public transport was dirty, overcrowded and tardy; there were no dining cars on trains, and the queues on the platforms were very long. The squatter movement – and the speed with which it spread across the country – took the newly elected Labour government by surprise.[60] Divorce rates drastically increased – so much so that the administrative offices could not cope with the demand this created.[61] Furthermore, women had taken over what was traditionally regarded as men's work and as a result gender divisions had become blurred.[62] Matt Houlbrook suggests that these social changes destabilised the critical interpretative categories – masculinity and nationhood – within which narratives of sexual difference and danger were framed. Established notions of Britishness seemed threatened from every direction. Therefore, homosexual urban culture was viewed as ever more dangerous, assuming a central symbolic position as a key threat to the establishment in the post-war politics of sexuality.[63]

Anxieties regarding homosexual corruption of society regularly surfaced in the many post-war debates regarding the perceived decline in moral standards in the UK. Those debates were concomitant with the wider apprehension regarding the nation's birth rate. The government took decisive action and there was a growing emphasis on propaganda to promote the importance of domesticity and family life in its traditional form.[64] The National Marriage Guidance Council (1948) and the Royal Commission on Marriage and Divorce (1951) were established to deal with this perceived crisis. Conventional gender roles were retrenched and strengthened. The closure of nurseries after the war has been seen as part of a policy to force women back into their homes and to 'reconstruct the family'.[65]

Sue March posits that film portrayals promoted the idea of the model family and the heterosexual couple.[66] Pre-war films such as *Design for Living*[67] in 1933, which tackles a sexually ambiguous love story between two men and a woman, and *Look Up and Laugh*[68] starring Gracie Fields in 1935 were replaced by post-war films such as *Brief Encounter* in 1945. Within this film, Celia Johnson played a middle-class housewife who falls in love with another man she meets by chance at a railway station. Overcome by guilt over a few clandestine meetings involving what may have been considered heavy 'petting'[69] at the time, she decides that the best course of action is to return to her stable but unexciting husband.

The language within this film also tacitly retrenched gender roles and upheld the idea of the model wife and husband. When the two lead characters were describing their spouses the male lead proudly described his wife as 'rather delicate' while the female lead equally proudly described her husband as 'unemotional and not delicate at all', therefore reinforcing the notion that the ideal husband should be masculine and impassive. Arguably, this ideal was threatened by the concept of effeminacy and transvestism. Indeed, many simply yielded to the prevailing attitude of heterosexual domesticity, which was promoted within the film. Albert Holliday recalls how the pressure of this 'propaganda' largely influenced his decision to get married:

> It seemed that every film I watched and book I read made marriage look like such an attractive option. Maybe I was brainwashed [. . .] I didn't want to be lonely and there were a lot of questions from my family regarding me getting married [. . .] I had met a girl at art school. She was hugely talented and I admired her creativity. I knew she loved me very much, so marriage seemed like the next step – it was the fashion, then.[70]

In 1945, the Archbishop of Canterbury gave a sermon in which he called upon Britons to reject 'wartime morality' and return to living

'Christian lives'.[71] In the House of Lords, Earl Winterton observed that 'few things lower the moral fibre and injure the physique of the nation more than tolerated and widespread homosexualism'.[72] Meanwhile, 'Anomaly's' *The Invert*, first published in 1927, was republished in 1948 and maintained that the homosexual was 'an abnormally lustful person of more or less insatiable and uncontrollable impulses . . . [a] moral leper, corrupt, obscene and monstrous'.[73] These shifts and changes amounted to a 'heterosexualization' of mainstream culture. In turn, London's homosexual scene became less 'blatant' and the flamboyant 'queans'[74] began to disappear from the streets.[75] The family was reaffirmed as the honoured site of sexual normality. Marriage was confirmed as the gateway to reputable adulthood. The message was clear: homosexual men were seen to be a contagious risk who undermined post-war social reconstruction, by turning their backs on family life.[76]

The Kinsey Report

The perception that homosexuality was a threat to the establishment was exacerbated with the publication of Alfred Kinsey's study – *Sexual Behaviour in the Human Male* – in 1948.[77] His data upturned all conventional notions of how the sexual universe was constructed by reporting that 37 per cent of American men had engaged in at least one homosexual experience to the point of orgasm since adolescence and that 4 per cent of males were exclusively homosexual all their lives. While there has been criticism of the reliability of the report,[78] Kinsey's data were difficult to refute. The study was based upon data obtained from 5,300 Americans carefully selected and balanced to attempt to give a representative picture of American male sexual behaviour. Parts of the data were based on as many as 12,000 cases. Indeed, Kinsey wrote:

> In brief, homosexuality is not the rare phenomenon which it is ordinarily considered to be, but a type of behaviour which ultimately may involve as much as half the male population.[79]

It was this aspect of the report that was considered most disquieting. Until then it was the generally accepted notion that homosexual men were a tiny minority. The idea that they were everywhere was particularly disconcerting. Perhaps even more unsettling was

Kinsey's development of the spectrum theory of sexuality, which ranged people in seven categories from zero to six according to where they stood on the continuum from exclusive heterosexuality to exclusive homosexuality. In reality, he argued, individuals not only occupied each of the seven categories but every gradation in between. This raised an even more perturbing idea: homosexuals were not a distinct group – everyone was slightly homosexual.[80]

Although the research was conducted in the USA, it did impact on the UK. In Doncaster, the local magistrates were so enraged by the publication of Kinsey's work that they decided to ban it on grounds of vulgarity. However, the Doncaster bench were later convinced by higher authorities not to go ahead with their decision when it became clear that it would be impossible to justify.[81] Further, in 1949, the British opinion organisation, Mass Observation, conducted the first large-scale sex survey in Britain, which used a mixture of national random surveys and qualitative interviews. In light of the publication of Alfred Kinsey's study, it became known as 'Little Kinsey'.

Its findings were not published until the 1990s when Liz Stanley brought out a contextualised edition.[82] It reported 'the isolationist manner in which homosexual groups appear to function; and a draft appendix described a 'homosexual group' on a trip to Brighton. The men had a 'distinctive outlook' and 'were not at all keen on the company of non-homosexuals except neuters, borderline cases and possible coverts'. It was also found that 60 per cent of the public sampled were antipathetic to homosexuality (it was 'absolutely detestable', said one respondent; 'I shouldn't think they're human', said another).[83] Indeed, Stanley argues that Little Kinsey had shown 'a more genuine feeling of disgust towards homosexuality . . . than towards any other subject tackled.'[84] The disdain of the public was more or less absolute. For the remainder, the burgeoning debate, analysis and press coverage of the 1950s would soon educate them about this type of person.

Reaction, 1952–1955

There was a brief explosive period of reaction to Kinsey's data during the early 1950s, which was expressed in three ways: via regulation by the police; by the publication of legal and sociological perspectives regarding sexual deviations; and through news media discourses.

There was a sense that something had to be done about the 'problem' of homosexuality and on 25 October 1952, the new head of the Metropolitan Police was appointed (Sir John Nott-Bower). The Home Secretary (Sir David Maxwell Fyfe) was noted to remark 'homosexuals make a nuisance of themselves'[85] and later went on to tell the House of Commons:

> Homosexuals ... are exhibitionists and proselytizers and a danger to others ... so long as I hold the office of Home Secretary, I shall give no countenance to the view that they should not be prevented from being such a danger.[86]

Nott-Bower was left in no doubt as to what his duties were and he made it clear that he was going to fulfil them with a 'ferocious zeal'.[87] On 25 October 1953, *The Sydney Morning Telegraph* published a cable from its London correspondent, Mr Donald Horne, about a 'Scotland Yard plan to smash homosexuality in London'.[88] Contemporary historians argue, however, that there was never any dedicated 'witch-hunt' against homosexuals.[89] Nevertheless, Jivani claims that the authorities during this time were more fervent in their persecution of gay men; arrests for homosexual offences did go up.[90] Furthermore, Elizabeth Povinelli and George Chauncey argue that there is still a need to account for what was a transitional anti-homosexual discourse in the post-war world.[91] Indeed, court cases involving sodomy, gross indecency and indecent assault had risen – from 719 in 1938 in England and Wales to 2,504 in 1955.[92]

As with Percival Thatcher, discussed in the Introduction, the police made arrests by developing an intimate and dynamic relationship with their suspects becoming agents provocateurs. In urinals and on the streets, such tactics were ubiquitous, leaving many homosexual men and transvestites feeling extremely fearful and cautious in the first half of the 1950s.[93] Houlbrook argues that many men transgressed bourgeois ideas of public and private through their dependence on public places, thus placing the homosexual within derogatory categories of sexual immorality. He goes on to suggest:

> Such representations centred around the apparent correlation between homosexual sex and the urinal – the most dismal and marginal of all public spaces, associated with intolerable bodily functions. The discursive production of person and place was a mutually constitutive process, in which

notions of the homosexuals' character were derived from the nature of that site at which he was most often arrested.[94]

Embedding the homosexual in the dirt and marginality of the urinal, the magistrate Harold Sturge defined homosexual sex as 'morally wrong, physically dirty and progressively degrading'.[95] Butcher took this to the extreme:

> Urinals have a certain odour . . . a staleness [which] . . . .excites [homosexual men] . . . When a urinal has been cleaned out with Dettol and scrubbed clean and smells clean they will not go anywhere near it . . . once the smell of cleanliness has worn off you can see these people . . . working themselves up to a frenzy . . . they are on heat . . . it is like the bitch, once they have the scent there is no holding them, they are oblivious to anything else.[96]

Houlbrook argues that Butcher neatly linked the dismal urinal to the supposed anonymity of the encounters that took place there, defining the homosexual as incapable of love and driven by inexorable, menacing lust.[97] The indecent assault and importuning charges generated by agents provocateurs only served to reinforce this construction.

Greta Gold who received aversion therapy in the 1960s for transvestism, recalls the climate at the time as 'very scary'.[98] Myrtle Pauncefoot remarked: 'I don't think the Isle of Man would have been a particularly nice place to be for a gay man in the 1950s and 60s.'[99] Oscar Mangle remembers being 'convinced' he 'was going to be arrested' and burning all his letters from his lover, Louis, as he 'didn't want anything that could incriminate' him.[100] Meanwhile, Colin Fox thought he was a 'bad person' and he 'lived in fear of going to jail'.[101] These testimonies demonstrate how the subjective experience is paramount. Whether there was an orchestrated campaign to target these individuals or not, it 'felt' like a witch-hunt to many. Indeed, numerous participants reflected on the negative impact that the unsupportive attitudes from the police had on them, and for Molly Millbury this provided the catalyst for her receiving treatment:

> I started dressing [wearing women's clothes] at 16. What I used to do was go for a walk in the early hours of the morning, dressed in a skirt and coat. Probably not a good idea for a young person to be out at that time in the morning, which was why the police stopped me. My instant reaction was to run away and to try to hide and avoid the police. The police caught me and took me to the police station. It was a blues and twos event. Lots of

people came in and saw me – it was like I was in a 'freak show'. I got quite a rough ride off the police. They seemed to think I was connected with rapes and sexual assaults, and all sorts, and I was quizzed and questioned about that for about three or four hours. [. . .] My family came to collect me and marched me to my GP the next day and I was referred to a psychiatrist.[102]

Anxieties were further exacerbated by the antipathy towards homosexuality by the then Director of Public Prosecutions (Sir Theobald Mathew).[103] In murder assault cases, defence councils frequently highlighted the provocation and insult of a homosexual approach. A 22-year-old Norwich sailor was acquitted after the judge told the jury they should be in no doubt that the 44-year-old murdered man was a 'pervert'.[104] Cook argues that roles were recast in courtrooms: the victim had got his just deserts, highlighting the dangers that could go with gay sex. Gay men were vulnerable to blackmail, theft and violence and, yet were unlikely to get much sympathy.[105]

News media

Newspapers became less taciturn and euphemistic in the 1950s, which may have been in response to competition from television. Waters argues that the decade after the war witnessed the emergence of what might best be termed a tabloid discourse of homosexuality.[106] During this period, the general public were exposed to more sensational depictions of the predatory homosexual, his sinister networks of vice, and also the idea of an intrepid police force and judiciary doing their best to combat the threat. Through such reports, medical aetiologies of sexual difference that distinguished between men on the basis of whom they had sex with permeated everyday life.[107] Homosexuals were highlighted by the *Sunday Pictorial* in 1951 when it exposed 'The Squalid Truth' that British spies Guy Burgess and Donald Maclean defected to the Union of Soviet Socialist Republics (USSR) having betrayed American secrets, were 'sex perverts', and asserted that 'homosexuals – men who indulge in unnatural love for another – are known to be bad security risks. They are easily won over as traitors.'[108]

Cook argues that the *Sunday Pictorial* tellingly defined the homosexual for a readership it assumed might be uncertain of the term, and returned to the enduring notion of homosexual treachery.[109] In 1952, the same paper warned parents of the 'pestilence' of 'Evil [homosexual] Men' who 'infest London and the social centres about many provincial cities'.[110] Indeed, many of the former patients in this book reflected on the negative impact that the media had on their lives and in some cases it motivated them to seek medical treatment. Greta Gold received aversion therapy in the 1960s, and her testimony below suggests that the media not only portrayed transvestites as individuals the public should be fearful of; but also that transvestism was an illness that could be cured:

> All I had to do was open the daily paper and it was rubbed in my face how evil and perverse I was. It made me feel like ending it all. I knew I had to do something; it was either kill myself or cure myself.[111]

This period also witnessed the very public arrest, trial and conviction of three influential individuals in 1954 – Lord Montagu, a peer of the realm, Peter Wildeblood, the diplomatic correspondent of the *Daily Mail*, and Michael Pitt-Rivers, a wealthy landowner and cousin of Montagu. The trio were convicted of conspiring to incite two RAF men – Edward McNally and John Reynolds – to 'commit unnatural offences'. The press reports made much of the case and of the precedent that had been set – this was the first time that a peer of the realm had been convicted in a criminal court since the right of peers to be tried by their fellow peers, in the House of Lords, was abolished in 1948. The case made legal history, but it was also a milestone in the history of Britain's attitude towards gay men.

The public curiosity towards the trial had been fed by the popular press who, argues Jivani, were 'agog'.[112] However, not all the general public had an unsympathetic interest towards the case: indeed, on 24 March 1954, the *Daily Sketch* mentioned in its report that, as the sentences were delivered to the suspects, an elderly woman in the public gallery gasped 'poor boys!'[113] Indeed, Wildeblood recalls the derision of some but also the support of others during his trial especially as he left the court after sentencing:

> It was some moments before I realised that they [the crowd outside the court] were not shouting insults, but words of encouragement. They tried to pat us on the back and told us to 'keep smiling', and when the doors were shut they went on talking through the windows and gave the thumbs-up sign and clapped their hands.[114]

As the accused had been treated very badly, Ughtred Lovis-Douglas believed that 'the Montagu trials actually worked in our favour'.[115] Not only did this trial mark the nadir of the persecution of gay men in the country: in retrospect it was hugely influential in persuading the liberal intelligentsia that something must be done regarding the 'problem' of homosexuality.[116]

Legal and sociological perspectives

A number of sociological studies were published during the 1950s which provided convincing accounts of the homosexual. However, these perspectives were in somewhat of a conflict regarding the debate on how best to deal with homosexuality. Tudor Rees and Harley Usill's *They Stand Apart: A Critical Survey of the Problem of Homosexuality* (1955) drew upon 'expert' opinion from legal and medical perspectives 'to examine the problem and to focus public attention to its gravity'.[117] Tudor Rees was a judge and came from a legal perspective. He argued that homosexuals should be dealt with by the law and the current law regarding homosexuality should remain. He went on to suggest that:

> Such a change in the law begs the whole moral issue, one which must be thought out carefully or there would be danger that it may have the effect of giving a legal *carte blanche* to all types of offenders.[118]

Conversely, Lindesay Neustatter, a consultant psychiatrist, wrote a more empathic chapter within the study, entitled 'Homosexuality: The Medical Perspective'.

> Those who lay down the law in regard to sex seem to take it for granted that we know, in fact, what is normal and healthy, whereas we only know what is customary . . . We plead, therefore, for more research, and for the recognition of the fact that the invert is not a villain to be punished, but a patient to be studied – to our own ultimate advantage.[119]

Michael Schofield produced a fairly sympathetic work – *Society and the Homosexual* (1952) (published under the pseudonym Gordon Westwood). Schofield's main aim was to bring the subject of homosexuality out into the open for public discourse: 'The secrecy and shame that surrounds the subject at present gives it the aura of forbidden fruit which is unwise and unhealthy.'[120] Underpinning this argument was his belief that treatment should replace punishment:

> The fate of the homosexual offender now depends upon the wisdom and discretion of the magistrate. Some of them have an intelligent understanding of the nature of the disease; others are not swayed by medical opinion even when it is available and their own interpretation of the law is their only guide.[121]

Despite their differing viewpoints regarding homosexuality, what both these works did was bring some of the debates regarding the subject out into the wider public consciousness. Elizabeth Granger, a nurse who undertook a degree-level nurse education, recalls reading both the books as a nursing student and the somewhat mixed message she was left with after reading them:

> I remember reading two books about homosexuality when I was at university. As I recall they were background reading to some sociology lectures. One was called 'Society and the Homosexual' by, erm . . . Gordon Westwood, I think. The other was 'They Stand Apart' – I can't remember the author of that, though. What I do remember, however, was that the Westwood book was a lot more supportive of homosexuals. It talked about treatments and these people being mentally ill. It had particular resonance for me as I wanted to be a psychiatric nurse, and I thought one day I may nurse a homosexual patient. However, the other book I felt had more of an antipathetic view of homosexuals, as I remember the author was arguing that prison was the best place for these people. I was left slightly confused about my position on the issue.[122]

Interestingly the Church of England was broadly sympathetic during this period, and focused on the misery and anxiety experienced by many gay people in their investigation into 'the problem of homosexuality'. The resulting report in 1954 advocated the legalisation of sex between consenting men and an equal age of consent, arguing that as it stood the law led to blackmail and suicide.[123] This notion was also promoted in new literary works, such as Rodney Garland's *The Heart in Exile* (1952) and Mary Renault's *The Charioteer* (1953). Both of these novels attempted to portray a respectable and discreet homosexual who should be tolerated and granted legal recognition. Moreover, each focused on the way in which the law regarding homosexuality had led to misery, isolation and even suicide. Una Drinkwater was a staff nurse during this period and recalled reading *The Heart in Exile*:

'Not only was it a well written book, but it gave me an understanding of the challenges homosexual men faced. I had never realised how difficult it must have been for them.'[124] The empathy Una gained towards homosexuals after reading this novel is explored later in the book, as this influenced her clinical practice when she nursed a patient receiving treatment for homosexuality. Houlbrook and Waters argue that *The Heart in Exile* should be 'read as an explicitly political intervention on behalf of the middle-class homosexual'.[125] More broadly, along with the film *Victim* (1961), a tragic tale of blackmail and suicide, all the above tacitly promoted the case for reform.

There had never been so much public discussion, coverage and analysis – both critical and supportive. However, public opinion was not slavishly following the line about 'evil men' pedalled by the *Sunday Pictorial* and other papers. Indeed, many of the participants recalled receiving mixed messages during this period. Zella Mullins was a state enrolled nurse (SEN) and recalls the perplexity she felt regarding her position on homosexuality and transvestism: 'I was terribly confused about the whole issue. The papers were saying this, the doctors and "experts" were saying that. I didn't know who to believe!'[126] There was considerable confusion and it was in this context that the *Sunday Times* called for an enquiry:

> The law [. . .] is not in accord with a large mass of public opinion [. . .] The case for a reform of the law as to acts committed in private between two adults is very strong [. . .] the case for an authoritative inquiry into it is overwhelming.[127]

The Wolfenden Committee, 1954

A proposal for a Royal Commission inquiry into homosexuality and prostitution had already been made to the Cabinet by Home Secretary Sir David Maxwell Fyfe. However, Prime Minister Winston Churchill was noted to remark:

> The Tory Party won't want to accept responsibility for making the law on homosexuality more lenient – or for *maisons tolerees*.
>
>   But without enquiry –
>   i) could we not limit publicity for homosexuality, as was done for divorce?

57

ii) persons convicted should have opportunity to apply for medical treatment.

Otherwise, I wouldn't touch the subject. Let it get worse – in a hope of a more united public pressure for some amendment.[128]

An interpretation of Churchill's opposition to the Commission has been suggested to be that any legal reform arising from this may have lost Tory votes.[129] As a compromise, Fyffe agreed to downgrade the level of investigation from Royal Commission to Departmental Committee.[130] Therefore, in response to the escalating anxieties about vice and public immorality in London, the Departmental Committee on Homosexual Offences and Prostitution, chaired by John Wolfenden, was set up on 4 August 1954 to appraise the law affecting homosexuality from the point of view of making it less draconian.[131]

Davidson argues that some of the fullest and most compelling evidence to the Wolfenden Committee in favour of homosexual law reform came from medical witnesses.[132] Drs Inch and Boyd from the Scottish Prisons and Borstal Services aired grave doubts as to the value of imprisonment in reforming sexual offenders and favoured the decriminalisation of homosexual behaviour for consenting adults over 21. They advocated that courts should have routine psychiatric reports on all homosexual offenders prior to sentencing, supplied by a properly staffed University or Regional Hospital Board Clinic. For the homosexual recidivist or 'homosexual psychopath' there should be a separate psychopathic institute. Finally, they stated that treatment regimes had to be more effectively monitored and sustained by means of improved staff resources for after-care and social work.[133]

Evidence submitted by Drs Winifred Rushford and W. P. Kreamer also favoured the decriminalisation of homosexual behaviour between consenting adults as integral to changing social attitudes and to refocusing public discourses on to issues of aetiology rather than punishment. Underlying their evidence was a belief that a less punitive policy would in fact produce a more liberal and sympathetic attitude to homosexuality in British society.[134] John Glaister contributed to the British Medical Association's evidence to the Wolfenden Committee. He combined a pathological view of homosexuality with support for its limited decriminalisation. He was a vigorous supporter of coercive measures, including segregation in colonies, for 'the inveterate and degenerate sodomist, the debauchers of youth, and those who resort[ed] to violence to meet their desires'. However, he did not feel that the incidence of homosexuality threatened the nation with 'racial decadence' and considered that consenting acts of adults in private (not including sodomy) were a matter 'of private ethics' and should be dealt with outside of the law. In his opinion, even though society's disapproval was 'inevitable and desirable' and while homosexuality was definitely not something to be encouraged, imprisonment was not the answer. Glaister viewed prison as 'the last place for homosexual treatment'.[135]

There were, however, attacks on the argument regarding the medicalisation of homosexuality. The most noteworthy refutation of this notion came from James Adair, a member of the Wolfenden Committee, and former procurator-fiscal. He was scathing of the tendency of psychiatrists to sentimentalise the problem of homosexuality and to downplay its paedophilic aspects and damage to physical health.[136] In his opinion, much of the evidence presented by 'mental specialists' was 'quite inexplicable and in not a few cases manifestly indefensible'. He believed that homosexuality had become the latest disease 'fashion' or 'craze' of 'medical men', and highlighted the uncertainties of medical and mental science 'and the limited knowledge and powers of the medical profession under existing circumstances to deal with homosexual patients'. Adair argued that a significant proportion of homosexuals seeking treatment were only doing so in order to evade the due process of law and were merely using medical therapy as a concealment for their perversion. Many, he posited, were already too old at 18 for treatment, with their sexuality and behaviour 'for all practical purposes immutable'.[137]

The committee only heard evidence from three professed homosexuals – all educated and middle class. Waters argues that these men did little to represent the diverse homosexual community, as access to the committee was highly exclusive, embedded in the materiality of power, class and privilege.[138] The three men were: Carl Winter the director of the Fitzwilliam Museum in Cambridge; Patrick Trevor-Roper, a Harley Street consultant; and Peter Wildeblood, the diplomatic correspondent for the *Daily Mail*.[139] All deliberately approached Wolfenden to counter what Winter termed the 'disproportionate emphasis on [homosexuality's] more morbid aspects' and the negative implications of the law's salience in shaping public knowledge of sexual difference.[140] While many other homosexual men's rights to speak were rejected, as they were perceived as 'disreputable cranks',[141] Winter, Trevor-Roper and Wildeblood were able to draw upon the privileges of social connection and status, thus enabling their voices to be heard.[142] Nevertheless, the committee believed that these men were adequately representative of Britain's diverse homosexual population.

The three men mapped the lifestyle of the homosexual in a way that the committee members could identify with. They positioned the homosexual within a middle-class home with a network of appropriate friendships. This ran parallel with the wider behavioural and emotional codes associated with respectability, particularly the emphasis on self-control, restraint and discretion.[143] This in turn condemned the effeminate homosexual, and other public homosexual practices, particularly the use of streets and parks for sex, as dangerous and immoral. Indeed, Trevor-Roper distanced himself from the effeminate homosexual, noting how 'most homosexuals dislike male effeminacy'.[144] Meanwhile, Wildeblood remarked such men were 'deplored' by homosexuals.[145]

Houlbrook argues that by surrounding the homosexual within this 'exclusive social and subjective geography and condemning those people and practices who dared to contravene the public domain', Wildeblood, Winter and Trevor-Roper contrived a political narrative for a particular audience.[146] While the Wolfenden Committee provided a space for homosexual politics, it privileged certain voices but silenced others. The legal reforms that the three men argued for were limited: they asked only that the words 'in private' be removed from the Labouchère Amendment of 1885, thereby decriminalising encounters that took place in the home. At no point did they advocate for the legislation of public practices, a reconfigured relationship between the state and homosexual commercial venues, or the right to be visibly different.[147] All agreed that the laws regulating *public* sexual behaviour should be retained, 'targeted at the disreputable "queer" who continued to transgress the public–private boundary'.[148] The conservative imperative of the law reform that followed angered some homosexual men, and is explored in Chapter 5.

Nevertheless, on 4 September 1957, the Committee published its report, in which it recommended that homosexual sex in private between consenting adults over 21 should be decriminalised; that buggery should be reclassified from a felony to a misdemeanour (reducing the potential length of sentences); and that sentences which were more than twelve months old should not be prosecuted, except in the case of indecent assault. The report also advocated further research into causes and treatment of homosexuality and suggested that oestrogen treatment should be made available to all prisoners who wanted to access it.[149]

The press response to the Wolfenden report was mixed. While the *Mail* feared legislation would 'certainly encourage an increase in perversion' and the *Express* wanted 'family life' to continue to be protected from 'these evils', *The Times, Mirror, Guardian* and the *Telegraph* were broadly sympathetic.[150] The press were also keen to report on the recommendation within the report relating to treatment of homosexuality, with the *Mirror* headline reading 'Planned to Help a Million'; the *Express* 'One Million Need This New Clinic'; and the *Sunday Pictorial* 'Sex Pills for Scots in Jail',[151] thus highlighting the message that homosexuality was an illness that could nevertheless be cured.

The therapeutic state: from Pavlov's dogs to the National Health Service

Psychiatrists were also keen to promote Wolfenden's recommendations regarding medically treating homosexuals, and during the 1950s and 1960s Jivani argues that the medical profession had a kind of authority enjoyed neither before nor since.[152] Waters has suggested that during those two decades Britain witnessed the 'therapeutic state', based on the belief that experts, with their 'modern knowledge', could assist in the eradication of any number of social maladies.[153] The medical profession were seen to be advocating for these stigmatised individuals. Indeed, in 1961, the *Glasgow Herald* ran an article entitled 'Treatment of Homosexuals: Public Opinion Hostile'. The paper reported excerpts from Dr Chesser's article earlier that week in the British Medical Association magazine *Family Doctor*. The newspaper reported that treatment of homosexuality was being 'gravely hindered by the hostility of public opinion . . . All the good work of the therapist is all in vain if society remains intolerant and uncooperative.'[154]

After World War II, Freudian arguments, which began in early twentieth century, came to play a pertinent role in much of the public discussion of homosexuality in Britain. Waters has attributed this status to the work of a generation of inter-war criminologists who had used Freud to further their own goals of reclaiming the delinquent.[155] Waters posits that Freudian dialogue could be found in *Against the Law* (1955), Wildeblood's book regarding his experiences and reflections of his trial and time in prison. He pondered whether his parents might have contributed to his 'condition'; he referred to friendships between boys that had an 'unconsciously homosexual basis'; he discussed adolescents who experienced a homosexual 'stage' before making 'the natural transition into normality'; and he claimed that homosexuality resulted from 'arrested development'.[156]

Westwood's *Society and the Homosexual* (1952) discussed above and D. J. West's *Homosexuality* (1955), were both indebted to a model of psychosexual development that originated with Freud. West's study was prefaced by Dr Hermann Mannheim, a psychoanalytically orientated criminologist, and also included contributions by Dr Edward Glover, who had established the Institute for the Scientific Treatment of Delinquency in 1932, which was a Freudian-inspired treatment centre.[157] However, Waters argues that many homosexual men were suspicious of Freud and preferred to conceive of themselves through the experience and language of others, as documented and made available in print like Havelock Ellis, discussed in the Introduction.[158]

Nevertheless, by the 1950s, popular reportage was also suspicious of the claims of Freudian psychoanalysis. The outcomes of treatment for sexual deviations by various psychoanalytical techniques were rather poor, despite the optimism expressed by some.[159] Indeed, David Curran and Daniel Parr found the rate of improvement to be no greater in twenty-five of their cases treated by psychoanalysis than in twenty-five others who received little or no treatment.[160] In 1958, Mary Woodward reported a series of homosexual patients referred by the courts and treated with psychoanalysis at the London Institute for the Study and Treatment of Delinquency. Out of 113 referred for treatment, data are reported for only sixty-four who either completed treatment or 'left for some good reason'. Only seven patients had no homosexual impulse and an increased heterosexual interest at the conclusion of their psychoanalysis. Attempts made to obtain follow-up data were somewhat vague and inconclusive.[161]

Furthermore, Charlie Rubinstein was cautious of the claims of psychoanalysis, stating: 'Psychoanalysis can help to a certain extent and for a fair number. Some improve well beyond the original expectation.'[162] This recalls Freud's statement in 1938: 'In a certain number of cases we succeed ... in the majority of cases it is no longer possible ... the result of our treatment cannot be predicted.'[163] A large-scale psychoanalytic study was reported by Irving Bieber.[164] Out of one hundred patients treated by full-scale psychoanalysis, 27 per cent were apparently solely heterosexual at the close of treatment. However, those patients who were reported as responding to the treatment had all had heterosexual experience up to intercourse at some stage prior to treatment. The authors report their results only at the close of treatment, however, and give no follow-up data.

The disillusionment with a psychoanalytical approach to the treatment of sexual deviations was accompanied by an increasing interest in behaviour therapy approaches; Joseph Wolpe was one of the key drivers of the therapy. His book *Psychotherapy by Reciprocal Inhibition* (1958) focused mainly on the treatment of disorders such as obsessions and phobias.[165] However, John Bancroft argued that this also had an influential effect in the field of sexual deviations and provided somewhat of a catalyst for utilising this approach to treat sexual deviations.[166]

There were several arguments in favour of applying learning theory techniques to the treatment of sexual deviations. First, there were the poor outcome results from psychoanalysis, as discussed above. Further, although the Wolfenden report had advocated for oestrogen treatment to be made available to all prisoners, and some studies had reported successful outcomes,[167] overall, little success had been seen with this intervention. Oestrogen treatment had, however, been used in Scottish prisons for consenting sexual offenders for some time (especially in Perth) before its recommendation within the Wolfenden report.[168] Nevertheless, according to Inch, oestrogen treatment had never been pushed 'to its limits' – 'to the extent of producing atrophy of the testicles or even gynaecomastis – but only to the point of eliminating or at least reducing libido'.[169] However, the tragic story of Alan Turing would refute Inch's argument. Turing opted for oestrogen rather than a prison sentence after his relationship with another man in Manchester was exposed and prosecuted. The injections lowered Turing's libido but also led to the growth of breasts and to depression. He was found dead in 1953, and although the coroner recorded an open verdict, it has been suggested that it was almost certainly suicide.[170]

Furthermore, an argument concerned the intrinsic interest of applying learning theory principles, derived in the laboratory, to a field in which the problem was one of real-life behaviour. It was believed that sexual behaviour could be described as consisting of two components: an intrinsic meditational component and an extrinsic behavioural component. The possibility of directly manipulating the latter and hence of influencing the former was theoretically, at any rate, quite evident.[171] Clearly, most of the operant responses involved in homosexual behaviour could not be reproduced in a laboratory setting, and were therefore not available for manipulation. Homosexual behaviour could, however, be considered as being frequently initiated by the visual response of looking at an attractive sexual object, while transvestism could be considered as being initiated by the visual and tactile response of wearing the opposite sex's clothes. Therefore, at least one sexual response was available for laboratory manipulation. In addition, there had been some success using aversion therapy to treat alcoholism.[172]

It was deemed that aversion therapy was the way forward in the bid to cure individuals suffering from homosexuality and transvestism. These treatments were largely based on 'behaviourism', which itself became less popular in the last decades of the twentieth century. Behaviourism has its origins in the psychological laboratories where the techniques developed were used as a basis for clinical work. The most influential drivers of this approach were Pavlov, Thorndike, Watson and Skinner.[173] Thorndike is recognised for devising laws of learning, whereas Watson was one of the initial proponents of the theory that emotions could be learnt.[174] Operant theory, the theory that deals with modification of voluntary behaviour, was initially posited by Skinner: this included the laws of reinforcement and punishment.[175] Most noteworthy in relation to the treatments developed for sexual deviation, however, was the work of Pavlov, who developed the theory of 'classical conditioning'.

Aversion therapy was the logical extension of Pavlov's classical conditioning.

Ivan Pavlov (1849–1936) was a Russian psychologist investigating digestive enzymes in saliva. He believed that if an animal could learn to associate a banal irrelevant event (the sound of bells ringing) with something critical and essential (eating), then it is possible that habits could be created or eradicated by applying pleasure or discomfort respectively. Basic instinctual responses to certain stimuli were labelled the 'unconditioned response'.[176] This includes salivating in the presence of a delicious meal, especially if one is hungry, becoming aroused at the sight of an attractive person, and running from a dangerous situation. Most other environmental stimuli are neutral, neither positive nor negative enough to affect the conditioning of an organism in and of itself. Nevertheless, when a neutral stimulus is paired with a powerful conditioned stimulus that evokes the unconditioned response, eventually the subject would react to the neutral stimulus (conditioned response) as strongly as the unconditioned one.[177] For example, at first Pavlov's dogs all salivated at the appearance of a plate of meat, but failed to respond to the sound of the bell ringing.[178] Pavlov would ring the bell and produce the meat simultaneously. After conditioning the dogs in that fashion, eventually, all the researcher would have to do was ring the bell in order to produce the salivation response in the dogs, as the sound of the bell ringing and the appearance of food had become linked in the dogs' minds. Therefore the response to the neutral stimulus was known as the 'conditioned response'. So, it is interesting that psychiatrists were able to make the links between previous experiments on dogs and the idea that human beings could be treated by similar interventions.

In the treatment of sexual deviants two powerful conditioned stimuli were used: chemical and electrical. Electrical aversive techniques consisted of giving electric shocks via electrodes fixed to the patient's wrists, calves or feet. Patients would be asked to fantasise as well as watch pictures of men in various states of dress. In some cases, electric shocks were paired with erections above a certain size, measured by a plethysmograph (a pressure transducer encircling the penis). Chemical aversion techniques utilised apomorphine, an emetic, which produced nausea and vomiting in the patient. When the medication had become effective, the patients were usually shown pictures of undressed men.[179]

As discussed in the Introduction, the first official report of aversion therapy being used to treat a homosexual was published in 1935 by Louis Max. He required a homosexual patient to fantasise about an attractive sexual stimulus in conjunction with a 'strong' electric shock, hence employing a classical conditioning approach.[180] He found it necessary to use an electric shock higher than that used in other laboratory studies on human subjects to cause a 'diminution of emotional value of the sexual stimulus'. Each treatment lasted several days, and over three months, the effect was cumulative. Max reported that four months after the end of the treatment, the patient said, 'The terrible neurosis has lost the battle, not completely but by 95 per cent of the way.'[181] No further details are given of the long-term effect of this revolutionary therapeutic intervention. This report was extremely brief, but the implication was that the author had been applying a method based on laboratory learning experiments. The fact that Max had used an electrical shock higher than that which was usual in laboratory studies displays the lack of regulation and the experimental nature of such treatments. The report, being an abstract of a paper read at a meeting, passed apparently unnoticed in the literature until the 1950s.

The next published case of aversion therapy being used to treat sexual deviation, following Max, was reported by Michael Raymond in 1956, and used a form of aversion therapy to treat a case of fetishism.[182] Freund followed in 1960 with a pioneering paper.[183] He administered to his patients a mixture of caffeine and apormophine in a number of treatment sessions, never exceeding twenty-four. When the emetic mixture became effective (and nausea overcame them), slides of dressed and undressed men were shown to the patient, and then the patient was shown films of nude or semi-nude women seven hours after the administration of testosterone propionate. Sixty-seven patients are reported on in this paper; treatment was refused to none. Out of twenty court referrals, only three achieved any kind of heterosexual adaptation, and in no case did this last for more than a few weeks. The first follow-up was undertaken after three years. Of the forty-seven patients who presented other than due to a court referral, twelve had shown some long-term heterosexual adaptation. A second follow-up two years later traced the histories of these twelve. At that time none of them could claim complete absence of homosexual desires, and only six could claim complete absence of homosexual behaviour. Three of the group were in fact engaging in homosexual behaviour fairly frequently. Ten of them had heterosexual intercourse at least every two weeks, but only three found females other than their wives sexually attractive. Clearly these results did not encourage an attitude of optimism, and Freund's series is the only one that included a satisfactory follow-up. Treatments, however, continued despite the lack of solid evidence-based outcomes.

In 1962, Basil James reported a case where he used apomorphine in the treatment of a 40-year-old homosexual.[184] The treatment was rather more invasive than that reported by Freund, and was carried out at two-hour intervals. It involved the patient being given an emetic dose of apomorphine and 57 ml of brandy. As soon as nausea occurred, a strong light was shone onto a large piece of cardboard on which were pasted several photographs of nude or semi-nude men. The patient was asked to select an attractive image, and recreate the experiences he had had with his current homosexual partner. This fantasy was verbally reinforced by the consultant on the first three occasions; thereafter, a tape recorder was played twice every two hours during the period of nausea. This consisted of an explanation of his homosexual behaviour, the adverse effects of this behaviour on him and its social repercussions. This was described in 'slow and graphic terms ending with words such as "sickening" and "nauseating", etc., followed by the noise of one vomiting'.[185]

The following night the patient was awakened every two hours and played a tape recording which optimistically explained the future consequences if he were no longer homosexual. During the three days following aversion therapy, photographs of 'sexually attractive young females' were placed in his room, and each morning he received an injection of testosterone propionate and was told to retire to his room whenever he felt any sexual excitement. The treatment was carried out in a darkened side room (see Figure 2) and continued without a break. It was only stopped after thirty hours because the patient developed acetonuria.[186] It was recommended following a twenty-four hour break for a further thirty-two hours. Five months after the treatment, the paper reported a highly satisfactory outcome, in

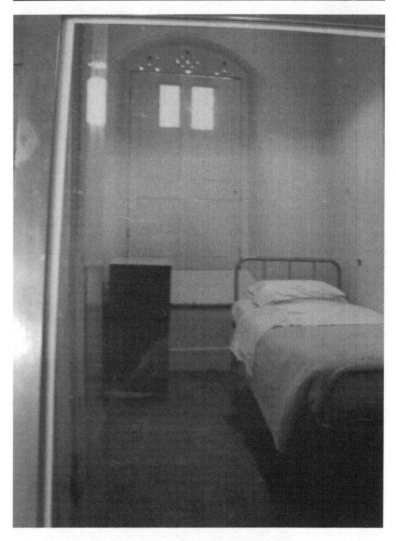

2 Side-room at Glenside Hospital, Bristol

that there was a complete change from homosexual to heterosexual behaviour. This paper displays a mixture of techniques involved in this treatment, without any discussion of the research base underpinning them.

The paper sparked some controversy, and in particular, opposition from a fellow doctor. In a letter to the editor published by the *British Medical Journal* on 31 March 1962, Sidney Crown wrote:

Sir – I was surprised to find in the paper by Dr. Basil James on aversion therapy in homosexuality that a method of treatment carried out on a single case followed up for such a short period was afforded the status of an article in one of the most widely read medical journals. Treatment in psychiatry is hindered by premature publication. As in other branches of medicine, a new therapy should be critically evaluated from the results of a controlled series of cases, with appropriate statistical analysis and adequate follow-up, before it is published. Scientific caution is, perhaps, particularly important in an emotionally toned subject such as homosexuality. Already the medical correspondent of an influential Sunday newspaper has, equally uncritically, featured the article in his column.[187]

Aversion therapy to treat homosexuality was not supported as a treatment option by the medical professional as a whole. In possible response to Crown, Basil James and his colleague Donal Early wrote a letter to the editor of the *British Medical Journal*, stating that they felt that 'a follow-up report would be of general interest'.[188] The follow-up report was given eighteen months post treatment, and despite the report stating that the patient's feelings for his current girlfriend did not have 'the same emotional component as his homosexual experiences'; the authors concluded that in their opinion, the 'patient remains a sexually normal person'.[189] Moreover, in the original paper by Basil James discussed above, James expressed his 'appreciation of the way in which the nursing staff co-operated so fully in the treatment'.[190] However, it is debatable whether this was cooperation, coercion or obedience to his orders, this will be explored in Chapter 3.

The majority (five) of the participants in this study received chemical aversion therapy. Conversely, in Smith and his colleagues' study, more of their participants received electrical aversion therapy.[191] This could attest the capricious nature of these treatments, as they varied throughout the country and had no general protocols or ethical guidelines.[192] Nevertheless, participants in both the studies recalled their experience of receiving this treatment in macabre detail:

I felt totally depersonalised. I had to give over my own clothes and was told to wear a hospital gown. [. . .] I can still taste the vile taste of stale sick in my mouth. All I wanted was to wash my mouth out with fresh water, but

I wasn't even allowed that. I remember trying to sneak out of my 'prison cell' one night to get some water, but the nurses caught me and literally threw me back in. I was not allowed out for three days. I went to the toilet in the bed; I had no basin, no toilet facilities – nothing. I had to lie in my own faeces, urine and vomit. I thought I must be dreaming at one point, it was like a torture scene by the Gestapo in Nazi Germany trying to extract information from me – I thought I was going to die.[193]

Oscar Mangle recalls: 'What was going through my mind was not that I was scared of being gay. I was petrified I would not come out of this mental hospital alive. I was a very frightened young man.'[194] Meanwhile Ughtred Lovis-Douglas casts further light on the depersonalisation process, 'I was admitted under a pseudonym, as it was of course illegal to be homosexual in those days and I would have directly incriminated myself.'[195]

The Sunday newspaper to which Crown was referring to previously was the *Observer* with an article entitled 'How Doctor Cured a Homosexual'.[196] This article appears to have played an influential role in encouraging individuals to seek these treatments. The patient described in a paper by John Thorpe and his colleagues sought treatment for his homosexuality, 'As a direct result of reading this newspaper article.'[197] Meanwhile Ughtred Lovis-Douglas, who was interviewed for this book recalls the *Observer* article in detail:

I was a veterinary student and, I am sure you can imagine it was a very masculine environment, spending a lot of time on farms. I knew I was 'queer' as they called it then, but I was desperate to be 'normal' and like all the other lads on my course. I remember we were in the common room one Sunday morning, slightly hung-over from the night before, and the lads were taking the 'piss' out of each other, as they had read an article in *The Observer* about a homosexual being cured. They were basically saying: 'Look **** [fellow student's surname] there is hope – you can be cured!' I remember joining in with the bravado to fit in. However, once they had all gone I took the paper to my room and read it properly. I remember feeling a sense of hope, as most of the other things I read about men like me were depreciatory to say the least! Anyway, I made an appointment to see my GP the next day to ask for this treatment.[198]

The influence of the media was often intensified by unsupportive attitudes from their friends, family and the police.[199] The *Sunday Pictorial* also ran a similar article the previous year entitled '"Twilight"

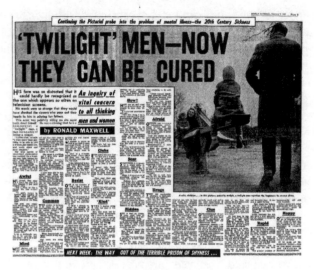

3 *The Sunday Pictorial*: '"Twilight" [homosexual] Men – Now
They Can Be Cured'

[homosexual] Men – Now They Can Be Cured' (see Figure 3),[200] thus
reinforcing the notion that homosexuality was an illness that could
be cured. It is interesting to note that the *Sunday Pictorial* article used
an image of a 'twilight' man looking furtively at children playing in
a park, with the tagline: 'A twilight man watches the happiness he
cannot share.' Arguably, this accentuated the familiar stereotype that
homosexuals had paedophilic tendencies.

The media reportage of these cases also appeared to have a positive
effect on some nurses' morality in regard to administering aversion
therapy. Ursula Vaughan remembers the press reportage of the patient
she had nursed and it serving as an affirmation of the work she was
doing:

> I remember the press discussing 'how a doctor had cured a homosexual'
> and although it didn't name names or places, I knew the report was refer-
> ring to the man I had nursed. It was my 'fifteen minutes of fame' as they say
> [laughs]. I suppose the fact it was printed for all to see was confirmation of
> the good work we were doing.[201]

A number of other papers followed on from James and included studies
by Isaac Oswald[202] and Angus Cooper.[203] Both also used noxious

(i.e. emetic) stimuli and treatment that continued without a break, and in some cases the patient was kept awake by means of amphetamines.[204] Some patients, who were deprived of sleep for long periods, felt temporarily cured, but some also experienced complete nervous breakdowns.[205] Health care staff also played tape recordings of contemptuous comments about the patient to them, and allowed them no food or drinks other than the prescribed alcohol. Psychiatrist M. J. Raymond remarked that 'modification of attitudes and psychological conversation are more easily obtained in states of exhaustion and hunger'.[206] Cooper suggested that the desired changes were 'more easily obtained in fatigued and debilitated subjects'.[207] Meanwhile, Oswald attempted to produce a 'maximal emotional crisis in order to facilitate conversion' in the case of a patient being treated for transvestism.[208]

In this case the patient was actually required to carry out the fetishistic acts. With the onset of nausea and vomiting, the patient was returned to bed and 'received intensive moral suggestion'. During the whole day he was not allowed to discard his female clothes, but was instructed to look at his reflection in the mirror and re-enact in his mind every detail of his 'disgusting perversion'. The patient was kept awake at night by means of amphetamine, and a tape recording played pejorative comments about him for twenty minutes every two hours. The patient finally broke down after seven days of this regime, having neither eaten nor slept for six days. Three days after treatment, a right ventricular stress was noted and this was considered to be due to a toxic myocarditis[209] produced by the emetic. Despite this being a potentially fatal condition, the treatment continued. This could give an indication of the medical attitude towards this patient group at the time.

It was fairly common to play the patient a pre-recorded audiotape as part of the treatment in chemical aversion therapy, which usually consisted of an explanation about the atrociousness of their behaviour and the goodness of stopping it. Maude Griffin recalls a consultant psychiatrist making such an audiotape:

> He [the consultant psychiatrist] was in his office for hours making this audiotape. Every time I walked past, you could see him rewinding and starting again. I could see he was taking a great deal of time to be as nasty as he possibly could on it. And he was. He really was. I was so upset when I heard the recording that I had to play the patient, it was awful. Truly awful.[210]

Sometimes, therapists asked patients to tape-record their own thoughts about their behaviour and why it was good or enjoyable, and then that audiotape was overlaid with messages repeatedly using pejorative words regarding their sexual desires such as 'sickening' and 'nauseating', and describing how the person needed to give it up to live a so-called normal life.[211] The effect of using a patient's own words and interests against them was depicted clearly in the film *A Clockwork Orange*. The now-classic 1971 film depicts a nightmarish version of aversion therapy called the Ludovico Treatment used on the main character, Alex, who is in prison for murder. He is placed in a straitjacket, his eyes are held open with a machine while a nurse drops liquid into his eyes, and doctors show him films with Nazis marching and destroying buildings. While this is happening, his beloved Beethoven music plays over the top. At one point he screams, 'Stop it, stop it, please I beg you.' The male doctor replies, 'I'm sorry, Alex. This is for your own good. You have to bear with us for a while.' Alex screams that he has seen the light and is cured, but the Nazi films continue in front of his artificially opened eyes. The idea that a patient who wanted to be cured of a particular desire must associate his most cherished feelings and experiences with atrocities was the reasoning of aversion therapy.[212]

As we have seen above, there were two types of noxious stimulus utilised for the treatments for sexual deviation – chemical and electrical. However, the literature appears to suggest that there was some contention regarding which was the most efficacious. Simon Rachman and John Barker both pointed out that chemical aversion was highly unpleasant, not only for the patient, but also for the therapist and nursing staff.[213] Therefore, psychiatrists in the late 1950s and early 1960s began to turn their attention to the usefulness of electric shock therapy as a replacement for nausea inducing drugs.

In 1963 John Thorpe and his colleagues reported the use of electric shock as the noxious stimulus.[214] Here the treatment was carried out in a room with a floor area of nine square feet, with the floor completely covered by an electric grid. 'Strong' and 'painful' electric shocks were delivered through the electric grid to the patient's bare feet. The patient was requested to bring one of his own photos of a nude male; this was fixed to the wall, and illumined by a bright light operated by a psychologist. The electric shocks were administered in response to increases in penile erection, measured by a plethysmograph. Within each treatment session, the picture was illuminated forty times. On nine of these occasions, the patient was randomly shocked.

Follow-up contact appears to have been through letter. The patient reported using heterosexual fantasy, and stated that he had made one attempt at heterosexual intercourse. Occasional homosexual patterns of behaviour had occurred, but the patient was not unduly worried about these, which he regarded as 'a safety valve'. The authors admitted that many would consider this patient to have technically relapsed. However, they predicted a satisfactory heterosexual adjustment for him, and they therefore considered his treatment to have been successful.

In 1964 Robert McGuire and Michael Vallance described what they state to be a classical conditioning technique.[215] The patient was required to signal to the therapist when the mental image of his usual fantasy was clear. When he did so, a shock was administered. The procedure was repeated throughout a thirty-minute session, which was held up to six times per day. The authors also designed a small and completely portable electrical apparatus to be used in the treatment, and this was usually handed over to the patient so that he could treat himself in his own home. He was told to use the apparatus whenever he was tempted to indulge in the fantasy concerned.

The people who received electrical aversion therapy found this equally unpleasant: 'In many respects the electric shocks were very, very painful [. . .] It was such a sharp bolt of pain shooting through my body.'[216] Meanwhile Greta Gold reflected on her treatment in graphic detail:

> I remember sitting in the room on a wooden chair 'dressed' [wearing women's clothes], but I had to be barefoot as my feet had to touch the metal electric grid. My penis was also wired up to something to measure if I got an erection – I felt totally violated. [. . .] I remember the excruciating pain of the initial shock; nothing could have prepared me for it. Tears began running down my face and the nurse said: 'What are you crying for? We have only just started!' . . . [Chokes] . . . I was speechless.[217]

Some nurses also found the therapy similarly distressing to witness:

> I remember the first time I witnessed it [electrical aversion therapy]. I thought it was barbaric, I mean I remember thinking: 'Where was the treatment?' The young lad nearly jumped out of his skin with the jolt of

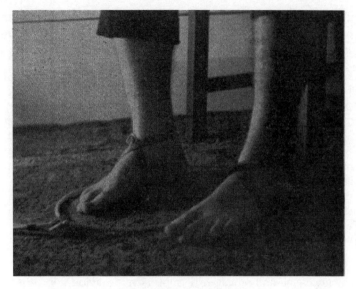

4 Electrical aversion therapy

the first shock. Then you could see it was almost mental torture waiting for the next one![218]

The medical press were keen to publish their studies and claim successful outcomes. However, King and Bartlett argue that there was no confirmation of successful outcomes beyond penile volume measurements in response to erotic stimuli, or the patient reporting that they now believed they were heterosexual or that they were repulsed at the thought of wearing the opposite sex's clothes.[219] In treatments that did not use a plethysmograph to measure penile volume measurements, the success of the treatment and, therefore, the patient's discharge was based mainly on self-reported outcomes from the patient.[220]

Some patients in this study were able to use this to their advantage and engaged in subversive behaviours in order to be discharged from the hospital. Indeed Percival Thatcher states that his aversion therapy was stopped, '. . . because I lied, and told them that it had worked'.[221] Greta Gold recalls a similar narrative:

> I suddenly had a 'eureka moment' and thought, how do the doctors actually know what I'm thinking? I knew I would have to start lying about my feelings if I ever wanted to get out.[222]

Both testimonies allude to the patients' ability to manipulate the system by feigning heterosexuality or repulsion with their transvestism. Benedict Henry muses on the self-reported nature of the treatments:

> I remember the consultant saying: 'How do you feel?' One of the best responses to the doctor at the time was to say: 'I feel repulsed by who I am.' That was always seen as a very good sign. Or: 'I have been thinking of some of the pictures you have shown me, and I realise now how distasteful that is.' That was always seen as a good response. As the patients were gaining insight, the patients were beginning to understand their own deviancy, and their own abnormality. Erm ... there was never actually any way of checking whether the patients actually believed in what they were saying. Or whether they were just saying it because they knew, you know, that this is what they ought to say. Because I do remember them being quite bright people, they were witty.[223]

It appears that Percival Thatcher and Greta Gold used this to their advantage and, engaged in subversive behaviours in order to speed up their discharge from hospital. This highlights how treatments varied throughout the country, as some consultants chose to utilise a plethysmograph to measure penile volume measurements, while others did not. There was a level of arbitrariness to the selection of treatments and a variety of methods were adopted, which lacked regularity and a sound evidence base. Furthermore, with no general protocol or ethical guidelines, the treatment of choice was often the unilateral decision of the consultant psychiatrist.[224] The treatments lacked rigour: in some cases the patients were able to feign the effectiveness of the treatment in order to be discharged.

Patients such as Percival Thatcher who were admitted to the hospital on a court order appear to have taken advantage of this. This could have been due to Percival already being 'fairly accepting'[225] of his sexuality, and his perception that the treatment 'was not going to make me straight, I didn't want it to'.[226] Nevertheless, many former patients self-referred for treatment owing to the turmoil they found themselves in regarding their sexual desires. Therefore, not all patients took advantage of the ability to subvert their health care professionals and many endured the unpleasantness of the treatments. In Albert Holliday's case he persisted with the treatment for over a year, in the otiose hope that it would be successful.[227]

Referral pathways

Many men were referred for these treatments by their general practitioner (GP). Indeed, seven of the men interviewed for this book approached their GPs about their problems and were referred to NHS professionals who specialised in this area. However, all reported that their GPs appeared perplexed by their disclosure and offered little empathy for their situation. Many men sought treatment because of the turmoil they found themselves in when they realised they were sexually attracted to other men:

> This was terrifying really because I was thrown into confusion and it made me very poorly because I had three children, little ones, and a wife, and we all loved each other, we had been happy building our lives, you know. I was very fond of my wife as well and everything was going okay and then all this began to happen and threw me into awful confusion and made me very, very poorly and so I thought I had to go to the doctor. So I did.[228]

Percival Thatcher was given an option of imprisonment or he could be remanded provided he was willing to undergo psychological treatment when he was entrapped and arrested by an undercover police officer in a public place for importuning:

> Well when I was given the option, prison or hospital, well I just thought if I go to prison . . . if the other inmates found out what I was in there for, well, I just thought they would kill me! I mean, I was fairly accepting of my sexuality, but in society and particularly within a prison, it was viewed in the same light as a paedophile. 'No, I'm not going to prison', that is all I could think. So I just said, 'Yeah, I'll go to hospital for the aversion therapy.' I knew it was not going to make me straight, I didn't want it to, but it seemed a better option than prison.[229]

Percival was tacitly coerced into receiving treatment, and although the other men in this book self-referred via their GPs, arguably they were all implicitly coerced into receiving aversion therapy by the media and the paternalistic attitudes of their GPs. These influences could all have led to the health care professionals not upholding the patients' autonomy in relation to their decision to consent to the treatment.

The late 1950s to the mid-1960s witnessed a marked refocusing of public debate with the transformation of sexual deviance from a 'crime' to a 'sickness'. Many of the former patients who participated in this study recalled their initial exuberance at this shift in ideology. For many, discovering that there was a 'cure' for their disorder gave them a sense of hope and legitimacy. Indeed, Oscar Mangle recalls: 'No longer was I an evil pervert. Now I believed I could be viewed as a patient with all the vulnerabilities and sympathy a patient demands.'[230] The press were keen to report this ideological shift; and when an anonymous donor gave Crumpsall Hospital, Manchester a donation of between £6,000 and £7,000 to set up a research and treatment unit for homosexuality, the *Birmingham Post*, the *Manchester Daily Telegraph*, the *Guardian*, *The Times* and *The Scotsman* all reported the case with a level of optimism.[231] Furthermore, the *New Statesman* published a letter from a former patient who had received treatment at the Portland Clinic at No. 8 Bourdon Street, London, following a 'homosexual offence'. The treatment in his case was so 'amazingly helpful' that he wanted to promote the clinic to others in his position.[232]

In spite of the popular reportage of these cases, some papers were still unsympathetic, with *The Scotsman* running headlines, 'Growing Problem of the Homosexual' and 'Control Must Come Before Cure'.[233] And, the *Guardian* peddled the headline 'Homosexuals Cured More Easily in Prison'.[234] Reports such as this left Cecil Asquith, who nursed patients who were receiving treatment for various sexual deviations, very confused:

> I felt like I was being given very mixed messages about the homosexuals I was nursing. I didn't know whether to believe the newspapers, the sociologists or the doctors I was working with. It really troubled me that there was such a lack of parity between these views.[235]

Conclusion

The period explored in this chapter witnessed many debates about the ideal way to manage the perceived problem of sexual deviation in men. Despite the liberal attitude expressed by many during World War II, this is also the period when the idea that homosexuality was a pathology was more popularised. There appeared to be a cultural shift after the war marking a drive for the nation to return to pre-war values with a growing emphasis on domesticity, family life and social order, with which it was believed that homosexual men were at odds. Although there was never any dedicated witch-hunt of homosexual men during the 1950s, the incidence of arrests and convictions did increase. This included some influential people. Homosexual men living through this period expressed hyper-vigilance towards the police and felt fearful and cautious. Homosexuality was being brought out into public rhetoric by the media, literary, medical, sociological and legal discussions. These played a role in shaping public knowledge about who the sexual deviant was and what he represented. However, these were all portraying mixed messages regarding homosexual men, leaving the recipients very confused.

Following Wolfenden, there was a distinct altering of notions regarding homosexuality from a criminal perspective to understandings of the subject as pathology. There was a shifting of control and power from the courts to the medical profession; many of whom were optimistically promoting their worth in being able to cure these individuals by reporting successful outcomes. Ideas regarding what was perceived to be the most efficacious therapy to cure these individuals changed through the period from psychoanalysis to oestrogen therapy and finally on to aversion therapy. These therapies were reported, it appears, somewhat sanguinely by the media and the medical profession, and by the late 1950s the desire to have sex with another man was being more universally seen to be the result of an ingrained condition that could now be cured.

However, there were still opponents to this view with some still believing that the sexual deviant should be dealt with under the auspices of the law. Therefore, despite this post-war propagation of writings regarding sexual deviations, no one explanatory system emerged victorious in the 1950s and 1960s. Through these traversing narratives of sexual danger and medical discourses, the sexual deviant was constructed beyond the boundaries of national citizenship and therefore, was a fitting subject for social exclusion, legal repression, or medical treatment. When nurses came on duty to care for patients receiving treatment for their sexual deviations during these years, they did so in a world in which tabloid, psychoanalytic, behavioural, legal, medical and other discourses of sexual deviations competed with each other for attention causing considerable confusion.

Notes

1 Benedict Henry, interviewed 23 June 2010.
2 Some progress was made in the 1940s in modifying the legal attitude to homosexuality. Under the Criminal Justice Act of 1948, the conditions of probation were extended and improved. Under the Act the court could now order treatment under a qualified medical practitioner; see also the National Archives (NA), Kew, H0345/9, Proceedings of the Wolfenden Committee on Homosexual Offences and Prostitution (PWC), Summary Record of 21st Meeting, March 1956.
3 John Costello, *Love, Sex & War: Changing Values, 1939–45* (London, 1985), p. 162; Peter Wildeblood, *Against the Law: The Classic Account of a Homosexual in 1950s Britain* (London, 1955).
4 Within the first year of the war, 2,000 male nurses left for military service and 600 women had left for war work: Chatterton, 'The Weakest Link in the Chain of Nursing?', p. 67. Peter Nolan, 'Jack's Story', *Royal College of Nursing. The History of Nursing Group* 2 (2) (1987), pp. 22–28.
5 Nolan, 'Jack's Story', pp. 22–28.
6 Peter Nolan, 'The Development of Mental Health Nursing', in Jerome Carson, Leonard Fagin and Susan A. Ritter (eds), *Stress and Coping in Mental Health Nursing* (London, 1995), p. 13.
7 Julian Wills, interviewed 4 January 2010.
8 Quentin Crisp, *The Naked Civil Servant* (London, 1968), p. 155.
9 Paul Jackson, *One of the Boys Homosexuality in the Military during World War II* (Montreal, 2010), p. 187.
10 Emma Vickers, *Queen and County Same-Sex Desire in the British Armed Forces, 1939–1945* (Manchester, 2013), p. 80.
11 'Roy's' testimony in Porter and Weeks, *Between the Acts*, p. 78.
12 Herbert Bliss, interviewed 2 January 2010; see, also Peter Wildeblood, *Against the Law: The Classic Account of a Homosexual in 1950s Britain* (London, 1955), pp. 19–21 (regarding the acceptance and tolerance to his homosexuality while he was in prison); Paul Jones, *Tales from Out in the City* (Manchester, 2009), pp. 91–93.
13 I have used Richard Dyer's definition of camp: 'a characteristically gay way of handling the products of a culture through irony, exaggeration, trivialization, theatricalization and an ambivalent making fun out of the serious and respectable'. Richard Dyer, *The Culture of Queers* (London, 2002), p. 250.
14 Vickers, *Queen and County*, p. 87.
15 Jivani, *It's Not Unusual*, p. 64.

16 Jivani, *It's Not Unusual*, p. 70.
17 For a more detailed exploration of class within homosexual urban culture: see, e.g. Houlbrook, *Queer London*, pp. 167–195.
18 Cook, *A Gay History of Britain*, p. 187.
19 Jivani, *It's Not Unusual*, p. 67.
20 Lesley Hall, *Sex Gender and Social Change Since 1880* (Basingstoke, 2000), p. 144.
21 Jivani, *It's Not Unusual*, p. 58.
22 Jivani, *It's Not Unusual*, p. 58.
23 Willaim T. Doidge and Wayne H. Holtzman, 'Implications of Homosexuality Among Air Force Trainees', *Journal of Consulting Psychology* 24 (1) (1940), p. 10.
24 Nicolai Giosca, 'The Gag Reflex and Fellatio', *American Journal of Psychiatry* 107 (1950), p. 380.
25 Jivani, *It's Not Unusual*, p. 58.
26 George Henry, 'Psychogenic Factors in Overt Homosexuality', *American Journal of Psychiatry* xiii (1940), p. 57. The describing of homosexual characteristics can be traced back to Mangus Hirschfeld who in 1897 founded the Scientific Humanitarian Committee. The motto of the Committee, 'Justice through Science', reflected Hirschfeld's belief that a better scientific understanding of homosexuality would eliminate hostility toward homosexuals.
27 Jivani, *It's Not Unusual*, p. 70.
28 Costello, *Love, Sex & Wars*. The original document is on p. 162.
29 Jivani, *It's Not Unusual*, p. 70.
30 Hall Carpenter Archives Gay Men's Oral History Group, *Walking After Midnight: Gay Men's Life Stories* (London, 1989), p. 33.
31 Crisp, *The Naked Civil Servant*, p. 156.
32 Crisp, *The Naked Civil Servant*, p. 156.
33 Vickers, *Queen and County*, pp. 40–45.
34 Costello, *Love, Sex & War*, p. 167.
35 Charles Anderson, 'On Certain Conscious and Unconscious Homosexual Responses to Warfare', *British Journal of Medical Psychology* 2 (1945), pp. 157–162; Costello, *Love, Sex & Wars*, p. 162.
36 Joanna Bourke, 'Disciplining The Emotions: Fear, Psychiatry and the Second World War', in Roger Cooter, Mark Harrison and Steve Sturdy (eds), *War, Medicine & Modernity* (Stroud, 1998), p. 231.
37 Philip S. Wagner, 'Psychiatric Activities During the Normandy Offensive', *Psychiatry* 9 (1946), pp. 348–356.
38 Cook, *A Gay History of Britain*, p. 149.
39 Once the concentration camps had been liberated, homosexual men were transferred to prison because homosexuality was still illegal. See, for example, Heinz Heger, *The Men with the Pink Triangle* (Boston, 1980).

40 Richard Plant, *The Pink Triangle* (New York, 1986), p. 51.

41 Hans Geissler, 'Homosexuellen-Gesetzgebung', in Plant, *The Pink Triangle*, p. 26.

42 Gad Beck, *An Underground Life: Memoirs of a Gay Jew in Nazi Berlin* (Wisconsin, 1999), p. 21.

43 Heger, *The Men with the Pink Triangle*, p. 56.

44 Plant, *The Pink Triangle*, p. 72.

45 While it never attained a firm enough constituency of support in the scientific community, it is important to note that there was also a eugenics movement in the UK during the inter-war years. This was powerfully illustrated by the campaign for the voluntary sterilisation of 'mental defectives', which developed in the 1920s, and reached a peak in the early 1930s. Voluntary sterilisation was the principle issue in the eugenics movement in the UK, and its implementation in legislation was seen as pertinent to the success of the movement. Indeed, one of the supporters of sterilisation was Havelock Ellis. See, e.g., John Macnicol, 'Eugenics and the Campaign for Voluntary Sterilization in Britain Between the Wars', *The Society for the History of Medicine* (1989), pp. 147–169; Matthew Thomson, 'Sterilization, Segregation and Community Care: Ideology and Solutions to the Problem of Mental Deficiency in Inter-War Britain', *History of Psychiatry* 3 (1992), pp. 473–498; Brickell, *Mates & Lovers*, p. 93.

46 Beck, *An Underground Life*, p. 89.

47 Heger, *The Men with the Pink Triangle*, p. 57.

48 Costello, *Love, Sex & War*, p. 161.

49 Costello, *Love, Sex & War*, p. 161.

50 Plant, *The Pink Triangle*, p. 21.

51 See, e.g., Pierre Seel, *I, Pierre Seel, Deported Homosexual* (New York, 1994); Heger, *The Men with the Pink Triangle*; Plant, *The Pink Triangle*.

52 Plant, *The Pink Triangle*, p. 14.

53 See, e.g., Seel, *Deported Homosexual*; Heger, *The Men with the Pink Triangle*; Plant, *The Pink Triangle*.

54 See, e.g., Susan Benedict and Jane M. Georges, 'Nurses and the Sterilization Experiments of Auschwitz: A Postmodernist Perspective', *Nursing Inquiry* 13 (4) (2006), pp. 227–288; Bronwyn Rebekah McFarland-Icke, *Nurses in Nazi Germany: A Moral Choice in History* (Princeton, 1999), p. 130; Francis Biley, 'Psychiatric Nursing: Living with the Legacy of the Holocaust', *Journal of Psychiatric and Mental Health Nursing* 9 (2002), p. 365; Hilde Steppe, 'Nursing in Nazi Germany', *Western Journal of Nursing Research* 14 (1991), p. 745.

55 Jivani, *It's Not Unusual*, p. 55.

56 Costello, *Love, Sex & War*, p. 173.

57 Crisp, *The Naked Civil Servant*, p. 160.

58 Houlbrook, *Queer London*, p. 236.

59 For a detailed discussion of the social changes following World War II: see, e.g., Harry Hopkins, *The New Look* (London, 1963).

60 Hopkins, *The New Look*, p. 57.

61 Weeks, *The World We Have Won*, p. 29; Jivani, *It's Not Unusual*, p. 89.

62 For a detailed discussion regarding women's wartime lives, see, e.g., Summerfield, *Reconstructing Women's Wartime Lives*; Juliette Pattinson, *Behind Enemy Lines: Gender, Passing and the Special Operations Executive in the Second World War* (Manchester, 2007).

63 Houlbrook, *Queer London*, p. 236.

64 Hall, *Sex, Gender and Social Change*, pp. 150–166.

65 Hall, *Sex, Gender and Social Change*, pp. 150–166; Weeks, *The World We Have Won*, p. 41.

66 Sue March, *Gay Liberation* (New York, 1974), p. 57.

67 *Design for Living* was the name of the original play by Noel Coward, and was first shown in 1932.

68 Throughout *Look Up and Laugh* there are clearly two gay male characters, played for laughs, but in a major musical sequence there is one unusual aspect. The number is 'Love is Everywhere' and Gracie is saying good-night to diverse characters, each in love in a different way – the miser with his money, the young couple, a spinster lady dreaming of love. She then approaches the gay couple, who are seen in silhouette behind a blind, as she approaches the two men she pauses and gives a warm smile as if in acknowledgement of their relationship.

69 Petting among unmarried individuals was strongly deplored in the later 1940s and 1950s and caused great concern for the Family Planning Association, as it was believed to be a slippery slope to illegitimate children or hasty marriages: Hall, *Sex, Gender and Social Change in Britain Since 1880*, pp. 156–157.

70 Albert Holliday, interviewed 2 January 2010.

71 Jivani, *It's Not Unusual*, p. 89.

72 Earl Winterton, in Montgomery Hyde, *The Other Love: An Historical and Contemporary Survey of Homosexuality in Britain* (London, 1970), p. 226–227.

73 'Anomaly' (pseudonym), *The Invert and His Social Adjustment* (London, 1948), pp. 7–8. It was written by Harry Baldwin, a Canadian civil servant.

74 Houlbrook uses this term to describe a flamboyant and striking figure in London's streets and commercial venues who was, for many Londoners, the very epitome of sexual difference. Quean is derived from the Middle English meaning a disreputable woman. While the spellings 'queen' and 'quean' were used interchangeably in the first half of the twentieth century, Houlbrook followed Eric Partridge's *Dictionary of the Underworld* (Wordsworth, 1995), pp. 545–549, and used 'quean' as the standard spelling in his book *Queer London*.

75 Weeks, *The World We Have Won*, p. 47; Houlbrook, *Queer London*, p. 236.

76 Cook, *A Gay History of Britain*, p. 167.

77 Alfred Kinsey, Warren Pomeroy and Clyde Martin, *Sexual Behaviour in the Human Male* (Philadelphia, 1948).

78 See, e.g., Donna J. Drucker, 'Male sexuality and Alfred Kinsey's 0–6 scale: Toward "a sound understanding of the realities of sex", *Journal of Homosexuality* 57 (2010), pp. 1105–1123; Peter Hegarty, *Gentlemen's Disagreement: Alfred Kinsey, Lewis Terman, and the Sexual Politics of Smart Men* (Chicago, 2013).

79 Kinsey, Pomeroy and Martin, *Sexual Behaviour in the Human Male*, p. 23.

80 Jivani, *It's Not Unusual*, pp. 96–97.

81 Jivani, *It's Not Unusual*, p. 96.

82 Liz Stanley, *Sex Surveyed 1949–1994: From Mass Observations: 'Little Kinsey' to the National Surveys and Hite Report* (London, 1995).

83 Stanley, *Sex Surveyed 1949–1994*, pp. 199–203.

84 Stanley, *Sex Surveyed 1949–1994*, p. 241.

85 Jivani, *It's Not Unusual*, p. 99.

86 NA, CAB/195/11, minutes of a meeting with Home Secretary and Prime Minister discussing issues around prostitution and homosexuality.

87 Jivani, *It's Not Unusual*, p. 99.

88 'Scotland Yard to Smash Homosexuality', *Sydney Morning Telegraph* (25 June 1953).

89 See, e.g., Houlbrook, *Queer London*, pp. 33–36; Higgins, *Heterosexual Dictatorship*.

90 Jivani, *It's Not Unusual*, p. 100.

91 Elizabeth A. Povinelli and George Chauncey, 'Thinking Sexually Transitionally: An Introduction', *Journal of Lesbian and Gay Studies* 5 (1999), pp. 439–449.

92 Statistics for sodomy also include bestiality cases: Jeffery Weeks, *Coming Out*, p. 158.

93 Jones, *Out in the City*, p. 31.

94 Houlbrook, *Queer London*, p. 63.

95 NA, HO 345 7: CHP II: memorandum submitted by Harold Sturge, Metropolitan Magistrate, Old Street.

96 NA, HO 345 12: CHP TRANS 8, Q633, 3.

97 Houlbrook, *Queer London*, p. 63.

98 Greta Gold, interviewed 24 March 2010.

99 Myrtle Pauncefoot, interviewed 20 February 2013.

100 Oscar Mangle, interviewed 21 June 2010.

101 Colin Fox interview on *Dark Secret: Sexual Aversion*, British Broadcasting Corporation (1996).

102 Molly Millbury, interviewed 31 December 2010.

103 Chris Waters, 'Disorders of the Mind, Disorders of the Body Social: Peter Wildeblood and the Making of the Modern Homosexual', in Becky Conekin, Frank Mort and Chris Waters (eds), *Moments of Modernity Reconstructing Britain 1945–1964* (London, 1999), p. 135.

104 'Sailor Cleared of Manslaughter', *News of the World* (26 October 1947).

105 Cook, *A Gay History of Britain*, p. 169.

106 Waters, 'Disorders of the Mind', p. 135.

107 Houlbrook, *Queer London*, p. 192.

108 'The Squalid Truth', *Sunday Pictorial* (25 September 1955).

109 Cook, *A Gay History of Britain*, p. 168.

110 'Evil Men', *Sunday Pictorial* (25 May 1952).

111 Greta Gold, interviewed 24 March 2010; Tommy Dickinson, Matt Cook, John Playle and Christine Hallett, '"Queer" Treatments: Giving a Voice to Former Patients who Received Treatments for their "Sexual Deviations"', *Journal of Clinical Nursing* 21 (9) (2012), p. 1349.

112 Jivani, *It's Not Unusual*, p. 110.

113 'Final Day of the Montagu Trial', *Daily Sketch* (24 March 1954).

114 Wildeblood, *Against the Law*, pp. 94–95.

115 Ughtred Lovis-Douglas, interviewed 4 January 2013.

116 March, *Gay Liberation*, p. 59.

117 Tudor Rees and Harley Usill, *They Stand Apart: A Critical Survey of the Problem of Homosexuality* (London, 1955).

118 Rees and Usill, *They Stand Apart*, p. viii.

119 Lindesay Neustatter, 'Homosexuality: The Medical Perspective', in Tudor Rees and Harley Usill (eds), *They Stand Apart: A Critical Survey of the Problem of Homosexuality* (London, 1955).

120 Gordon Westwood, *Society and the Homosexual* (New York, 1952), p. 178.

121 Westwood, *Society and the Homosexual*, p. 168.

122 Elizabeth Granger, interviewed 3 May 2010.

123 'The Problem of Homosexuality: Report by Clergy and Doctors', *The Times* (26 February 1954).

124 Una Drinkwater, interviewed 29 December 2009.

125 Matt Houlbrook and Chris Waters, 'The Heart in Exile: Detachment and Desire in 1950s London', *History Workshop Journal* 62 (2006), p. 145.

126 Zella Mullins, interviewed 14 July 2010.

127 *Sunday Times*, 28 March, 1954.

128 NA, CAB/195/11, minutes of meeting with Home Secretary and Prime Minister discussing issues around prostitution and homosexuality.

129 'An Uneasy History', *Attitude Magazine* (March 2010).

130 Frank Mort, *Capital Affairs: London and the Making of the Permissive Society* (New Haven, 2010), p. 140.

131 Mort, *Capital Affairs*, p. 139.

132 Roger Davidson, 'Law, Medicine and the Treatment of Homosexual Offenders in Scotland, 1950–1980', in Ingrid Goold and Charles Kelly (eds), *Lawyers' Medicine: The Legislature, the Courts & Medical Practice, 1760–2000* (Oxford, 2009), p. 129.

133 NA, HO345/15, CHP/TRANS/41, PWC, evidence of W Boyd, 1 November 1955; see, also Davidson, 'Law, Medicine and the Treatment of Homosexual Offenders', pp. 129–130.

134 Davidson, 'Law, Medicine and the Treatment of Homosexual Offenders', p. 130.

135 British Medical Association Archives, B/107/1/2, memo. By Professor John Glaister, 30 June 1955.

136 Davidson, 'Law, Medicine and the Treatment of Homosexual Offenders', pp. 133–134.

137 NA, HO345/12 and /16, PWC, 15th October 1954, 10th April 1956; HO345/2, J Adair to WC Roberts, 4 October 1956; HO345/10, note on WC discussion meetings, 11 and 12 September 1956.

138 Waters, 'Disorders of the Mind', p. 149.

139 Cook, *A Gay History of Britain*, p. 172.

140 NA, HO 345 14, CHP TRANS 32: two witnesses called by chairman (28 July 1955).

141 Houlbrook, *Queer London*, p. 255.

142 Waters, 'Disorders of the Mind', p. 149.

143 Houlbrook, *Queer London*, p. 259.

144 NA, HO 345 8, CHP 53.

145 Wildeblood, *Against the Law*, p. 57; Waters, 'Disorders of the Mind', p. 145.

146 Houlbrook, *Queer London*, p. 259.

147 Cook, *A Gay History of Britain*, p. 172.

148 Houlbrook, *Queer London*, p. 261.

149 Despite this recommendation, it would take until 1967 for the government to decriminalise homosexuality in England and Wales with the passing of the Sexual Offences Act 1967. The reasons for this ten-year gap are discussed in Chapter 5, along with the implications of the conservative imperative the new Act.

150 'What the Papers Say about the Report', *Evening News* (5 September 1957).

151 'Planned to Help a Million', *Mail* (6 September 1957); 'One Million Need This New Clinic', *Express* (23 August 1957); 'Sex Pills for Scots in Jail', *Sunday Pictorial* (16 February 1958).

152 Jivani, *It's Not Unusual*, p. 123.

153 Waters, 'Disorders of the Mind', p. 151.

154 'Treatment of Homosexuals: Public Opinion Hostile', *Glasgow Herald* (28 September 1961).

155 Waters, 'Havelock Ellis, Sigmund Freud and the State', pp. 173–174.

156 Wildeblood, *Against the Law*, pp. 19–21; Waters, 'Havelock Ellis, Sigmund Freud and the State', pp. 173–174.

157 Westwood, *Homosexuality* (London, 1955).

158 Waters, 'Havelock Ellis, Sigmund Freud and the State', p. 174.

159 Callen Allan, 'The Treatment of Homosexuality', *Medical Press* 235 (1956), p. 141; Alan Ellis, 'The Effectiveness of Psychotherapy with Individuals who have Severe Homosexual Problems', *Journal of Consulting Psychology* 20 (1956), pp. 58–60.

160 David Curran and Daniel Parr, 'Homosexuality: An Analysis of 100 Male Cases seen in Private', *British Medical Journal* 1 (1957), pp. 797–801.

161 Mary Woodward, 'The Diagnosis and Treatment of Homosexual Offenders', *British Journal of Delinquency* 9 (1958), pp. 44–59.

162 Charlie, R. Rubenstein, 'Psychotherapeutic Aspects of Male Homosexuality', *British Journal of Medical Psychology* 31 (1958), pp. 14–18.

163 Ernest Jones, *The Life and Work of Sigmund Freud* (London, 1964), p. 43.

164 Irving Bieber, *Homosexuality* (New York, 1965), p. 78.

165 Joseph Wolpe, *Psychotherapy by Reciprocal Inhibition* (Stanford, 1958), p. 54.

166 See, e.g., Bancroft, *Deviant Sexual Behaviour*.

167 See, e.g., Francis Golla and Robert Sessions-Hodge, 'Hormone Treatment of the Sexual Offender', *The Lancet* 11 (1949), pp. 1006 – 1007; Joshua Bierer, 'Stilboestrol in Out-Patient Treatment of Sexual Offenders: A Case Report', *British Medical Journal* (1950), pp. 935–936.

168 Davidson, 'Law, Medicine and the Treatment of Homosexual Offenders', p. 129.

169 NA, HO345/15, CHP/TRANS/42, PWC, evidence of TD Inch, 'Sexual Offenders: Treatment in Prisons'.

170 Cook, *A Gay History of Britain*, p. 166.

171 David H. Barlow, 'Increasing Heterosexual Responsiveness in the Treatment of Sexual Deviation: A Review of the Clinical and Experimental Evidence', *Behaviour Therapy* 4 (1973), p. 655.

172 See, e.g., Nvzia V. Kantrovich, 'An Attempt at Associate Reflex Therapy in Alcoholism', *Psychology Abstracts* 4282 (1930), p. 26.

173 John Sugden, Andrew Bessant, Mike Eastland and Ray Field, *A Handbook for Psychiatric Nurses* (London, 1986), pp. 219–220.

174 John Watson and Rosaline Rayner, 'Conditioned Emotional Reactions', *Journal of Experimental Psychology* 3 (1920), pp. 1–14.

175 Brian F. Skinner, *Science and the Human Behaviour* (New York, 1953), pp. 34–37.

176 Diane Coon and Jane O. Mitterer, *Introduction to Psychology: Gateways to Mind and Behaviour* (New York, 2009), p. 36.

177 Sugden, Bessant, Eastland and Field, *A Handbook for Psychiatric Nurses*, pp. 219–220.

178 Lyn Y. Abramson, 'Relevance of Animal Learning Models to Behavioural Psychotherapy', *British Association for Behavioural and Cognitive Psychotherapies* 4 (1976), p. 2.

179 Stanley Rachman, 'Aversion Therapy: Chemical or Electrical?', *Behaviour Research and Therapy* 2 (1965), p. 289.

180 Max, 'Breaking up a Homosexual Fixation', p. 734.

181 Max, 'Breaking up a Homosexual Fixation', p. 734.

182 Max, 'Breaking up a Homosexual Fixation', p. 734; Michael Raymond, 'Case of Fetishism Treated by Aversion Therapy', *British Medical Journal* 2 (1956), pp. 854–857.

183 Kevin Freund, 'Some Problems in the Treatment of Homosexuality', in Henry J. Eysenck (ed.), *Experiments in Behaviour Therapy* (London, 1960), p. 79.

184 Basil James, 'Case of Homosexuality Treated by Aversion Therapy', *British Medical Journal* 17 (1962), p. 768.

185 James, 'Case of Homosexuality', p. 768.

186 Acetonuria: the excretion in the urine of excessive amounts of acetone, an indication of incomplete oxidation of large amounts of fat; common in diabetic acidosis and starvation.

187 Sidney Crown, 'Aversion Therapy for Homosexuality', *British Medical Journal* 31 (1962), p. 943.

188 Basil James and Donal F. Early, 'Aversion Therapy for Homosexuality', *British Medical Journal* 23 (1963), p. 538.

189 James and Early, 'Aversion Therapy for Homosexuality', p. 538.

190 James, 'Case of Homosexuality Treated by Aversion Therapy', p. 770.

191 Smith, King and Bartlett, 'Treatments of Homosexuality in Britain since the 1950s', p. 1.

192 Smith, King and Bartlett, 'Treatments of Homosexuality in Britain since the 1950s', p. 3.

193 Percival Thatcher, interviewed 29 April 2010; Dickinson, Cook, Playle and Hallett, 'Queer Treatments', p. 5.

194 Oscar Mangle, interviewed 21 June 2010.

195 Ughtred Lovis-Douglas, interviewed 4 January 2013.

196 'How Doctor Cured a Homosexual', *Observer* (18 March 1962).

197 John G. Thorpe, Edward Schmidt and David Castell, 'Comparison of Positive and Negative (Aversive) Conditioning in the Treatment of Homosexuality', *Behaviour Research and Therapy* 1 (1963), p. 357.

198 Ughtred Lovis-Douglas, interviewed 4 January 2013.

199 Dickinson, Cook, Playle and Hallett, '"Queer" Treatments':, p. 1349.

200 '"Twilight [homosexual]" Men Can Be Cured', *Sunday Pictorial* (5 February 1961).

201 Ursula Vaughan, interviewed 12 February 2010.

202 Isaac Oswald, 'Induction of Illusory and Hallucinatory Voices with Consideration of Behaviour Therapy', *Journal of Mental Science* 108 (1962), pp. 196–212.

203 Angus J. Cooper, 'A Case of Fetishism and Impotence Treated by Behaviour Therapy', *British Journal of Psychiatry* 109 (1963), pp. 649–653.

204 John C. Barker, 'Behavioural Therapy for Transvestism: A Comparison of Pharmacological and Electrical Aversion Techniques', *British Journal of Psychiatry* 111 (1965), p. 270.

205 Donna J. Drucker, *The Machines of Sex Research* (Amsterdam, 2014), p. 30.

206 Raymond, 'Case of Fetishism Treated by Aversion Therapy', p. 857.

207 Cooper, 'A Case of Fetishism and Impotence Treated by Behaviour Therapy', p. 650.

208 Oswald, 'Induction of Illusory, p. 210.

209 Toxic myocarditis: inflammation of the heart muscle, which if not treated can be fatal.

210 Maude Griffin, interviewed 8 March 2013.

211 Drucker, *The Machines of Sex Research*, p. 30.

212 Drucker, *The Machines of Sex Research*, p. 29.

213 Simon Rachman, 'Aversion Therapy: Chemical or Electrical', *Behavioural Research Therapy* 2 (1965), pp. 289–299; Barker, 'Behavioural Therapy for Transvestism', pp. 268–276.

214 Thorpe, Schmidt and Castell, 'Comparison of Positive and Negative (Aversive) Conditioning', pp. 357–362.

215 Robert J. McGuire and Michael Vallance, 'Aversion Therapy by Electric Shock: A Simple Technique', *British Medical Journal* 1 (1964), pp. 151–153.

216 Colin Fox interview on *Dark Secret: Sexual Aversion*, British Broadcasting Corporation (1996).

217 Greta Gold, interviewed 24 March 2010; Dickinson, Cook, Playle and Hallett, '"Queer" Treatments', p. 5.

218 Benedict Henry, interviewed 23 June 2010; Tommy Dickinson, Matt Cook, John Playle, Christine Hallett, 'Nurses and Subordination: A Historical Study of Mental Nurses Perceptions on Administering Aversion Therapy for "Sexual Deviations"', *Nursing Inquiry*, pp. 1–11. DOI: 10.1111/nin.12044

219 King and Bartlett, 'British Psychiatry and Homosexuality', p. 47.

220 Smith, King and Bartlett, 'Treatments of Homosexuality in Britain since the 1950s', p. 4.

221 Percival Thatcher, interviewed 29 April 2010.

222 Greta Gold, interviewed 24 March 2010.

223 Benedict Henry, interviewed 23 June 2010.

224 Dickinson, Cook, Playle and Hallett, '"Queer" Treatments', p. 1350.

225 Percival Thatcher, interviewed 29 April 2010.

226 Percival Thatcher, interviewed 29 April 2010.

227 Albert Holliday, interviewed 27 January 2010.

228 Albert Holliday, interviewed 27 January 2010; Dickinson, Cook, Playle and Hallett, '"Queer" Treatments', p. 5.

229 Percival Thatcher, interviewed 29 April 2010; Dickinson, Cook, Playle and Hallett, '"Queer" Treatments', p. 5.

230 Oscar Mangle, interviewed 21 June 2010.

231 'Homosexuality Research Unit', *Birmingham Post* (25 November 1964); 'Gift to Start Homosexuality Research Unit', *Manchester Daily Telegraph* (25 November 1964); '£6,000 Gift for Research into Homosexuality', *Guardian* (25 November 1964); *The Times*, 25 November, 1964; 'Offer for Study of Homosexuality', *The Scotsman* (26 November 1964).

232 *New Statesman* (31 January 1959).

233 'Growing Problem of the Homosexual', *The Scotsman* (5 June 1959); 'Control Must Come Before Cure.' *The Scotsman* (6 June 1959).

234 'Homosexuals Cured More Easily in Prison', *Guardian* (10 October 1965).

235 Cecil Asquith, interviewed 5 December 2010.

2

Work and practice of mental nurses, 1930–1959

It seemed like the order of the day was to do things to patients, whether that was shock them into next week, pump them full of insulin or carve away at their brains. Although we can all look back on this in horror – at the time, it was exciting; we believed we could actually cure patients, whereas before such treatments, there was little hope of it. It was just what we did; we didn't really think to question it.[1]

Introduction

Nurses were introduced to two new legislative frameworks brought in by the Mental Treatment Act 1930, which was geared towards a model of treatment, where patients would have greater autonomy; and the Mental Health Act 1959 that put a new emphasis on community care. In the period between these two Acts, nurses witnessed what has been described as 'therapeutic optimism'; as new therapeutic options particularly somatic (physical) therapies for treating psychiatric patients were introduced.[2] The introduction of these new approaches raised expectations of curative treatment, in keeping with the nomenclature of the new 1930 Act. This chapter explores these innovative therapies in a bid to gain an insight into the culture and practices within which the mental hospitals' nurses were working during the 1930s to the 1950s. In doing so, it offers a framework to explain how nurses became accustomed to administering treatments which caused pain and distress to patients. The chapter also explores the hitherto hidden history of gay life among male homosexual nurses within mental hospitals and deconstructs the contentious dichotomy of these nurses administering treatments for patients 'suffering' from the same 'condition' as themselves.

The Mental Treatment Act 1930: from therapeutic pessimism to therapeutic optimism

The Mental Treatment Act 1930 was the first major revision of mental health policy since the Lunacy Act 1890, and with the introduction of this new Act, asylums became hospitals.[3] The 1930 Act was introduced following, among other things, a book by Montagu Lomax, *The Experiences of an Asylum Doctor* (1921).[4] The book led to stories in the national press, questions in the House of Commons and an internal investigation. The investigation scrutinised evidence from thirty-eight witnesses, including five inmates, and later led to a report of this inquiry. John Hopton argues that this report was generally hostile to Lomax, however, it recommended 'improvement of diet, the introduction of formal training for nursing staff and improvement in care'.[5]

The internal inquiry, which followed the publication of Lomax's book, led to a Royal Commission on Lunacy and Mental Disorder (The Macmillan Commission, 1924–1926). The published report by the committee dismissed many of Lomax's allegations and claims but agreed with his overall recommendation that psychiatry was in need of reform.[6] The specific recommendations of the report were that the population of each mental hospital should not exceed one thousand patients; only formally qualified specialists in psychiatry should become superintendents of psychiatric hospitals; seclusion should only be used in clearly defined situations and its use monitored closely; the quality of food and type of employment for patients should be reviewed; and aftercare facilities for the rehabilitation of patients should be developed.[7]

The Royal Commission on Lunacy and Mental Disorder led to the 1930 Mental Treatment Act. Kathleen Jones suggests that the new 1930 Act did four things: it reorganised the Board of Control; it made provisions for voluntary treatment; it gave official approval to the establishment of psychiatric outpatient clinics and observations wards; and, in line with the Local Government Act of 1929, it abolished outmoded terminology, and brought the official expressions used in conjunction with mental illness into line with the modern approach to the subject.[8]

The Local Government Act 1929, which reformed the Poor Law system and created Public Assistance Boards that had the statutory duty to provide extramural services for the mentally ill, had already swept away such terms as 'pauper' and 'Poor Law'.[9] The 1930 Act abolished other outdated words that were still being used officially in connection with mental illness. 'Asylum' was replaced by 'mental hospital' or simply 'hospital'; and 'lunatic' – except 'criminal lunatic' (where the individual had been in contact with the criminal justice system) – 'was replaced by a variety of phrases such as "patient" or "person of unsound mind" as the context might require'.[10]

The Macmillan Report had considered only two categories of patients: 'Voluntary' and 'Involuntary'. The 1930 Act established three: 'Voluntary', 'Temporary' and 'Certified'. The procedure for certified patients was already established under the Lunacy Act 1890.[11] The broadening of the categories of patients reflected the philosophy of the new Act, which was geared towards a model of treatment where patients would have greater autonomy.

Valerie Harrington argues, however, that these changes were not unprecedented. The Maudsley Hospital, funded mainly by Dr Henry Maudsley, had opened in 1915 with the express intention of providing care to early and acute cases (much of its work was on an outpatient basis).[12] A number of voluntary hospitals had also started to offer outpatient facilities, initially in response to the number of soldiers returning from World War I suffering from 'shell-shock'.[13] These facilities were usually under the supervision of asylum superintendents and located on general hospital premises. However, these innovations were limited: before the 1930 Act the vast majority of people in receipt of publicly funded psychiatric care were the legally committed inmates of asylums.[14] With the passing of the Act, by the late 1930s, just over a third of all asylum admissions were of voluntary status and a total of 177 outpatient clinics were in existence.[15]

New therapeutic options

By the 1930s, psychiatrists were left caring for patients for whom in many cases there was no effective treatment;[16] the treatment offered amounted to little beyond custodial care, particularly for patients with an ill-defined diagnosis such as dementia praecox.[17] Psychiatrists wanted effective therapies and an improved understanding of mental patients.[18] In keeping with the ethos of the new Act, they were seeking to treat and cure patients, enabling them to return to their homes and into employment.[19] Not only were there changes in the legislative framework, the therapeutic options for treating psychiatric patients were being transformed during the 1930s. There was a spirit of optimism within psychiatry, as new somatic treatments were introduced, which provided hope to psychiatrists – and nurses – who had previously had few effective treatments to draw on. One important consequence of these new treatments was that they helped to undermine any remaining belief (which had been so important to the initial establishment of the asylums), that a stay in the institution had therapeutic value in itself. Nevertheless, ironically these new and distinctly unpleasant somatic treatments were being introduced at a time when patients were being given greater legal rights to accept or reject treatment. The four most significant were: insulin treatment, Cardiazol treatment, electroconvulsive therapy (ECT) and leucotomy.[20] Thus, from having no therapeutic interventions beyond sedation for the mentally ill, four treatments were now available and a 'wave of enthusiasm resulted in the adoption of these therapies before proper evaluation'.[21]

Patients undergoing such treatments required varying degrees of nursing care in its more medical sense. This led to some nurses taking on new roles. There was also a change in uniform culture, with male nurses starting to wear white coats like doctors and female nurses dressing more like their counterparts in the general hospitals; this was due in part to the new closer working relationship between doctors and nurses which was emerging during this period.[22] The introduction of somatic treatments did two things: it not only shifted the nurses' roles towards a more medical focus, but also impacted on their work in other ways. Some treatments provided opportunities for staff to engage in one-to-one care of patients, and owing to their effectiveness, some treatments gave nurses hope that their patients could be cured or at least achieve early discharge from hospital. A more negative impact of the treatments, however, was the coercive role expected of nurses.[23]

Insulin treatment

Insulin was first prepared and used in Toronto by Banting and Best in 1922 for the treatment of diabetes mellitus; this was life changing for patients suffering from the condition, as it virtually freed them from a death sentence. The clinical observations that led to the use of insulin in psychiatry were the return of patients' weight to within normal limits and the induction of sleepiness and coma from insulin overdose.[24] Manfred Shakel first noted the effects of insulin coma on schizophrenia symptoms in 1933, but it had gained popularity since a Swiss researcher, Max Muller, had arranged a conference on new therapies in 1937.[25] The first cases of insulin treatment in the UK were directed by Dr Pullar-Streckerin, who worked under the supervision of Professor Henderson in Edinburgh.[26]

Insulin treatment was first used in England in Moorcroft House, a private psychiatric hospital, where the help of Dr Freudenberg from Vienna was enlisted.[27] Francis James argues this was partly due to the fact that 'private licensed mental hospitals were less subject to control by central and local government than asylums or other institutions administered by local authorities'.[28] For two years, Dr William Sargant[29] was endeavouring to persuade Professor Mapother[30] to try the treatment at the Maudsley Hospital. However, Edward Mapother considered the treatment too risky, particularly given that 'the local coroner was fierce and ready to pounce on the psychiatrists at the slightest provocation'.[31] Nevertheless, in 1938, Dr Sargant treated the first patients at the Maudsley Hospital suffering from schizophrenia using insulin treatment. Once introduced, this treatment was rapidly adopted and utilised at most mental hospitals. However, the conditions in many hospitals were far from ideal.

The treatment involved daily injections of insulin, which were gradually increased until the patient's blood sugar was so low that he or she fell into a deep coma. The patient would be kept in an unconscious state for approximately four hours and would then be brought back to consciousness by tube feeding with a glucose solution or, in an emergency, by being given intravenous glucose. Patients were treated daily over a period of five to six weeks.[32] Una Drinkwater recalls that insulin was administered every day except Sundays, when patients were allowed to, 'rest and stock up on food mainly carbohydrates'.[33] There were serious risks involved in this procedure and these included respiratory difficulties, projectile vomiting, seizures, irreversible coma, collapse and delayed coma. Insulin therapy was considered to be 'intricate and exacting and unremitting medical and nursing attention [was] required for its success'.[34]

In the treatment of anxiety, hysteria and anorexia nervosa, a less intensive form of insulin treatment – 'sub-coma shock treatment' – was sometimes used. This intervention involved administration of insulin at high enough doses to produce symptoms such as hunger, drowsiness, weakness and sweating. Because the patient did not go into a coma it was not considered as risky.[35]

Insulin treatment was usually administered on a specialised unit to a small group of patients by experienced medical and nursing staff. This ensured the maintenance of enthusiasm and high standards of care.[36] The treatment had to be supplemented by other forms of therapeutic interventions. Not only were nurses required to provide physical care, monitor symptoms and regulate the patients' diets; they also had to consider psychological factors. They had to manage agitated behaviour and listen sympathetically when patients emerged from unconsciousness – such intensive psychological support was not something they could usually give on the wards. Insulin treatment appeared to create enthusiasm among nurses; as the challenging environment of these specialist units was a welcome change for them compared to the dull routines of ward work. Monitoring and care for patients receiving insulin was usually reserved for the senior nurses.[37] However, even they did not appear to have a deep knowledge of the theoretical underpinning for their interventions, as Elspeth Whitbread recalls:

> I was only a student and the senior staff nurse would give the heavy dose of insulin but before she did that she would pass a tube down into her [the patient's] stomach, and then after she was out, put out with insulin for so long, they would pour some liquid glucose, and that would bring her round. And when she was fully round, you used to have to take her down into the shower, give her a hot shower for a while and suddenly switch it round to the cold, now whatever that was for I don't know. I couldn't see sense of that. When I asked the staff nurse she said: 'It's just what Sister says we have to do'.[38]

During World War II, the availability of insulin treatment was affected by the reductions in medical and nursing staff and in the availability of insulin and glucose. After 1945, it was noted to pick up again. However, it was severely criticised in a 1953 paper in the *Lancet* entitled 'The Insulin Myth' in which good results were ascribed to the strong suggestive effect of the technique together with enthusiasm of a dedicated staff, the inculcation of a group morale in a special unit and the 'total push' adjuvant treatment.[39] The treatment appeared to decline after the publication of this article. Further reasons for its decline were ascribed to poor selection of patients, neglect of technique and limited rehabilitation of patients.[40]

Cardiazol treatment

In 1938 Ladislas von Meduna started treating patients suffering from psychosis with Cardiazol to chemically induce convulsions; this was on the mistaken basis that those with epilepsy did not develop schizophrenia.[41] Cardiazol was initially used as a cardiac or respiratory stimulant, but in psychiatry Cardiazol was given in large doses to induce an epileptic convulsion. Cardiazol was given mainly to people suffering from schizophrenia in a series of 12–20 intravenous injections. The treatment was usually commenced between 7 a.m. and 10 a.m. The patient would be placed on their back in bed with arms and legs stretched out. A pillow was placed under the patient's head and a folded pillow put under the shoulders to prevent injuries due to the violent seizures that the treatment induced. Roughly ten seconds after the Cardiazol had been administered, the doctor in charge of the treatment would take hold of the patient's wrists with one hand and press down on the patient's shoulders with his other hand. In the following 50 seconds, the time the convulsions normally lasted, the patient had tonic seizures[42] with stiffening of the body and subsequently clonic seizures.[43] The patient would generally turn blue, and their arms and legs would rapidly and rhythmically jerk until they eventually passed out.[44]

In the majority of cases, treatment was administered twice and sometimes three times weekly.[45] It was considered less problematic than insulin treatment and required less time each day. However, it still had its risks and many patients feared the powerful effect of Cardiazol. Indeed, one former patient who received the treatment recalled:

> About 10 seconds after having received the injection, it is as if you are pulled out of yourself and into another world, but you can still see the persons around you as if in a limpid fog. It is utterly unbearable and quite impossible to get out of. Sometimes the effect is stronger, sometimes weaker; when it is strong you have hallucinations . . . The room you are lying in begins to look like Hell, and it is as if you are burned by an invisible fire. It is scary. But luckily it is over now.[46]

Another patient was noted to remark 'they shock me with terror'.[47] Despite this, former nurse Gilbert Davies commented, 'Even if they were kicking and screaming they still got the jab.'[48]

Electroconvulsive therapy

In 1937 Cerletti and Bini introduced electroconvulsive shocks, which were perceived to be safer and less unpleasant than Cardiazol treatment.[49] Shortly after the start of World War II, Flemming, Golla and Walter published the first British trial of ECT in the *Lancet*.[50] The authors concluded that 'no untoward results have been observed; the claims of Cerletti and Bini are confirmed; the method is technically effective, simple and safe and arouses no fear or hostility in the patients'.[51] German Berrios argues that the *Lancet* paper is significant, 'because its views on the safety and feasibility of ECT reassured the British psychiatric brotherhood that a more controllable method of inducing seizures had been found'.[52]

The electroshock machine occasioned great enthusiasm among psychiatrists, and the machine was introduced widely into most psychiatric hospitals during the 1940s. It was favoured by psychiatrists because it produced instant unconsciousness, induced less fear from the patients, elicited no physical upset after the convulsion and was deemed safer than Cardiazol. Indeed, Elliot Whitman was noted to remark 'ECT was like the Prozac of today – everyone had it!'[53] However, there were risks, mostly fractures of limbs and vertebrae, particularly in the elderly. These dangers began to be mitigated when a new procedure called 'modified ECT' was introduced. This procedure used succinylcholine, a muscle relaxant, to cause paralysis a few moments before seizure, and a short-acting anaesthetic, methyohexital ('Brevital').[54]

Nurses were involved in the administration of shock treatment, as with the other treatments. They were responsible for preparing the patients, guaranteeing they had nil by mouth prior to the treatment and attempting to alleviate any fears the patient may have had regarding the treatment. To reduce the possibility of fractures, the treatment was given on a firm mattress placed on top of a fracture board and four to six nurses held the patient down firmly during the convulsion. A gag was placed in the patient's mouth to prevent biting of the tongue. Usually a nurse applied the paddles to the patient's temples while the doctor switched on the current. Post treatment, they observed and reported any side effects.[55]

Electroconvulsive therapy features fairly frequently in the testimonies of former nurses and patients who tell of their experiences of mental hospitals during the 1940s to the 1950s.[56] Many nurses recall its inception as a major breakthrough for mania and clinical depression. Furthermore, it appeared to make a positive impact on the nurses' working environment; as increased rate of discharge, success with severely depressed patients and shortening of manic episodes all forged a pathway for nursing staff to begin working in a rehabilitative manner with some patients.[57] Nevertheless, some nurses were also perturbed about aspects of ECT administration:

> We literally had to throw ourselves over the patient to stop them thrashing about. It would usually take five of us: one nurse would hold the patients head and try to compress the jaw; one would hold the feet, while two would be on either side of the patient holding the patients shoulders with one hand and the patient's hand with another, meanwhile another would press down on the pelvis. I remember thinking it was awful. I could see the benefit for really depressed people, but for schizophrenia, I really couldn't see its worth.[58]

Meanwhile, Cecil Asquith recalls the education he received regarding ECT:

> I can almost visualise the lecture on ECT by this psychiatrist: he said you won't understand this, so it was a good place to start with students, and he drew this diagram of a skull, and this skull was full of arrows and they were all pointing the same way, and he said now this is me and you. Now people with schizophrenia, and he drew all these arrows all over the place – that's schizophrenia, give them ECT and all the arrows go the same way as you and me . . . you kind of think, that's a very good theory, but it didn't hold water, it was 'crap'. It was one of those happy accident discoveries really. So it was extensively used, really quite extensively, particularly in acute care.[59]

Most nurses recall feeling tense or horror-struck when they first witnessed ECT, especially before the introduction of modified ECT. Furthermore, despite psychiatrists perceiving that it was less feared than Cardiazol, many patients were petrified of ECT, they suffered unwanted side effects such as memory loss, and some took great lengths to avoid it; some went as far as attempting suicide.[60] Indeed, from a patient's point of view, Janet Frame described the ward atmosphere on ECT days as resembling that in a prison on execution day.[61]

There was tangible evidence of the efficacy of ECT for severe affective disorders. However, electroconvulsive therapy was also used to control behaviour, and to treat disorders for which it had questionable efficacy, particularly schizophrenia.[62] Leith Cavill recalled such incidences of ECT being used to control behaviour: 'If they were as you might describe "unmanageable", these people were unmanageable, then they might go for half a dozen ECT's.'[63] It was the nurses' responsibility to ensure that patients came for their treatments, and all the nurses interviewed for this book recalled this aspect of their role in relation to ECT. However, their views seemed embedded in vagueness about their ability to question this. Thaddeus Chester commented, 'It was fairly common to have to drag the patient, kicking, screaming and biting for ECT. Looking back, that is awful, at the time, it was what we did – doctors' orders.'[64] Reflecting back, one nurse in Prebble's study summed up his attitudes to the use of unmodified ECT: 'When you didn't have anything else, what did you use?'[65] Although pharmacological advances in psychiatry have lessened the need for ECT, it still has a place in the psychiatric armamentarium today.

Frontal leucotomy

Arguably the most invasive of all the somatic treatments was the prefrontal leucotomy (known as lobotomy in the USA), which for upwards of twenty years was used in the UK, and by 1954 had been performed on upwards of twelve thousand people; although the final figure may never be known.[66] The treatment involved brain surgery to cut the nerve fibres leading back from the prefrontal lobes. The objective was to interfere with negative, ingrained emotional and psychological patterns.[67] The procedure was usually performed using local anaesthetic. This reduced the overall risk of a general anaesthetic and enabled the surgeon to monitor the immediate effects of leucotomy by engaging the patient in what must have been an overwrought dialogue.[68] Some of these conversations were recorded, and were rather macabre:

> SURGEON: What is going through your mind now?
> PATIENT: A knife.[69]

The prefrontal leucotomy was introduced by Egas Moniz in 1936 for aggressive or seriously disturbed patients.[70] However, this was popularised by an American neurologist Walter Freeman (pictured in figure 5) in collaboration with neurosurgeon, James Watts.[71] They published a book called *Psychosurgery* in 1942 that detailed the pre-operative care, operative technique and post-operative care.[72] There had been a paucity of academic discussion regarding psychosurgery in Britain prior to 1942, when eight patients were operated on, the first of whom had a leucotomy preformed in Bristol in December 1940.[73] The *Lancet* published the results of these procedures in July 1941

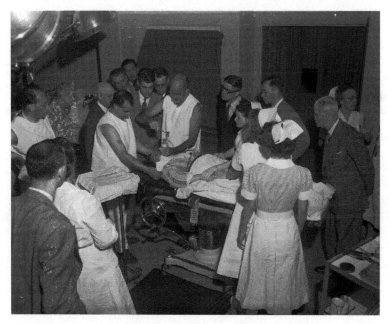

5 Walter Freeman performing a leucotomy in 1949

and noted that they were 'encouraging', and went on to claim that 'improvement could be hoped for in every type of case'.[74] Given the adequate conceptual ground, leucotomy developed rapidly in the UK. The original aims of the leucotomy programme at one mental hospital, as stated in its 1943 Annual Report, were that it would 'hasten recovery' and help the 'hospital stay to be curtailed'.[75] Early reports in the British medical press posited that leucotomy could offer relief from anxiety, apprehension, obsessional symptoms and 'tension states' and also control distressing behaviour. A central assertion by the medical profession was that it could resocialise a subcategory of individuals otherwise predestined to institutional care. A common view was that the operation was indicated more by symptoms and behaviour than by diagnosis per se.[76]

Nurses had an implicit but fairly influential role in the selection of patients for leucotomy, as it appears that the selection of patients at the North Wales Psychiatric Hospital, Denbigh, was influenced by the degree of behavioural disturbance and nursing supervision required. In at least half of the original twenty-four patients operated on there, nursing challenges were explicitly stated. Indeed, the supervising psychiatrist made the following plan for one patient: 'leucotomy [has been] carried out largely with an eye on easing nursing care [in a patient who is] a low grade imbecile, destructive, unclean and cannot apply himself to anything'.[77] This selection criterion was publicly accredited in the psychiatric literature of the time. Leucotomy may be prescribed for patients 'who require a great deal of nursing supervision, who [are] a constant source of trouble'.[78]

The testimonies of some of the participants in this study corroborate this notion. Gilbert Davies recalled this implicit power nurses appeared to have had in relation to leucotomy: 'If a patient was hard work we could express this to the doctor, and this could have a big impact on whether they went under the knife or not.'[79] Meanwhile, Claudine de Valois recalled an incident where a patient was given a leucotomy because of their behaviour:

I remember **** ****** [name of her nursing colleague]. Well a patient bit him. He took a working party out from *** [name of the ward]. It was at a time when *** [name of the ward] was full of rough ones. Well one of the patients hacked **** ****** [name of her nursing colleague] head – took a massive chunk out of it! So they did a leucotomy on this patient. And he was like a vegetable, after the leucotomy.[80]

There is no documentary evidence to suggest, however, that leucotomy was ever carried out for disciplinary reasons or solely to control behaviour.[81] Indeed, Una Drinkwater commented, 'It was always seen as a last resort and never considered as an inconsequential intervention, as there were definite risks involved.'[82] Nevertheless, some psychiatrists were advocating for leucotomy to be deliberated for any patient who had been in hospital for more than a year.[83]

Prebble suggests that nurses were involved in all aspects of the procedure: pre-operatively, they had to ensure the patient had nil by mouth, shave the patients' head, and also escort them, sometimes in restraints, for the procedure. They were required to restrain the patient during the procedure too if required and hand instruments to the doctor (see figure 5). Prebble goes on to argue that post-operatively the patients required intensive nursing care, since they were usually confused and disorientated, uncooperative and incontinent; they had to be toileted frequently to help them regain bladder control. The patients usually suffered from fatigue, apathy and inattention in the early stages post-surgery and required intensive retraining in basic living skills, such as table manners and self-care. In most cases, patients were found to require, 'long-term aftercare by nursing staff experienced in details of rehabilitation and habit training', and improvement was slow.[84] Julian Wills recalls patients' presentation post-surgery, 'They were completely disorientated. There was no feeling or expression in the face and they would often be sat drooling in a corner on the floor for weeks'.[85]

It is interesting to note that in figure 5 there are eighteen people observing the doctor conducing the procedure. This could demonstrate their idealisation, trust and confidence vested in him. While the picture was taken in a hospital in the USA, there have always been medical interchanges between the UK and USA.[86] The testimonies of the participants in this book demonstrate that such idealisation and faith in doctors was also evident in UK hospitals. This could offer a context to explain why some nurses participated in this clinical practice and did not think to question it: nurses appeared to assume that the doctors' knowledge, morals and values were superior to their own.

Chlorpromazine arrived in Britain in the early part of 1954 and its introduction had a huge influence in reducing the use of leucotomies and other somatic treatments.[87] Crossley argues that the relief of suffering following a leucotomy was brought at a price of 'accepting a level of existence qualitatively different from and usually below that which the patient had enjoyed before onset of their illness'.[88] Following leucotomy, 25 per cent of patients received no benefit at all, for 3 per cent their condition was exacerbated and a further 3–4 per cent were killed by it.[89] Psychosurgery is still performed in contemporary medical practice; however, it is under much tighter social and legislative controls. Una Drinkwater sums up this aspect of her nursing career:

> Looking back it was a barbaric procedure fuelled by desperation. However, at the time there was so much enthusiasm for it. A lot of nurses, especially some of the more ambitious 'career nurses' you might call them, were desperate to get involved with it. I can just imagine what their CVs would have said: 'I have assisted with Brain Surgery'! . . . [Rolls eyes] . . . I on the other hand, a nurse who happily stayed at the patients' bedside my entire career, found the procedure brutal to say the least. It was so disturbing; at least before the procedure the patient had life, and the majority of patients were a mess after it. It really was heartrending. Pathetic.[90]

During the 1950s, psychiatrists and nurses continued to use a variety of somatic treatments, depending heavily on a combination of insulin treatment, ECT, and to a lesser degree, leucotomy, all of which became standard treatments for suitable cases. If one treatment was ineffective, another was tried.[91] Great emphasis was placed on these innovative treatments and all became orthodox, despite them being highly experimental in nature and lacking regulation. There was a spirit of optimism, particularly during the 1930s, regarding somatic treatments, and nurses were taking on new and more advanced roles. Optimism was premature. By the end of the decade, another war had erupted causing intolerable strain on a system that was already seriously stressed. World War II delayed the widespread use of both ECT and psychosurgery in Britain and it was not until the end of the 1940s and the early 1950s that their use became common.[92] Nevertheless, nurses' exposure to somatic treatments arguably normalised them to administering treatments which were unpleasant, painful and distressing for the patients receiving them. This could provide a possible interpretation for some nurses' acceptance of aversion therapy in later years.

The World War II years

In the early 1940s, many nurses were called up, including some who were still in training, and assigned to the Royal Army Medical Corps.[93] Nationwide, psychiatric hospitals were cleared of patients in order to accommodate the large numbers of soldiers with war-induced mental health problems. Some mental hospitals were completely emptied and their patients were transferred to other hospitals, which soon became severely overcrowded.[94] The population of psychiatric hospitals rose so sharply during World War II that it became imperative to relieve the pressure on them. The subsequent overcrowding coupled with low staffing levels increased the barely contained discontent among mental nurses.[95]

In some hospitals, up to a quarter of the nursing staff had gone. In response to this staffing crisis, the Mental Health Association lobbied for all male nurses with either GNC registration or the RMPA certificate to be exempted from military service, and in August 1941, the Ministry of Health acted. They produced the Mental Nurses (Employment and Offences) Order, which was known colloquially as the 'Standstill'. Claire Chatterton highlights that this prohibited any member of the nursing staff who had worked in their hospital for more than a year from leaving, without the permission of the Visiting Committee. If they did so, they could be imprisoned or fined.[96]

The war had a positive impact on mental nursing. During their time in military service, nurses learned to handle medical emergencies and acquired psychotherapeutic skills, which they would not have covered in training. Mental nurses on the home front were also developing new skills, as the Maudsley Hospital was overwhelmed with soldiers suffering from neurasthenia and conversion hysteria, so these nurses were also involved in dynamic and innovative new approaches to the care of very disturbed patients.[97] Many nurses transferred these skills to their practice when they returned to their hospitals after the war.[98] Chapter 4 considers how some nurses' wartime experiences also had a positive impact and influence on the care they delivered to sexually deviant patients in later years. Conversely, the militarisation of nursing during and following the war may have had a negative effect on some nurses, by reinforcing the notion of obedience to authority.

In 1943 the Rushcliffe Report, more properly entitled 'The Report of the Nurses' Salaries Committee', appeared and provided a bedrock for discussions on nurses' pay and conditions. This led to the setting up of the Nurses' and Midwives' Whitley Council in 1948, which aimed to improve the status of nursing and the quality of nurse training. The report also recommended that the working fortnight be reduced to ninety-six hours and that continuous night duty should not exceed three months for student nurses and six months for trained staff. It also suggested that all nurses should have twenty-eight days' holiday a year and one off-duty day per week, with sick pay graded according to the length of service.[99]

Penny Starns argues that there was no distinction between registered and assistant nurses during the late 1930s and early 1940s, which polarised status issues in nursing.[100] This was compounded during the war years with the introduction of the controversial 'Nurses Act' passed in 1943, which was an attempt to alleviate the chronic nursing shortage, particularly for tuberculosis, mental and chronic hospitals.[101] The Act created a new level of nurse who was enrolled rather than registered, and allowed 'bona fide' assistant nurses to apply to the GNC for enrolment.

A roll was established and advertisements encouraging nursing orderlies and auxiliaries to apply to the GNC for enrolment on the basis of experience were placed around hospitals. This was noted to cause some anger among registered nurses as nursing auxiliaries were being given a nursing qualification based purely on experience, without sitting an exam or receiving assessment, as the criteria needed to apply were, 'two years whole time training or experience of nursing the sick under trained nursing staff in hospital'.[102] Those whose names were entered on this roll, which was overseen by the GNC, were entitled to call themselves State Enrolled Assistant Nurses (SEANs). These nurses remained known as SEANs until the Nurses Amendment Act 1961 shortened the title to State Enrolled Nurse (SEN).[103]

Despite publicity campaigns launched by the government, only the maternity field saw an improvement in the number of applicants.[104] Nolan argues that the introduction of the enrolled nurse had the effect of substantially increasing the number of trained nurses at no extra cost.[105] However, enrolled nurses were not introduced into mental nursing until 1964.[106] These new SENs were also known as 'subordinate' nurses.[107] Four former SENs were interviewed as part of this study, three of whom are also, interestingly, homosexual; their testimony is explored later in the chapter.

Mental health and the National Health Service

The UK was spiritually and economically drained by the two world wars, and the creation of a National Health Service (NHS) in July 1948, free at the point of entry to every citizen, represented the ultimate act of national altruism.[108] However, the inclusion of mental health services into the NHS was by no means a foregone conclusion. Mental health services were not included in early plans for the NHS, and first featured in the 1944 Plan.[109] Aneurin Bevan, the Minister of Health in the new Labour government, supported their inclusion, echoing the 1926 Royal Commission Report in his statement: 'The separation of mental from physical treatment is a survival from the primitive conceptions and is a source of endless cruelty and neglect.'[110]

The major restructuring in 1948, following the creation of the NHS, brought the former county asylums under the control of the new Regional Hospital Boards (RHBs), while local authorities were charged with providing after-care facilities for patients. They in turn delegated local management functions to new hospital management committees.[111] The new arrangements did not diminish the role of the mental hospitals' board of control, which remained an important influence on management, and the hierarchy within the institutions went largely unchanged.[112] Despite the advent of a nationwide health service structure, the self-containment and remoteness of the mental health hospitals, located as they often were in the countryside, meant that they were difficult to incorporate into the NHS and were able to continue with many of their traditional practices.[113]

Hospital culture: daily life in psychiatric hospitals

Despite the absorption of mental health services into the NHS and the medical rhetoric of curative treatment within psychiatry, the mental hospitals from the 1930s to the mid-1970s, where the patients would have received treatments for their sexual deviations, more closely resembled nineteenth-century asylums than they did twentieth-century general hospitals.[114] Although the mental deficiency and mental illness hospitals accounted for nearly half the beds within the new health service, they were still seen very much as the 'poor relation'.[115] Further, according to Nolan, job satisfaction among nurses during this period was poor, owing to overcrowding in hospitals, the hierarchical structure of mental hospitals, and nurses being used as domestics.[116] There appeared to be a mismatch between the idealism of mental hospital administrators and the reality of conditions. Administrators' aims to provide comfortable, home-like conditions often went unrealised because they were battling against their Victorian legacy of resource constraint, overcrowding and understaffing. The pace of integration of mental health services into the NHS was disrupted by the relative isolation of the Hospital Management Committee (HMC). Unlike the general hospitals that were grouped together, the mental hospital HMCs operated separately, which resulted in their peculiar methods and culture remaining little changed for some years to come.[117]

In 1946, there were 147,000 mental patients in institutional care. The government had recommended the maximum number of patients in any mental hospital should be 1,000. However, by 1947, 67 of the nation's 140 mental hospitals housed more and some had as many as 3,000 patients.[118] By 1952, nearly all regions reported overcrowding. In some cases, no new beds had been created since 1948, despite a rapid increase in voluntary admissions and older people. Furthermore, the mental hospitals were old, poorly maintained, under-resourced with amenities, geographically isolated and 'mostly too large to provide an appropriate caring environment for highly vulnerable people'.[119] The growth of mental hospital populations was not accompanied by an equivalent increase in accommodation. Shortages of labour and building materials during and after the war inhibited building projects. Many hospitals, especially in London,

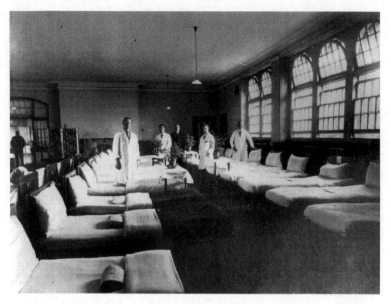

6 Male ward c.1946

had been bombed during World War II, but had never recuperated to the point where they were providing the equivalent level of service as before.[120]

An article in the *Nursing Mirror* in 1945 described: 'Overcrowding as the worst problem'. They depict a vivid image of conditions with hospitals akin to 'stables' where, 'Beds are sometimes so close together that patients have to climb over each other's beds to reach their own and privacy is impossible.'[121] In addition, in 1953, the *Nursing Times* published an exposé of the conditions at Menston Hospital, near Leeds, where they reported a ward for 103 patients had only five toilets and mattresses were laid on the floor between beds to accommodate extra patients.[122] Overcrowding had an intense effect on nursing care. Day rooms often had to be converted to dormitories, so there was little indoor space for recreational or social activities, and patients had minimal privacy (see figure 6).[123] The beds are very close together and there are no curtains around the beds for privacy.

Despite the advent of the NHS, there was still the ongoing problem of staffing the mental hospitals. The overcrowding and low staffing levels meant that large wards were sometimes left with only one nurse on duty. In 1945 a speaker at the 22nd meeting of the National Advisory Council for the Recruitment and Distribution of Nurses and Midwives pointed to the 'loneliness and responsibility of ward duty'.[124] Una Drinkwater recalls how she was often the only nurse on night duty: 'There'd only be me on duty sometimes for about fifty patients, it was difficult when you had patients on insulin treatment; sometimes they would go into a coma and not come out of it.'[125] Chatterton posits several reasons for the shortage of mental nurses. These included: the isolation of the mental hospitals; stigma and low status; the negative attitude of the general public; prejudices from general nurses; low pay; female nurse wastage due to marriage; poor working conditions; shifts; strict discipline; competition from other fields (i.e. teaching and clerical work); and lack of promotion.[126] This enduring staffing problem can begin to 'explain how nursing staff on some of the more overcrowded wards began to develop time-saving practices which compromised the dignity of those in their care'.[127]

One of the main priorities of nursing care was to manage large numbers of patients, with the least risk of harm. Hospital routines and hierarchical systems of supervision allowed the nurses to process large numbers of patients with comparative safety.[128] Bathing, for example, was a very organised activity:

> It was like a production line in a factory at bath time – there were naked bodies everywhere. Staff in one room would undress the patients and pass them through the door to me in the bathroom. I would bathe them, wash their hair and pull them out of the bath. I'd then push them through the door to another set of nurses who would dry them and check them for any injuries. The next lot was usually in before the dirty water had fully drained out of the bath. Everything was ultra, ultra safety and routine and very little personal dignity or whatever. But because it was the norm you didn't question it.[129]
>
> On the 'back' wards nearly all the patients were incontinent, and you were on the go all night, changing beds and toileting patients. We used to put buckets all around the ward so the patients could urinate in them. It would make me heave [almost vomit] having to empty those out in the morning.[130]

Hopton argues that some of these practices may have been implemented to facilitate nurses to cope with chronic staff shortages.

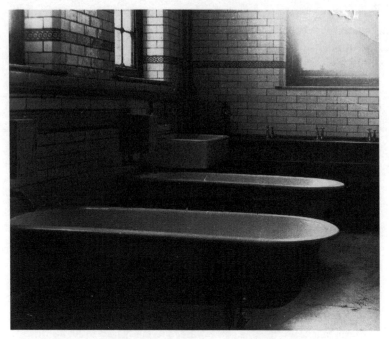

7 Communal bathroom at Glenside Hospital, Bristol circa 1950s

He goes on to suggest that they may have continued for longer than was required because staff were suffering from 'burnout'.[131] He also suggests, that it is important to note, that as late as 1957 the only remark the Commissioners of the Board of Control made about the modernisation of the central male bathroom at Prestwich Hospital, Manchester, was to express reservations about the use of showers.[132] This could be interpreted as an implicit endorsement of sustained use of the communal bathroom, such as that pictured in figure 7.

Many of the things that have been described above are evidence of an immense gulf between the prescriptions of theory, the intentions of policy and the realities of practice. For example, even though dignity, compassion and privacy were not accentuated in mental health nursing literature until much later, the 1923 edition of *The Handbook for Mental Nurses* stated that 'bathing should not be too hurried'.[133]

111

Hopton argues, however, that in situations where up to forty individuals were expected to bathe in a matter of a few hours using only five or six baths, it was impossible to conform to the demands of this injunction.[134] Prebble suggests that "'Conveyer belt care", at its best, achieved standardisation and protection from harm".[135] Mental nurses took pride in their standard of care of severely infirm patients, which included conducting regular bed changes and toileting to prevent pressure sores. Nevertheless, such practices rarely upheld an individual's privacy or dignity.[136]

Mental nurses' working lives were conducted within a comprehensive and custodial framework where a breach of discipline could lead to instant dismissal. When staff joined the asylum payroll they were typically issued with a long list of rules and also asked to sign 'obligation forms'.[137] The rules tightly circumscribed staff actions when managing high-risk situations such as bathing, mealtimes, fires and 'constant observations'. Infringement could lead to instant dismissal. Leith Cavill recalls an incident involving a suicidal patient:

> I remember this one bloke on a suicidal caution card who went missing along with a dinner knife. Christ! Panic stations. You'd have thought the Cuban missile was heading our way. He'd previously tried to cut his wrists a couple of times. Well, we eventually found him in the hospital grounds. He was fine, but the nurse who'd let him escape while on his constant observations was immediately sacked. He didn't have the knife on him. I'm telling you it couldn't cut butter, but we stripped **** [name of ward] from top to bottom to try to find this dinner knife in case he'd hidden it somewhere. Anyway, we eventually found it in the bin after about two hours of searching.[138]

Mick Carpenter argues that living in and working long hours allowed the medical superintendents 'almost absolute power' over their nursing staff, and the superintendent was seen as a figure of great prestige and power.[139] The majority of nurses in this study established a subordinate relationship with medical staff and this notion is explored later in the book. Carpenter goes on to posit that 'nursing is, of course, an occupation noted for its authoritarian management'.[140] Within mental hospitals the matron or chief male nurse (CMN) was at the top of the nursing hierarchy. Furthermore, wards were the undisputed territory of their individual charge nurse or sister who might have worked there for decades and thereby defined its culture.

Indeed, the *Report of the Committee of Inquiry into Whittingham Hospital* condemned the finding that one nurse, who became the ward sister, had remained on the same ward for 47 years, ever since her qualification.[141] If such a person became embittered or 'burnt out', their indifference to those in their care could be 'infectious':[142]

> The Charge Nurses were in complete control of their wards and nobody ever challenged them. Many of them spoke in a bullying way to patients; they were arrogant and always spoke down to staff. They were men who were familiar with violence because of the War and took it for granted. I was a coward – I should have done something about it, but those to whom I would have had to complain were part of the same system. Patients who were beaten were seen by the Medical Superintendent who invariably accepted the account of the incident given by the Charge Nurse which was always untrue.[143]

Towards the end of the 1940s, there was a status divide, in so far as the female matron was senior to the CMN. She was in charge of nurse training; she was a member of the Hospital Management Committee, and there were instances where she earned £120 a year more in pay than her male counterpart.[144] This was markedly different from other professions, as before 1970, it was common practice in the private sector and some parts of the public sector for there to be separate and lower rates of pay for women.[145] In the pre-Rushcliffe era, the CMN was known as the Head Attendant. Nolan argues that the person who held this position was 'resplendent in braid and brass buttons' and was expected to 'produce other male "nurses" who could move beds and bodies about, fill coal bunkers, empty dustbins, and any other job which required strength rather than skill'.[146] But the CMNs began to feel isolated, as unlike the matron they were not involved with the training of nurses or in policy making. Furthermore, they could not join the Royal College of Nursing (RCN) and were refused entry to the Matrons' Association meetings. This led to the establishment of the National Association of Chief Male Nurses.

Poor treatment of patients

The treatment of patients was sometimes poor. Some were not discharged after improvement, and were kept in complete suspense about whether or not they would ever be discharged. Other patients appeared entirely sane to some nurses. However, they were not discharged, as they were perceived to be good workers. Cecil Asquith recalls how many nurses felt scared to spend time speaking to their patients:

> You were just frightened to sit down and talk to them, because if you weren't stood up busy doing something physical; or running round tidying the laundry cupboard that didn't need tidying; or doing the washing; mopping the floor; or something like that, you were just considered lazy. I learnt the hard way, you see, I got banished to a 'back' ward once. Sister caught me playing cards and talking with some patients, and it wasn't the thing so, I got banished.[147]

There were staff who were aggressive towards patients and others who took a delight in teasing and provoking the most vulnerable of patents.[148] Nolan found that some participants in his study had disapproved of the treatment of patients. However, behaviours such as senior nurses announcing that they were coming on to wards by tapping on pipes to give a warning, in order to avoid getting a true impression of what was going on, affirmed to the participants that complaints would not be properly investigated, if at all.[149]

Alexander Walk and Richard Hunter have argued, however, that some mental nurses had a very influential role in effecting the positive changes that occurred during this time period.[150] In 1959, Teodoro Allyon and Jack Michael reported on a project in which mental nurses were utilised as 'behavioural engineers' to change patients who 'failed to engage in normal activities'. These activities included not tending to their personal hygiene needs and expressing their anger in 'inappropriate' ways.[151] Furthermore, following a transformation at the Glasgow Royal Mental Hospital, it was noticed that those patients:

> Paid more attention to their appearance, and some began to sew, draw, or make rugs. Most of them took over small jobs which they jealously insisted on doing themselves. Thus, at tea-time, one patient made the tea, another laid out the cups, a third put the sugar on the table, another the milk, yet another spread the table-cloth, and so on.[152]

The transformation discussed above was initiated by doctors and involved patients and nurses spending time together. Nurses were allocated to the same patients each day and gradually the patients began to know them and relax in their company. Patients were encouraged to read, talk to each other and do things for themselves. Therefore, some nurses were possibly beginning to identify themselves as autonomous therapeutic practitioners, who could have a positive effect on their patients' recovery, as opposed to merely containing them.[153]

However, for the majority of nurses there was little room for independent decision-making, as Elliot Whitman recalled: 'The Charge Nurse told you what you were doing that day, you just did what you were told.'[154] Evander Orchard recalls the minimal thinking he did while practising as a nurse: 'My thinking was done for me by the doctors, because I had no evidence to counter it.'[155] Most were guided almost entirely by verbal instructions from ward charges or the next most senior nurse:

> It seemed as if we were marooned in time – nothing much ever happened, nothing much ever changed – and every task was repeated each day over and over again.[156]

> I didn't find the staff that knowledgeable – management, control, reduction of conflict, running a smooth ward – that was the order of the day. I remember saying: 'Tell me more about mental illness, and what can I do about it?' They were very good on describing mental illness, but I don't think they were terribly clever on what to do about it.[157]

Within most mental hospitals the order of the day was for nurses to get on with their jobs in an unquestioning and unreflective manner. Hopton argues that there was an entrenched ideology by nurses in mental hospitals, which held that nursing was learnt 'by watching the example of others, based on "common sense" assumptions and concern with neatness rather than on research-based theory'.[158]

Mental nursing was hard work both physically and mentally. In addition to the physical work involved in caring for patients, much of the nurses' time was also taken up with domestic duties:

> There is usually no domestic staff for these wards, and it is not uncommon for nurses to do all the domestic work that patients are unable to do. This has so often been stressed that we will not labour it, but some jobs which

nurses do are not so commonly spoken of, such as hauling large bales of laundry without trucks or baskets, emptying pig-swills etc. The male staff are in an even worse case. They do farming, gardening and work of the crudest types, with squads of patients.[159]

Benedict Henry recalled the preoccupation with cleanliness: 'The staff were obsessed with cleanliness and hygiene – obsessed with patients being up at a certain time and being washed, the washing ritual in the morning was terribly important.'[160] As well as being physically demanding, the work could also be emotionally distressing. Thaddeus Chester recalls his time on a male long-stay ward where patients were expected to spend most mornings walking without purpose around 'airing courts' (enclosed courtyards adjacent to wards): 'It upset me to see those poor lads wandering around the airing courts in the morning. I could not see the point of it. Snow, ice, rain, desert heat: they were out there.'[161] The Minister for Health, in 1952, portrayed a very different picture of therapeutic approaches being implemented in mental hospitals, which he said meant that, 'like the general nurse, the mental nurse has the satisfaction of seeing a large proportion of patients cured of their ailments and returned to happy and useful lives'.[162] There was a dissonance between reality and rhetoric.

'Dirty work'

Everett Hughes first coined the term 'dirty work' in 1951. He expanded this further in 1958 when he referred to occupations that were considered socially, morally or physically degrading or disgusting.[163] These occupations are not inherently 'dirty' but carry the social construction of 'dirtiness'. Prebble suggests that the definition can usefully be applied to mental hospital nursing. Physically, the nurses were intimately involved with the generally unpleasant aspects of bodily function: toileting, washing and hand-feeding.[164] Socially, they were marred by their regular interactions with stigmatised people; this has been known as 'courtesy stigma'.[165] Indeed, Maude Griffin recalls: 'In those days some people seemed to think that if you went into a mental hospital [as a patient] you were some sort of freak, and they were very wary of the people who worked there too.'[166] Dutifully, mental nurses were expected to control and contain others; tasks which society demanded but also regarded with vacillation.[167]

Blake Ashforth and Glen Kreiner argue that members of a group who carry out 'dirty work' come to personify the work itself, and therefore become 'dirty workers'. They go on to posit that people involved in dirty work employ a range of strategies to construct an affirmative shared identity.[168] Prebble suggests that one of the central strategies is that of social cohesion and the emergence of a strong occupational and work group. She argues that mental nurses developed strong networks that traversed work, sport and social activities. These networks were strengthened by the social isolation engendered by physical distance and shift work.[169] Nurses were expected to care for people in severe psychological distress whom society had turned their back on. They were exposed to extraordinary sights, sounds, smells, and by patients presenting with bizarre behaviour. Myrtle Pauncefoot recalls an incident that happened only a few weeks into her nurse training, 'I was barely eighteen and Sister sent me down to the bathroom. Well this man came running out with not a stitch on. I was petrified I'd never seen a naked man before.'[170] Claudine de Valois recalls the first patient that she met as a student nurse:

> I will never forget her. She was like a skeleton, her knees were up under her chin and she was lying in her own urine and faeces. I felt so nauseous, as I'd never been exposed to another person's elimination before. She used to cry out when you used to change her. I remember getting very upset the first time I changed her, as I thought I'd hurt her.[171]

Both the former patients and nurses in this book reflected on the 'mismatch' of patients on the wards where they worked or received their treatment. Herbert Bliss recalls, 'I remember thinking: "Am I mad like these other people?" There were depressed people, schizophrenics, and a young boy with anorexia nervosa. It was crazy.'[172] Endeavouring to generate a 'therapeutic environment' in these conditions created a sense of incongruity. For nurses to survive, they had to become resilient and view their work as normal.[173]

The hidden history of gay life in mental hospitals

Not only was there great disparity in the mix of patients within mental hospitals, the staff who worked within them also came from diverse sections of society.[174] By virtue of their position on the fringes of 'respectable society', mental hospitals appeared to represent a space where variation not only within the patients, but also within the workforce could be relatively accepted. For some staff, their difference was their 'counter-cultural'[175] lifestyle, or a problem with substance misuse.[176] However, for others it was their sexual orientation. For some nurses, deciding to place themselves among an already stigmatised population was a fairly easy choice, as one nurse in Diana Gittins's study of Severalls Hospital in Colchester, Essex reflected, 'Where better to hide the stigma than in a stigmatised population?'[177]

There is evidence to suggest that there was a lesbian nurse sub-culture within some mental hospitals.[178] However, there is a dearth of literature that discusses the sub-culture of homosexual male nurses in mental hospitals. Indeed, Prebble found that homosexual male nurses were not as visible as lesbian nurses in the psychiatric nursing community of New Zealand in the 1960s, and that the dominant culture on the male nursing side was 'blokey' and, on the whole, not supportive of sexual difference.[179] Conversely, despite the culture of toughness and sporting prowess among some male staff in UK mental hospitals,[180] and the pathologising attitudes towards homosexuality discussed in Chapter 1, on analysis of the testimonies of the nurses interviewed for this book, it appears that there may have been an overt homosexual male sub-culture among nurses in some mental hospitals in the UK, and that these men were generally accepted. Indeed, four of the nurses interviewed identified themselves as gay men.

While the nature of this study may have attracted more gay volunteers, and given a distorted impression of the proportion of gay men in the workforce, Cecil Asquith who is heterosexual deliberated:

> There was a very strong gay contingent of staff. Moreover, their behaviours were quite overly gay most of the time too, but because it was an enclosed community and, you know, in the sense that it was ten miles from town in the middle of a forest, it didn't matter, nobody bothered that much about it.[181]

A mental hospital could be a refuge, a workplace or a holiday camp,[182] and as such within these hospitals, some gay men found a lively atmosphere, a culture and a community to belong to. With their network of wards, underground tunnels and departments, mental hospitals created an ideal space and a unique environment where homosexual male nurses could meet lovers and enjoy a social climate of fleeting love, romance and sexuality. The homosexual male sub-culture within the mental hospitals was multifaceted, with different types of nurses having their own implicit rules and behaviours; this included status distinctions, for example, between the lower ranking SENs and the nursing officers in the higher ranks. The level of acceptance these men experienced has important implications for this book and there appears to be a dichotomy as Elspeth Whitbread reflects:

> It was a very, very odd contradiction. Mental hospitals were a refuge for male gay nurses, but looking back, quite horrendous for gay patients. Ironically, I don't ever recall any of them [gay male nurses] refusing to administer the treatments either. Very interesting.[183]

Concurring with the above testimony, all the homosexual nurses interviewed for this book administered distressing treatments to 'cure' homosexual patients in their care, and this contradiction warrants further examination. In parallel with Barker and Stanley's work exploring gay life at sea, there are three important points that need to be understood in order to examine what life was like for homosexual male nurses in mental hospitals. First, it is important to note that each nurse experienced these institutions differently. The nurse's openness regarding his homosexuality, his social class and the job he did were important factors. Second, mental hospitals offered a special kind of culture, even a community. Finally, they also offered spaces that homosexual (and heterosexual) nurses could use to their advantage.[184]

Identity boundaries

In order to understand the relationship between these nurses and their mental hospitals, we need to first consider the level of openness that individual nurses displayed regarding their sexuality. Like the higher-ranking officers in the army during World War II, discussed in Chapter 1, the homosexual nursing officers within mental hospitals also had to be very covert regarding their sexuality. Meanwhile, lower-ranking nurses such as nursing auxiliaries and SENs could be more overt regarding theirs and still be accepted. In addition, mental hospitals were very hierarchical places to work and many gay nursing officers felt that they could not mix with gay men of lower rank.[185] Thaddeus Chester, who was a nursing officer, recalls:

> I remember thinking that it would ruin everything I had worked so hard to achieve if I came out as gay to my colleagues. I could get quite jealous sometimes at some of the nursing auxiliaries' and SENs' freedom, and their ability to be blatantly homosexual. I mean some of them, looking back, were totally outrageous! There were others, however, that I actually found very attractive, but I knew if I was seen chatting to them in the hospital social club, for instance, it could incriminate me.[186]

Carol Warren defined the polarities between covert and openly gay men, which correspond with the situation we see among the homosexual male nurses in this study. She recognised men who perceived themselves as 'essentially normal, deviating only in the choice of sexual partner, a deviance that they could conceptually minimise'.[187] Arguably, this was the arrangement for the homosexual nursing officers. Conversely, Warren identified gay men on the opposite end of the spectrum, who saw 'themselves as completely outside society . . . [They] organise their entire lives, including the working lives, around the self-definition and the deviance.'[188] In essence, she suggests that these individuals cope with being part of a frequently stigmatised group by flaunting their differences. These traits tended to be most popular with the lower-ranking staff, as Leith Cavill, a SEN, recalls:

> We [other homosexual lower ranking nurses] had a fabulous time and I was never ashamed of my sexuality. We were at it like rabbits too; there were lots of places to have fun in a mental hospital without others seeing . . . [Laughs] . . . I also remember me and some other SENs, who I had been friends with since we were pupil nurses together, used to get 'dragged up' when the hospital social club was having a fancy dress party. We were the 'belles of the ball' . . . [Laughs] . . . We always went down a storm and I don't really remember anyone complaining.[189]

The lower-ranking nurses could be very open in the way they expressed their sexuality, however, the higher-ranking nursing officers appeared to have believed that they had to be exceptionally furtive regarding theirs. This echoes the behaviour of homosexual men in the armed forces during World War II. Houlbrook argues that working-class culture enabled individuals to be more accustomed to sexual openness. Young workingmen were not labelled 'queer' or 'pansies' because they had sex with men. He argues that such encounters were sufficiently accepted, and that 'men could openly look for, enjoy, and talk about male partners without worrying about any potential reper-cussions'.[190] This offers a context to explain why lower-ranking 'work-ing-class' nurses may have been more overt in how they expressed their sexuality.

The mental hospital as a community

The insularity of the mental hospitals, coupled with the fact that many nurses lived within the confines of the hospital walls, created a lifestyle in which social networks were strong and the boundaries between work and 'home' were porous.[191] Mental hospitals could offer a homosexual male nurse a community where they could be open regarding their sexuality and sometimes very overt in how they dem-onstrated this. Baker and Stanley also found this with gay men at sea, as they were able to express feelings, explore outlawed desires, gain new knowledge, and belong to a culture as well as a community.[192] Within the mental hospitals, this culture had its own rules regarding how one should behave, as we have seen. It also had its own rituals. One such ritual was for the homosexual nurses to try to have their breaks together while they were on duty:

> There was a table in the staff canteen. It was known as 'The Queens' Table' . . . [Laughs] . . . That is because we [other homosexual lower ranking gay nurses] all used to sit together on it at break times. We would go to great lengths so we could all have a break at the same time.[193]

Furthermore, twelve of the nurses included in this book commented on the emphasis that many homosexual male nurses placed on domesticity, particularly on their wards:

> I remember **** [Name of nurse], he was an SEN on ** [Name of ward]. It was a female ward and he took great pride in it. He would use the ward funds to buy flowers to put round the ward and at meal times, he insisted on arranging napkins on the tables. When it was time for the staff to sit down and have a 'brew' together, the best china would come out with a matching teapot. It had a very homely feeling and I loved working there.[194]

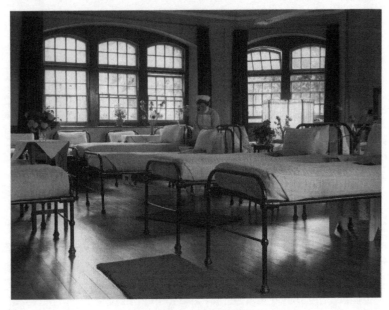

8 Female ward c.1960s

Despite the ward in figure 8 looking rather institutionalised with the beds all in line, there is some attempt to domesticate it with the flowers arranged around the ward.

For some homosexual male nurses, to be open regarding their sexuality within a mental hospital meant that they could not only express their personal feelings, but they also joined a collective that emphasised the importance – moreover the normality – of being homosexual. Newly gay male nurses, as with newly gay seafarers, became part of the process of making publicly visible what was ashore, or outside the hospital boundaries, illegal and offensive. It was an affirmation both of the individual and the newly visible culture of which he was part.[195]

However, not all men who had homosexual sex within mental hospitals became part of this culture, as we have seen with the testimony of Thaddeus Chester. Others may also have had a wife or a girlfriend outside, or even inside, the hospital. Therefore, their membership status within this culture may have only been temporary or non-existent. Houlbrook argues that opportunistic 'homosex'[196] and intimacy was very common prior to the gay liberation movement in the 1970s. He goes on to indicate that 'homosex and intimacy were integrated within erotic and affective lives that encompassed male *and* female partners'.[197] This could have been exacerbated by the fact that in the early asylums, male nurses often occupied all-male residential, labour, or leisure spaces. Also the strict segregation between males and females in mental hospitals meant that their interactions with women were limited.[198]

Contradictions

Arguably, one of the most interesting paradoxes with this finding is the fact that all the homosexual male nurses interviewed administered treatments to cure patients of the same 'illness' they had. Leith Cavill offers his reasons for this simply saying: 'I was different to most of them. I was at ease with my sexuality; they weren't. My job was to help them.'[199] Meanwhile, Evander Orchard offered the following explanation:

> The men I nursed had all been referred from their GP or another psychiatrist. So I thought they must have already been asked to explore the notion of accepting their sexuality. I just assumed, therefore, that they couldn't do that. I then thought: 'Well I have got to try and help that person.' Because you have to realise, they were usually very distressed about it. I guess that was the different thing between me and them. I wasn't distressed by my sexuality. These men included priests for whom their sexuality was a great contention with their religious beliefs. Or there were married men who were willing to try anything to get rid of their homosexual desires. All of these men were willing to do or try anything to make them straight. Although my experience of being gay was very different, I suppose I just thought: 'I've got to help them.' There were others on a court order so they had to have the treatments really. I have to be honest too, only being an SEN I don't really know how I would have been able to get out of doing it anyway. I didn't really want to question my superiors.[200]

Thaddeus Chester believed that objecting to the treatments, or refusal to assist with them might bring his sexuality in to question:

> Being a nursing officer my time doing 'hands-on' nursing care was limited. However, I remember the winter of 1961. We had a lot of staff sickness that year and we were really short-staffed on the wards, so I was helping out on one of them. That is where I nursed the young chap who was being treated for homosexuality. Some of the nurses appeared to enjoy what they were

doing to him. This confirmed what I probably already knew: some of the nurses were very homophobic. This made me even more determined not to draw any attention to myself. I remember feeling sickened by what we did to him, and it still haunts me to this day. I was a coward and selfish. I just didn't want anyone to know I was gay so I just went along with it.[201]

The irony is that he was just as willing to do anything to hide his sexuality as some of his patients were willing to do anything to change theirs. For Evander Orchard and Leith Cavill, their justifications for partaking in the administration of the aversion therapy appear to be embedded in the notion of beneficence (the good of the patient as a person) and the inability to question their superiors.

Homosexual male nurses appear to have been broadly accepted within mental hospitals. Prebble proposes that the marginalisation of the mental nursing community created an environment in which difference could be both understood and accommodated. By choosing to work with people who were on the margins of 'respectable society', she argues, mental nurses made room for their own 'queer folk'.[202] The mental hospital appeared to provide a bastion for the homosexual male nurses in this study. The sense of community and acceptance these nurses experienced within them was in stark contrast to the oppression faced by many homosexual men who lived beyond the hospital boundaries. By questioning the value of aversion therapy, the homosexual nurses featured in this book may have thought that they would jeopardise their place within this accepting community, and the following chapters explore how nurses who questioned practice were often constructively dismissed. This could offer a context, at least in part, to why they participated in aversion therapy and did not overtly question its efficacy.

Mental nurse training, 1925–1951

As discussed in the Introduction, the GNC introduced their own alternative training programme leading to registration as a registered mental nurse (RMN) in the early 1920s. Between the early 1920s and 1951, there were two routes'leading to mental nurse registration, provided by the MPA (RMPA from 1926) and the GNC. But, there was a bitter conflict throughout this period between the two organisations regarding who should have overall responsibility for training mental nurses.

In June 1925, after the end of the 'period of grace' discussed in the Introduction, the GNC stated that they would no longer recognise the MPA certificate for the purpose of registration, although members of the MPA would still be instrumental in acting as examiners for them.[203] The rationale behind this decision was that 'the time had come for a statutory body, such as the GNC, to stand on its own two feet and not delegate any of its work or responsibilities to another body'.[204] However, the MPA/RMPA refused to renounce their role and the two organisations 'kept up a bitter conflict through the pages of various journals and committees of enquiry throughout the 1920s and 1930s'.[205] Harrington suggests that gender differences contributed to the opposition between the two organisations. She argues that the GNC were keen to promote the image of the nurse as predominately middle class and female. Conversely, mental nurses were mainly male and were perceived to be lower in regard to both general calibre and professional status, and 'thus trailed behind their "Sisters" in general hospitals'.[206]

On 4 November 1943, the Society of Mental Nurses was founded. Initially it consisted of seventy mental nurses and they met under the auspices of the RCN's London Branch to discuss organisational and educational matters.[207] The notes of the first meeting suggest that there was a widely held view among the nurses present that training should be controlled by a single nursing body – the GNC; it was also hoped that general trained nurses could be attracted to work in psychiatric and mental handicap hospitals, thus raising the standards and status of nursing therein.[208]

However, the majority of nurses appeared to choose the RMPA's training course. Nolan argues that this was because it was a more practical course and more prestigious due to it being controlled by doctors.[209] The society favoured the GNC's training scheme, leading to RMN status, on the grounds that it was a more rigorous course, and more like the training of general nurses. The RMPA course was seen as inferior and lacking credibility:

> The quality of those recruits [for the RMPA] makes it doubtful if they would be accepted for training by the General Nursing Council, even as Enrolled

Nurses. If the RMPA stopped examining, we should be left with a group of nurses for whom no training was possible.[210]

The Interdepartmental Nursing Committee, chaired by Lord Athlone, had been set up in 1937 by the government in response to concern about shortages and wastage of nurses, and had a subcommittee specifically to examine mental nursing. However, owing to the war, the Committee's report was delayed until 1946 when it recommended the cessation of the two systems of training.[211] In May and June 1946 the GNC and the RMPA both held meetings, and agreement was finally reached that the RMPA would discontinue their training scheme. The last cohort of students to qualify under the RMPA's scheme started their training in 1948, and by 1951, training for mental nurses had passed entirely into the hands of the GNC.[212] In addition, the GNC agreed to recognise holders of the RMPA certificate for admission to the register. They also agreed to the inclusion of psychology in the syllabus at the request of the RMPA.[213]

Training mental nurses regarding 'sexual deviations'
There is a dearth of literature in nursing textbooks during this period which discuss sexual deviations. The texts that do mention homosexuality and transvestism do so under the categories of 'Sexual Perversions', 'Sexual Anomalies' or 'Sexual Disorders'.[214] Furthermore, the emphasis in these texts appears to be on describing these disorders rather than training nurses how to actually care for this patient group. Some of the nurses in the study recalled the training they received about homosexuality and transvestism, and its limitations in regard to equipping them with the skills required to actually nurse these patients. Zella Mullins recalls: 'They were very good at describing sexual deviants, but not so good at giving us the skills to actually nurse these patients.'[215] Other nurses recalled their training regarding sexual deviants:

In lectures the tutors would lump abnormal sexuality into a common pot, so the fact that you might have paedophile tendencies, or you might be gay, was all the same, it was all deemed to be wrong. They would be lumped into this bag of, you know, deviants if you like.[216]

I do remember a lecture that was given at the ******** [name of the hospital]. This lecture was on deviancy, and as part of deviancy, homosexuality and transvestism came up. It was talked about in the same vein as criminality. Homosexuality and transvestism were included in a bunch of lectures that were given by a consultant. Now how it was presented to us was that these behaviours were deviancies, and they came as part of a package of deviancies. They were seen as a denial of who you were, an adoption of a lifestyle that you chose, rather than had to. There was also gain to be had from behaving and acting as a homosexual or a transvestite, but they were not normal – that was the point that was trying to be got across.[217]

The training nurses received with regard to homosexuality and transvestism had a clear emphasis on viewing these people as abnormal, with little importance paid to actually training nurses on how to care for these individuals. Indeed, Ursula Vaughan recalled: 'I remember my colleagues and I being totally unprepared for dealing with and talking to them [homosexuals and transvestites] when they arrived on the ward.'[218] This was emphasised by the wider debate around how to view the sexual deviant that was being promoted by the media and literary works. Nurses were not receiving any training that presented a coherent and robust knowledge about these individuals.

The 1950s: mental hospitals under attack

During the 1950s, the tradition of caring for the mentally ill within large institutions came under intense criticism both from inside and outside the system. Karen Jones posits that the 1950s was a hopeful period for the mentally ill. During this period new drugs, particularly Chlorpromazine, came on to the scene; the open-door policy became established in mental hospitals and a Royal Commission was appointed to review the law relating to mental illness.[219] However, for staff working within these institutions, the greater emphasis on community care and pharmacological advances meant that there could be a threat to their jobs.

The first public acknowledgement by the government that psychiatry was under scrutiny came from Enoch Powell as Minister of Health at the annual conference of the National Association of Mental Health in 1961. He stated that mental hospitals were part of a bygone age and these 'doomed institutions' must disappear. What was required to remove them was a completely new approach to the mentally ill and their welfare.[220] On 31 May 1961, Powell officiated at the opening of a Nurse Training School at Littlemore Hospital, Oxford. According to Nolan, he again emphasised here the government's intention to cut the number of psychiatric beds, especially on long-stay wards. Powell is noted to have stressed that this was not part of a campaign to undermine psychiatry, but to strengthen it. He stated that more resources would be spent on improving the training of mental nurses, and this would lead to an improved standard of care for patients. He saw nurses as having the opportunity to play a leading role in the exciting changes ahead.[221] However, Nolan goes on to posit that, despite this upbeat political rhetoric, mental nurses were not convinced that their lot was likely to improve.[222]

Community care

The population in mental hospitals had continued to increase and by 1955 there were over 150,000 patients within the UK's mental hospital system.[223] Had this number been allowed to increase, it would have threatened the NHS, as doctors and administrators seemed unable to stem this rising tide of patients.[224] Something had to be done and caring for patients beyond the boundaries of the hospital was high on the political agenda. Community care, in this context, is an elusive concept whose meaning changes over time. It is most simply defined as the policy of treating mental disorder outside the mental hospital, and in 1950s Britain, when it was adopted as national policy, this was the dominant overriding meaning.[225]

Community care was primarily about services for people who could be discharged from the mental hospital and about expanding these services so that more people, especially those with chronic problems, could be discharged at an earlier stage. The contemporary interpretations of community care in this period had, according to Busfield, three facets: it meant services outside the mental hospital, it particularly meant after-care services for those with long-standing problems, and it meant services provided in the public sector.[226]

The policy shift away from the mental hospital was accentuated by the introduction of anti-psychotic drugs in the 1950s. The new drugs reawakened assumptions about the curability of mental illness and led to an (over-) optimistic discussion about the abolition of the old long-stay patients.[227] It was believed that patients with chronic disorders would disappear in time as they died, and many claimed that there would be no new generations of long-stay patients. Mental hospitals would no longer be needed and could arguably be closed.[228] Furthermore, Nolan argues that some mental nurses were apprehensive about the new psychotropic drugs and worried that they might spell the end for nursing care for mentally ill patients, or at least drastically reduce the need for nursing input.[229] Myrtle Pauncefoot concurs and noted: 'A lot of the older staff were suspicious of the new meds, as they believed they were part of a larger conspiracy to get rid of the institutions completely.'[230]

The Royal Commission on Mental Illness and Mental Deficiency, which would become known as 'The Percy Commission', was developed to review the legislation surrounding the admission, certification and detention of the mentally ill in 1954. Harrington argues that the commission was tasked with examining the relationships between hospital and community, health service and local authority. The commission advocated a less legalistic framework for admissions, with more responsibility on doctors implementing compulsory detentions, rather than the courts, and its recommendations were embedded into the Mental Health Act 1959.[231]

The Act placed a new emphasis on community care, and its aims were to reduce the number of inpatients immediately and, in the long term, to change the course of mental health care provision. The Act unreservedly damned overcrowding as an organisational malpractice, that produced in itself a great deal of ill health. Furthermore, it introduced the concept of 'informal' patients; these were to be treated in outpatient clinics, by GPs and in the community.[232] Nolan has argued that the impetus for the Act was definitely economic, however, it also embodied the dissatisfaction that had been mounting for years among those concerned with the care of the mentally ill.[233]

The introduction of the new Act witnessed changes in the balance of power between professional groups. Within the mental hospitals themselves the overriding power of the medical superintendent was diminished and the post began to be phased out. Additionally, integration of psychiatry with other parts of medicine often led to a loss of power to other health bodies. The development of community mental health services arguably led to a diffusion and gradual diminution of psychiatry's power as mental health facilities became more widespread. Within these facilities, psychiatrists were often in more direct competition with other mental health professionals, such as social workers. All of the above were deemed a threat to psychiatrists.[234] Nurses' jobs were also under increasing threat. This was due in part to two new professional disciplines assuming direct responsibility for mental patients: social workers and occupational therapists, whose numbers were increasing rapidly.[235] In this precarious climate with its emphasis on reducing patient numbers, it is inevitable that both the medical and nursing professionals feared for their job security, which may have prompted them to turn their attention to 'fixing' 'social maladies'.[236]

Jo Phelan and her colleagues argue that the definitions and conceptions of mental illness were broadened during the 1950s. This included a greater proportion of neurotic or non-psychotic disorders being treated, such as alcoholism.[237] In 1949, the sixth edition of the World Health Organization's *International Statistical Classification of Diseases, Injuries and Causes of Death* was published.[238] This included a section on mental disorder for the first time. Prior to this edition, it had only been a manual of causes of death (mortality): *International Classification of Causes of Death*. The American Psychiatric Association (APA) followed suit in 1952 and issued the first version of the Diagnostic Statistical Manual (DSM), which listed and categorised mental disorders.[239] Both these diagnostic tools began to be utilised interchangeably in the UK and both listed homosexuality and transvestism as mental disorders. Some of the nurses in this book recalled such broadening of the definitions of mental illness and offered their own interpretations for the reasons behind this:

> I recall psychiatry in the mid to late 1960s as a branch of medicine that was desperately in need of some sort of affirmation, opting for anything or anyone that it could take on. And the more it could please the government, and the more it could be seen to get people to conform, the better. That is why I believe it took on sexual deviants and drug addicts, the government were at a loss at what to do with both of them at the time. Psychiatry held the notion that they were social fixers – that they could fix the problem for society. But what they were about essentially was about identifying and labelling, and once people had these labels, they had done their job as far as they were concerned.[240]

Ida Ashley perceived that psychiatry used homosexuals to gain credibility with the government:

> I think psychiatry made a stance following the introduction of the Mental Health Act 1959, which was insistent on reducing patient numbers in mental hospitals. I think that they felt that their credibility as a profession was being undermined, and they felt threatened. So, I think, psychiatry saw a niche in the market [treating homosexuals] of how they could get back in the government's good books.[241]

Meanwhile, Una Drinkwater recalls how some nurses' salaries were based on the occupancy of the hospital and the pressure that reducing patients numbers could have on these nurses:

> Doctors were convincing in how they were thinking and behaving at the time. On the one hand, we were made very much aware that admitting people now had to be the last resort, as community care was coming into force; however, not many people, myself included, actually knew what community care was. And of course, there was a fear in some of the senior staff that if the numbers were going to reduce, that would affect their salary. Particularly the Chief Male Nurse, the Assistant Chief Male Nurse, and the Matron: they were paid on the number of beds that they had. So there was this fearing that if you start reducing the numbers, their pay would reduce. So there was a surge I think . . . I don't know whether it was done consciously, although it seemed to happen around the same time, that there were other forms of mental illness being created.[242]

Indeed, Philip Thomas and Patrick Bracken argue that the government influenced psychiatry to cast its gaze on 'antisocial and immoral behaviours'.[243] Some psychiatrists responded to the government's uncertainty, regarding the most effective way of dealing with sexual deviants, by developing and implementing treatments to 'cure' these individuals. This could have been a tacit, but pragmatic way of bringing 'new' patients into hospital at a time when patient numbers were ever decreasing. Meanwhile, mental nurses were worried that new psychotropic drugs and the introduction of social workers and occupational therapists might reduce the need for nursing input. It may have seemed that developing and implementing treatments for sexual deviations would prove their worth to the government; who at the time were reducing spending on mental health services.[244]

Conclusion

The period this chapter explored witnessed many changes for practising mental nurses in both legislation and practice. The Mental Treatment Act 1930 brought with it a therapeutic optimism, owing to the possibility of curative treatment for mental patients. This led to the introduction of new somatic treatments, which meant that nurses were taking on more advanced roles. However, the vast majority had no theoretical underpinning for the interventions they were implementing. Essentially, nurses were unaware that what passed for treatment in their workplace might represent no more than the penchant of their particular medical superintendent, based on no firm evidence at all. Moreover, by exposing nurses to these somatic treatments, it arguably normalised the implementation of 'therapeutic' interventions that caused pain and distress to the patients who received them. This could offer a context to explain some nurses' later acceptance of aversion therapies.

During this period, mental nursing attempted to improve its public image but was generally aggravated by lack of resources. Its direction was primarily transformed by the absorption of psychiatry into the NHS and the RMPA's relinquishing responsibility for training of mental nurses. Mental nursing was also significantly affected by World War II. The rapid and ill-organised discharge of large numbers of patients from one hospital to another, in order to make way for wounded soldiers, led to mass overcrowding. This was compounded by gross understaffing as many nurses were called up for military service.

Furthermore, with the inception of the Mental Health Act 1959, oratory around community care, the introduction of new health and social care practitioners and diminishing patient numbers, many nurses and psychiatrists felt that their profession was under threat. When we revisit the rhetoric in Chapter 1 regarding the lack of consensus on the optimal way to deal with the problem of sexual deviants, it could be argued that some psychiatrists – and nurses – developed and implemented treatments for the these individuals as a tacit way of bringing 'new' patients into the mental hospital. This could have been a pragmatic, and perhaps unacknowledged, attempt to protect their jobs and increase their profile positively with the government. It further marked out a specialism and a specialist discourse.

Within some mental hospitals there also appeared to be a homosexual male nurse sub-culture. These men developed their own routines, community and rituals, and appear to have been accepted by their heterosexual colleagues. The finding that all of the homosexual nurses in this study also administered treatments to 'cure' patients suffering from the same 'illness' as themselves appeared to be justified under the notions of beneficence and subservience. This combined with the sense of community and acceptance these nurses experienced in mental hospitals may have also prevented them from objecting to the treatments, as they would have had a lot to lose if they were no longer part of this community.

Finally, while there is some evidence of nurses implementing dynamic new approaches to care for patients during this period, the vast majority of nurses were not party to the wider debate about treatments, which was taking place outside mental hospitals. Nor, in fact within their hospitals, as they did not generally participate in case conferences, discuss patients' treatments or diagnoses, or assess the progress of patients. The culture of many mental hospitals – and their nurses – was still custodial, ritualised and impersonal. Nurses working within such establishments were expected to provide therapeutic interventions with little, if any, consideration of their efficacy or theoretical underpinning. The majority of nurses accepted that their role was to carry out, uncritically and without question, whatever medical staff or their nursing superiors had prescribed. It is to these 'subordinate' nurses that we now turn.

Notes

1 Gilbert Davies, interviewed 10 February 2010.
2 Nolan, 'Mental Health Nursing – Origins and Developments', p. 254.
3 Kathleen Jones, *A History of Mental Health Services* (London, 1972).
4 Montagu Lomax, *The Experiences of an Asylum Doctor* (London, 1921). Lomax wrote his book after working at Prestwich Asylum in Manchester as a *locum tenens* during the World War I. He stated his rationale for writing the book was, that under the legislation then in force, the psychiatric system for the pauper insane was defective and open to abuse. The book itself was an indictment of the regime at Prestwich Asylum, in particular, and

psychiatric care in general. He described the asylum as gloomy, dilapidated, barrack-like and dirty; considered the patients' clothing and diet to be of poor quality; described the regime as dull and monotonous; and criticised the lack of a system for assessing and categorising patients according to their needs. He also considered that many attendants were lazy, vain, unjust, mean and tyrannical, but attributed this to long hours, low pay, lack of prospects and generally being treated with contempt by hospital management: Hopton, 'Prestwich Hospital in the Twentieth Century', p. 351; Tom Butler, *Mental Health, Social Policy and the Law* (Basingstoke, 1985), p. 83.

5　Hopton, 'Prestwich Hospital in the Twentieth Century', p. 351; Kathleen Jones, *Mental Health & Social Policy, 1845–1959* (London, 1960), p. 94.

6　Nolan, *A History of Mental Health Nursing*, pp. 82–83.

7　Hopton, 'Prestwich Hospital in the Twentieth Century', p. 352.

8　Jones, *Mental Health & Social Policy*, p. 94.

9　Busfield, *Managing Madness*, pp. 319–320; Nolan, *Psychiatric Nursing Past and Present*, p. 137.

10　Pamela Dale and Joseph Melling, *Mental Illness and Learning Disability Since 1850: Finding a Place From Mental Disorder in the United Kingdom* (London, 2006), p. 112; Jones, *Mental Health & Social Policy*, p. 121.

11　Jones, *Mental Health & Social Policy*, p. 120.

12　Valerie Harrington, 'Death of the Asylum: The Run-Down and Closure of Prestwich Mental Hospital' (unpublished MSc thesis, University of Manchester, Manchester, 2004), p. 18. See also Joan Busfield, 'Restructuring Mental Health Services', in Marijke Gijswijt-Hofstra and Roy Porter (eds), *Cultures of Psychiatric and Mental Health Care in Post-War Britain and the Netherlands* (Amsterdam, 1998), p. 16.

13　The phenomenon of shell-shock had a profound influence on conceptions of mental illness and on psychiatric practice. Doctors and nurses within psychiatry were expected to treat men suffering from shell-shock and return them, cured and ready for military service, as quickly as possible. Shell-shock was an ill-defined but demonstrably 'real' condition which psychiatrists were able to address. Respectable people – men of 'good character' – appeared to go mad. Society was forced to take madness more seriously and to redraw the line between that condition and sanity: Harrington, *Death of the Asylum*, p. 18; Nolan, 'Mental Health Nursing – Origins and Developments', pp. 253–254; See also Tracey Longhran, 'Hysteria and Neurasthenia in pre-1914 British Medical Discourse and in Histories of Shell-Shock', *History of Psychiatry* 19 (2008), pp. 25–46.

14　Harrington, *Death of the Asylum*, p. 19.

15　Joan Busfield, *Managing Madness: Changing Ideas and Practice* (London, 1986) pp. 295–300.

16　Francis E. James, 'Insulin Treatment in Psychiatry', *History of Psychiatry* iii (1992), p. 221; Before the 1930s, unpleasant and ineffective treatments included: 'the bath of surprise' a reservoir of water into which the patient was suddenly precipitated while standing on its movable and treacherous cover, cold showers and 'the swivel chair', which involved spinning the patient around continually in a swivel chair.

17 Dementia praecox (a 'premature dementia' or 'precocious madness') referred to a chronic, deteriorating psychotic disorder. It was characterised by rapid cognitive breakdown, which usually began in the late teens or early adulthood. It was eventually reframed into a substantially different disease concept and relabelled as schizophrenia.

18 Andrew Scull, 'Desperate Remedies: A Gothic Tale of Madness and Modern Medicine', *Psychological Medicine* 17 (1987), p. 562; David Crossley, 'The Introduction of Leucotomy: A British Case History', *History of Psychiatry* iv (1993), p. 557.

19 Jack D. Pressman, *Last Resort: Psychosurgery and the Limits of Medicine* (Cambridge, 1998), p. 41.

20 Edward Shorter, *History of Psychiatry: From the Era of Asylum to the Age of Prozac* (New York, 1997), pp. 522–530.

21 James, 'Insulin Treatment in Psychiatry', p. 222.

22 Nolan, 'The Development of Mental Health Nursing', p. 12.

23 Prebble, 'Ordinary Men and Uncommon Women', p. 119.

24 James, 'Insulin Treatment in Psychiatry', p. 222.

25 Wilfred L. Jones, *Ministering to Minds Diseased: A History of Psychiatric Treatment* (London, 1983), p. 21; James, 'Insulin Treatment in Psychiatry', p. 221.

26 James, 'Insulin Treatment in Psychiatry', p. 222.

27 Shorter, *History of Psychiatry*, p. 522.

28 James, 'Insulin Treatment in Psychiatry', p. 222.

29 'William Sargant (1907–1988) was a pioneer during the war years in the introduction of physical treatment in psychiatry. Following the war he served his association with the Maudsley Hospital and became physician in charge of psychological medicine at St. Thomas' Hospital until his retirement in 1971': James, 'Insulin Treatment in Psychiatry', p. 235.

30 'Edward Mapother (1881–1940) first came to psychiatry when he joined the staff of Longrove Hospital, Epsom. Later, he became the first Superintendent of the Maudsley Hospital and in 1937 the first professor in clinical psychiatry in the University of London': James, 'Insulin Treatment in Psychiatry', p. 235.

31 James, 'Insulin Treatment in Psychiatry', p. 223.

32 Adams, *Challenge and Change in a Cinderella Service*, p. 128; Prebble, 'Ordinary Men and Uncommon Women', p. 119.

33 Una Drinkwater, interviewed 29 December 2009.

34 Prebble, 'Ordinary Men and Uncommon Women', p. 119.

35 Prebble, 'Ordinary Men and Uncommon Women', p. 119.

36 Adams, *Challenge and Change in a Cinderella Service*, p. 128.

37   Prebble, 'Ordinary Men and Uncommon Women', p. 119; Adams, *Challenge and Change in a Cinderella Service*, pp. 129–130.
38   Elspeth Whitbread, interviewed 7 January 2010.
39   Harold Bourne, 'The Insulin Myth', *Lancet* ii (1953), p. 964.
40   Jones, *Ministering to Minds Diseased*, p. 23.
41   Meduna of Hungry had made the 'discovery' that the brains of people with schizophrenia and those with epilepsy were different. He first experimented with producing seizures by administering camphor, but when this was found to be unreliable, he changed to using Cardiazol: German E. Berrios, 'The Scientific Origins of Electroconvulsive Therapy: A Conceptual History', *History of Psychiatry* viii (1997), p. 106.
42   This type of seizure causes a person's body to stiffen, because all the body's muscles contract. The person may sound like they are crying out as air is pushed out of their lungs and they may lose control of their bladder or bowels.
43   A seizure characterised by rhythmic or semi-rhythmic contractions of a group of muscles. The arms, neck and facial muscles are most commonly involved.
44   Jesper Vaczy Kragh, 'Shock Therapy in Danish Psychiatry', *Medical History* 54 (2010), p. 348.
45   Adams, *Challenge and Change in a Cinderella Service*, p. 129.
46   Testimony of a former patient who received Cardiazol cited in Kragh, 'Shock Therapy in Danish Psychiatry', p. 351.
47   Testimony of Martha Sherman, a former patient cited in Joel Braslow, *Mental Ills and Bodily Cures* (London, 1997), p. 110.
48   Gilbert Davies, interviewed 10 February 2010.
49   Braslow, *Mental Ills and Bodily Cures*, 57.
50   Gerald W. T. H. Flemming, Fredrick L. Golla and William Walter, 'Electric-Convulsion Therapy of Schizophrenia', Lancet II (1939), pp. 1353–1355. Flemming et al. 'administered 75 electrical shocks of the brain, as a result of which there have been 50 major convulsions and 25 minor seizures. The major convulsions are similar to spontaneous ones and are followed by complete amnesia for the shock'.
51   Flemming, Golla and Walter, 'Electric-Convulsion Therapy of Schizophrenia', p. 1355.
52   Berrios, 'The Scientific Origins of Electroconvulsive Therapy: A Conceptual History', p. 107.
53   Elliot Whitman, interviewed 20 March 2010.
54   Adams, *Challenge and Change in a Cinderella Service*, p. 126.
55   Prebble, 'Ordinary Men and Uncommon Women', p. 121.
56   See, e.g., Michael King, *Wrestling with the Angel: A Life of Janet Frame* (Auckland, 2000); Diana Gittins, *Madness in its Place: Narratives of Severalls Hospital, 1913–1997* (London, 1997); Prebble, 'Ordinary Men

and Uncommon Women', pp. 122–123; Adams, *Challenge and Change in a Cinderella Service*, pp. 124–127.

57 Prebble, 'Ordinary Men and Uncommon Women', pp. 122.

58 Ursula Vaughan, interviewed 12 February 2010.

59 Cecil Asquith, interviewed 5 December 2010.

60 Adams, *Challenge and Change in a Cinderella Service*, p. 127; Prebble, 'Ordinary Men and Uncommon Women', p. 123.

61 King, Wrestling with the Angel, p. 97.

62 Braslow, *Mental Ills and Bodily Cures*, p. 97; Adams, *Challenge and Change in a Cinderella Service*, p. 126.

63 Leith Cavill, interviewed 25 March 2010.

64 Thaddeus Chester, interviewed 8 August 2010.

65 Prebble, 'Ordinary Men and Uncommon Women', p. 124.

66 Crossley, 'The Introduction of Leucotomy', p. 554.

67 Pressman, *Last Resort*, p. 36.

68 Crossley, 'The Introduction of Leucotomy', p. 555.

69 Walter Freeman and James Watts, *Psychosurgery: Intelligence, Emotion and Social Behaviour Following Prefrontal Lobotomy for Mental Disorders* (Illinois, 1942), p. 109.

70 Along with neurosurgeon Almeida Lima, Moniz resected part of the prefrontal lobes of twenty patients transferred from the Bombarda asylum to the neurology service of the Santa Marta Hospital in Lisbon. Seven had been 'cured', seven improved, and in six there was no change: Shorter, *History of Psychiatry*, p. 226.

71 Crossley, 'The Introduction of Leucotomy', p 553.

72 By 1942 Freeman and Watts had operated on eighty cases: Crossley, 'The Introduction of Leucotomy', p. 554.

73 Crossley, 'The Introduction of Leucotomy', p. 554.

74 Emanon L. Hutton and Gerald W. T. H. Fox, 'Early Results of Prefrontal Leucotomy', *The Lancet* ccxli (1941), pp. 3–7.

75 Medical Superintendent's Annual Report to the Committee of Visitors of the North Wales Countries Mental Hospital for 1943, p. 25 cited in Crossley, 'The Introduction of Leucotomy, p. 561.

76 Crossley, 'The Introduction of Leucotomy, p. 555.

77 Crossley, 'The Introduction of Leucotomy, p. 556.

78 Roger Strom-Olsen, 'Results of Prefrontal leucotomy', *Journal of Mental Science* lxxxix (1943), p. 491.

79 Gilbert Davies, interviewed 10 February 2010.

80 Claudine de Valois, interviewed 30 December 2009.

81 Crossley, 'The Introduction of Leucotomy, p. 553.

82 Una Drinkwater, interviewed 29 December 2009.

83 Percy T. Rees, 'Symposium on Prefrontal Leucotomy', *Journal of Mental Science* xc (1943), p. 161.

84 Prebble, *'Ordinary Men and Uncommon Women'*, pp. 124.
85 Julian Wills, interviewed 4 January 2010.
86 See, e.g. Peter Neushul, 'Fighting Research: Army Participation in the Clinical Testing and Mass Production of Penicillin during the Second World War', in Roger Cooter, Mark Harrison and Steve Sturdy (eds), *War, Medicine & Modernity* (Stroud, 1998), pp. 203–224.
87 Adams, *Challenge and Change in a Cinderella Service*, pp. 138–143.
88 Crossley, 'The Introduction of Leucotomy, p. 562.
89 George C. Tooth and Michael P. Newton, *'Leucotomy in England and Wales, 1942–1954', Great Britain Ministry of Health Reports on Public Health and Medical Subjects No. 104* (London, 1961), p. 21.
90 Una Drinkwater, interviewed 29 December 2009.
91 Adams, *Challenge and Change in a Cinderella Service*, pp. 154–155; Prebble, 'Ordinary Men and Uncommon Women', p. 124.
92 Busfield, 'Restructuring Mental Health Services', p. 17.
93 It appears that male RNs called up for military service were not given commissions in the British army, as it was not considered appropriate for male officers to deal with unpleasant aspects of bodily function, particularly elimination.
94 Nolan, *A History of Mental Health Nursing*, p. 98.
95 Nolan, 'The Development of Mental Health Nursing', p. 12.
96 Chatterton, 'The Weakest Link in the Chain of Nursing?', p. 67.
97 Nolan, 'The Development of Mental Health Nursing', p. 12; Christine M. Silverstein, 'From the Front Lines to the Home Front: A History of the Development of Psychiatric Nursing in the U.S. During the World War II Era', *Issues in Mental Health Nursing* 29 (2008), pp. 719–737.
98 Nolan, *Psychiatric Nursing Past and Present*, p. 203.
99 Stella Bingham, *Ministering Angels* (Over Wallop, 1979), p. 194.
100 Penny Starns, 'Fighting Militarism? British Nursing During The Second World War', in Roger Cooter, Mark Harrison and Steve Sturdy (eds), *War, Medicine & Modernity* (Stroud, 1998), p. 192.
101 Bingham, *Ministering Angels*, p. 196.
102 Chatterton, 'The Weakest Link in the Chain of Nursing?', p. 131.
103 Chatterton, 'The Weakest Link in the Chain of Nursing?', p. 131.
104 Bingham, *Ministering Angels*, p. 196.
105 Nolan, *A History of Mental Health Nursing*, p. 102.
106 Chatterton, 'The Weakest Link in the Chain of Nursing?', p. 143.
107 Eileen Baggott, 'The SEN in Psychiatric Hospitals', *Nursing Times* 29 (1965), p. 1478; Chatterton 'The Weakest Link in the Chain of Nursing?', p. 129.
108 Nolan, 'Mental Health Nursing – origins and developments', p. 254.
109 Busfield, 'Restructuring Mental Health Services', p. 16.
110 Quoted in Michael Foot, *Aneurin Bevan, 1945–1960* (St Albans, 1975), p. 137.

111 Under the 1948 regulations the RHBs were responsible for 'guiding and controlling the planning, conduct and development of services in their Regions; Hospital Management Committees, as the Board's agents, for administering these services': Harrington, *Death of the Asylum*, p. 21.
112 See also Monica E. Baly, 'The National Health Service', in Monica E. Baly (ed.), *Nursing & Social Change* (New York, 1995), pp. 180–196.
113 Peter Nolan, 'Swing and Roundabouts: Mental Health Nursing and the Birth of the NHS', *Mental Health Care* 1 (1998), pp. 371–374.
114 Hopton, 'Prestwich Hospital in the Twentieth Century', pp. 349–369.
115 Harrington, *Death of the Asylum*, p. 21.
116 Nolan, *Psychiatric Nursing Past and Present*, p. 193.
117 Harrington, *Death of the Asylum*, p. 22.
118 Charles Webster, 'Nursing and the Early Crisis of the National Health Service', *Bulletin of The History of Nursing Group at the RCN* 7 (1985), p. 12–24.
119 Peter Nolan and Barone Hopper, 'Mental Health Nursing in the 1950s and 1960s Revisited', *Journal of Psychiatric and Mental Health Nursing* 4 (1997), p. 334.
120 Nolan and Hopper, 'Mental Health Nursing in the 1950s and 1960s Revisited', p. 334.
121 Olive Griffiths, Norman Reid and Margaret Scott, 'Reconstruction Scheme for Mental Nursing', *Nursing Mirror* October 27, pp. 46–47.
122 *Nursing Times*, 'Friends of Menston Hospital', *Nursing Times* (28 November 1953), pp. 1215–1216.
123 Adams, *Challenge and Change in a Cinderella Service*, p. 87.
124 Chatterton, 'The Weakest Link in the Chain of Nursing?', p. 67.
125 Una Drinkwater, interviewed 29 December 2009.
126 Chatterton, 'The Weakest Link in the Chain of Nursing?', pp. 77–103.
127 Hopton, 'Prestwich Hospital in the Twentieth Century', p. 349.
128 Prebble, 'Ordinary Men and Uncommon Women', p. 120.
129 Claudine de Valois, interviewed 30 December 2009.
130 Thaddeus Chester, interviewed 8 August 2010.
131 'Burnout' can be described as physical and emotional exhaustion and loss of compassion and empathy owing to intense involvement with other people over a prolonged period of time: Hopton, 'Prestwich Hospital in the Twentieth Century', p. 355.
132 City of Salford Local History Library, Manchester Regional Hospital Board Minutes, Report of Buildings and Works Committee, 3 May 1957, in Hopton, 'Prestwich Hospital in the Twentieth Century'.
133 Royal Medico-Psychological Association, *Handbook for Mental Nurses* (London, 1923/1939).
134 John Hopton, 'Daily Life in a 20th Century Psychiatric Hospital: An Oral History of Prestwich Hospital', *International History of Nursing Journal* 2 (3) (1997), p. 33.

135 Prebble, 'Ordinary Men and Uncommon Women', p. 113.
136 Prebble, 'Ordinary Men and Uncommon Women', p. 113.
137 Mick Carpenter, *They Still Go Marching On* (London, 1985), p. 12.
138 Leith Cavill, interviewed 25 March 2010.
139 Carpenter, *They Still Go Marching On*, p. 10.
140 Carpenter, *They Still Go Marching On*, p. 15.
141 National Health Service, *Report of the Committee of Inquiry into Whittingham Hospital* (London, 1972).
142 Hopton, 'Daily Life in a 20th Century Psychiatric Hospital', p. 33.
143 Testimony of a male nurse in: Nolan, *Psychiatric Nursing Past and Present*, p. 215.
144 Nolan, *Psychiatric Nursing Past and Present*, p. 204.
145 For example, at the Ford Motor Company, before a new pay structure was introduced in 1967, there were four grades for production workers: male – skilled; male – semi-skilled; male – unskilled; and female: National Union of Teachers, *Equal Pay & The Equal Pay Act 1970*, available at: www.teachers. org.uk/node/12977 (last accessed 27 January 2012).
146 Nolan, *Psychiatric Nursing Past and Present*, p. 205.
147 Cecil Asquith, interviewed 5 December 2010.
148 Nolan, *Psychiatric Nursing Past and Present*, p. 216.
149 Nolan, *Psychiatric Nursing Past and Present*, p. 217.
150 Richard Hunter, 'The Rise and Fall of Mental Nursing', *The Lancet* 1 (1956), p. 3; Walk, 'The History of Mental Nursing', pp. 1–17.
151 Teodoro Allyon and Jack Michael, 'The Psychiatric Nurse as Behavioral Engineer', *Journal of Experimental Analysis of Behavior*, 2 (1959), pp. 323–333.
152 John L. Cameron and Robert D. Laing, 'Effects of Environmental Change in the Care of Chronic Schizophrenics', *The Lancet* (1955), pp. 1384–1386.
153 See also Peter Nolan, 'Reflections of a Mental Nurse in the 1950s', *Royal College of Nursing History of Nursing Journal* 5 (1994), pp. 150–156.
154 Elliot Whitman, interviewed 20 March 2010.
155 Evander Orchard, interviewed 10 August 2010.
156 Testimony of a male nurse in: Nolan, *Psychiatric Nursing Past and Present*, p. 205.
157 Benedict Henry, interviewed 23 June 2010.
158 Hopton, 'Prestwich Hospital in the Twentieth Century', p. 360.
159 Griffiths, Reid and Scott, 'Reconstruction Scheme for Mental Nursing', p. 46.
160 Benedict Henry, interviewed 23 June 2010.
161 Thaddeus Chester, interviewed 8 August 2010.
162 *British Journal of Nursing*, 'Conference of Mental Hospital Authorities', *British Journal of Nursing* (25 April 1952), p. 26.

163 Everett C. Hughes, *Men and their Work* (Glencoe, 1958); Everett C. Hughes, 'Work and the Self', in John H. Rohrer and Muzafer Sherif (eds), *Social Psychology at the Crossroads* (New York, 1951), pp. 313–323.

164 Prebble, 'Ordinary Men and Uncommon Women', p. 199.

165 The phrase 'courtesy stigma' was first posited by Erving Goffman. It refers to the stigma experienced by family, friends and health professionals who closely associate with a person from a stigmatised group: Erving Goffman, *Stigma: Notes on the Management of Spoiled Identity* (Harmondsworth, 1963).

166 Maude Griffin, interviewed 8 March 2013.

167 Prebble, 'Ordinary Men and Uncommon Women', p. 199.

168 Blake E. Ashforth and Glen E. Kreiner, "How Can they Do It?' Dirty Work and the Challenge of Constricting a Positiver Identity', *Academy of Management Review* 24 (1999), pp. 413–434.

169 Prebble, 'Ordinary Men and Uncommon Women', p. 200.

170 Myrtle Pauncefoot, interviewed 20 February 2013.

171 Claudine de Valois, interviewed 30 December 2009.

172 Herbert Bliss, interviewed 2 January 2010.

173 Prebble, 'Ordinary Men and Uncommon Women', p. 202.

174 See, e.g., Chatterton, 'The Weakest Link in the Chain of Nursing?'; Gittins, *Madness in its Place*.

175 'Counter-culture' is a sociological term used to describe the values and norms of behaviour of a cultural group, or sub-culture, that run counter to those of the social mainstream of the day. Counterculture can also be described as a group whose behaviour deviates from the societal norm.

176 Prebble, 'Ordinary Men and Uncommon Women', p. 203.

177 Gittins, *Madness in its Place*, pp. 155–156.

178 See, e.g., Jivani, *It's Not Unusual*, pp. 71–72; Prebble, 'Ordinary Men and Uncommon Women', pp. 203–207.

179 Prebble, 'Ordinary Men and Uncommon Women', pp. 197 and 204.

180 Tommy Dickinson and Karen M. Wright, 'Stress and Burnout in Forensic Mental Health Nursing: A Review of the Literature', *British Journal of Nursing* 17 (2) (2008), p. 85.

181 Cecil Asquith, interviewed 5 December 2010.

182 It has been argued that the introduction of holiday-camp type activities within mental hospitals, which included the formation of cricket and football teams among staff and patients in the 1920s and 1930s, can be attributed to the holiday camps which were becoming popular at the time. See e.g. Nolan, *A History of Mental Health Nursing*, p. 96.

183 Elspeth Whitbread, interviewed 7 January 2010.

184 Baker and Stanley, *Hello Sailor!*, p. 66.

185 A similar pattern has been noted in gay men at sea. Robert, a purser, knew it would be 'career suicide' if he were found chatting up a crewman he fancied.

On his first ship he noticed that 'the strange thing was in the Merchant Navy [that] . . . while it was quite accepted for stewards and cooks and all those people to be gay, as an officer you really had to keep it covered up': Baker & Stanley, *Hello Sailor!*, pp. 62–63.

186 Thaddeus Chester, interviewed 8 August 2010.

187 Carol A. B. Warren, *Identity and Community in the Gay World* (New York, 1974), p. 39.

188 Warren, *Identity and Community in the Gay World*, p. 43.

189 Leith Cavill, interviewed 25 March 2010.

190 For a more detailed exploration of class within homosexual urban culture: see, e.g., Houlbrook, *Queer London*, pp. 167–195.

191 Prebble, '*Ordinary Men and Uncommon Women*', p. 192.

192 Baker and Stanley, *Hello Sailor!*, pp. 65.

193 Elliot Whitman, interviewed 20 March 2010.

194 Julian Wills interviewed, 4 January 2010.

195 Baker and Stanley, *Hello Sailor!*, p. 66.

196 Houlbrook uses the term 'homosex' as an amalgam that indicates sexual activities of various sorts between two males without making any assumptions about the motivations of those activities – without, for example, viewing the individuals who engaged in such acts as 'gay'.

197 Houlbrook, *Queer London*, p. 168.

198 The strict division of the asylum on gender lines, with a female and a male side was prompted by Victorian fears about sexual misbehaviour by male staff towards female patients and concerns that female patients might become pregnant by male staff or patients. This was a pertinent issue in an era when mental illness was perceived as hereditary. See, e.g., Claire Chatterton, '"An Unsuitable Job for a Woman?": Gender and Mental Health Nursing', *The Bulletin of the UK Association for the History of Nursing* 2 (2013), pp. 4–49.

199 Leith Cavill, interviewed 25 March 2010.

200 Evander Orchard, interviewed 10 August 2010.

201 Thaddeus Chester, interviewed 8 August 2010.

202 Prebble, '*Ordinary Men and Uncommon Women*', p. 192.

203 Chatterton, 'Caught in the Middle?', p. 32.

204 General Nursing Council for England and Wales, minutes of Mental Nurses Sub Committee, 1st December 1926, in Chatterton, 'Caught in the Middle?', p. 32.

205 Robert Dingwall, Anne Marie Rafferty and Charles Webster, *An Introduction to the Social History of Nursing* (London, 1988), p. 125.

206 Harrington, *Voices Beyond the Asylum*, p. 8.

207 The birth of the Society of Mental Nurses was symptomatic of the fact that in 1943, some mental nurses felt they had no forum in which to voice their opinions. However, as the years passed, membership began to fall, and in

1972, the society was terminated. The rationale behind this was that it was felt that there was no longer any need to have a separate organisation for mental nurses, as the RCN had adopted a more open policy towards them: Nolan, *Psychiatric Nursing Past and Present*, pp. 197–198.

208 Arton, *The Professionalization of Mental Nursing*, p. 71; Nolan, *Psychiatric Nursing Past and Present*, pp. 195–196.

209 Peter Nolan, 'Mental Nurse Training in the 1920s', *History of Nursing Group of the Royal College of Nursing* 10 (1986), p. 18.

210 'A Brief History of The Society of Mental Nurses, 1943–1972', in Nolan, *Psychiatric Nursing Past and Present*, p. 197.

211 Chatterton, 'Caught in the Middle?', p. 32.

212 Nolan, *A History of Mental Health Nursing*, p. 104.

213 Chatterton, 'Caught in the Middle?', p. 34.

214 See, e.g., Brain Ackner, *Handbook for Psychiatric Nurses* (London, 1964), pp. 108–116; Ivor R. C. Bachelor, *Henderson and Gillespie's Textbook of Psychiatry* (Oxford, 1962), pp. 197–209.

215 Zella Mullins, interviewed 14 July 2010.

216 Elspeth Whitbread, interviewed 7 January 2010; Dickinson, Cook, Playle and Hallett, 'Nurses and Subordination', p. 6.

217 Benedict Henry, interviewed 23 June 2010; Dickinson, Cook, Playle and Hallett, 'Nurses and Subordination', p. 6.

218 Ursula Vaughan, interviewed 12 February 2010.

219 Karen Jones, 'The Culture of the Mental Hospital', in German E. Berrios and Hugh Freeman (eds), 150 *Years of British Psychiatry 1841–1991* (London, 1991), p. 124. For a detailed discussion regarding a personal history of the demise of the asylums see Barbara Taylor, 'The Demise of the Asylum in Late Twentieth-Century Britain: A Personal History', *Transactions of the Royal Historical Society* XXI (2011), pp. 193–216.

220 Enoch J. Powell, *Speech by the Minister of Health, the Rt Hon. Enoch Powell. Report of the Annual Conference of the National Association for Mental Health* (London, 1961).

221 Nolan, *A History of Mental Health Nursing*, p. 125.

222 Nolan, *A History of Mental Health Nursing*, p. 125.

223 Harrington, *Death of the Asylum*, p. 27.

224 Nolan, *A History of Mental Health Nursing*, p. 120.

225 Adams, *Challenge and Change in a Cinderella Service*, pp. 308–309; Busfield, 'Restructuring Mental Health Services', p. 18.

226 Busfield, 'Restructuring Mental Health Services', p. 19.

227 Shorter, *History of Psychiatry*, p. 387.

228 Harrington, *Death of the Asylum*, p. 25; Busfield, 'Restructuring Mental Health Services', p. 19.

229 Nolan, *A History of Mental Health Nursing*, p. 123.

230 Myrtle Pauncefoot, interviewed 20 February 2013.

231 Harrington, *Voices Beyond the Asylum*, p. 39.

232 Jones, *A History of Mental Health Services*, p. 307.

233 Nolan, *A History of Mental Health Nursing*, p. 120.

234 Busfield, 'Restructuring Mental Health Services', p. 19.

235 Nolan, *A History of Mental Health Nursing*, p. 118.

236 Waters, 'Disorders of the Mind', p. 151.

237 Jo C. Phelan, Bruce G. Link, Ann Stueve and Bernice A. Pescosolido, 'Public Conceptions of Mental Illness in 1950: What is Mental Illness and is it to be Feared?', *Journal of Health and Social Behaviour* 41 (2) (2000), p. 188.

238 World Health Organization, *The International Statistical Classification of Diseases, Injuries and Causes of Death* (Geneva, 1949).

239 American Psychiatric Association, *Diagnostic Statistical Manual Version I* (Arlington, 1952).

240 Benedict Henry, interviewed 23 June 2010.

241 Ida Ashley, interviewed 17 July 2010.

242 Una Drinkwater, interviewed 29 December 2009.

243 Philip Thomas and Patrick Bracken, 'Critical Psychiatry in Practice', *Advances in Psychiatric Treatment* 10 (2004), p. 366.

244 It is interesting to note that a similar phenomenon to this had already occurred in psychiatry in the late nineteenth century. During this period, asylum doctors' professional status remained distinctly questionable. They were very eager to have their medical (psychiatric) skills recognised by their hospital-based colleagues as equal in status to that of general medicine. In order for asylum doctors to achieve their aim, an attempt was made to 'hospitalise' the asylums. This included proving their worth by deliberately changing the names of the institutions into hospitals, and by labelling and defining mental illnesses and developing 'treatments' to 'cure' the insane: See, e.g., Andrew Scull, *The Most Solitary of Afflictions: Madness and Society in Britain, 1700–1900* (New Haven, 1993). Michael Arton argues that a further aspect as this 'hospitalisation' was the transformation of the attendants into a body of trained asylum nurses who would have the same relationship to these 'hospitals for the insane' as general trained nurses had to the general hospitals: Arton, *The Professionalization of Mental Nursing*, p. 14.

3

'Subordinate nurses'

I didn't really understand what we were doing, none of us nurses did. We knew we were trying to get him to go for women instead of the men, but that was about it. The doctor brought the young man in and told us what we were going to do. I didn't really think any more about it, just got on with it – it was my job. I thought the doctor knows what he is doing, so it must be in the patient's best interests. In those days you didn't really ask questions, and you just did what the doctor told you to do really. When I think about it, we did not have any real knowledge to base this practice on . . . not like you have now: my granddaughter is a nursing student and is trained to 'question practice' [laughs], even doctors! My god! You would never do that in my day, you would not have dared. They had overall superior knowledge. [. . .] We did what they said, because they could not possibly have been wrong.[1]

Introduction

The motivations of the majority of nurses in this study to administer treatments for sexual deviation appeared to rest on the notion of obedience to authority. Some nurses sensed that there was something wrong in what they were doing but participated because they were 'following orders', and appeared to salve their conscience by diffusing the individual responsibility that they could take for their actions. Some used humour to do this, while others assumed that the doctors' knowledge was superior to their own. Meanwhile, other nurses actually believed that the treatments were helpful and genuinely believed that they were acting beneficently. This chapter seeks to explore these notions further in an attempt to offer an interpretation of some nurses' acceptance of and participation in aversion therapy for sexual deviations.

Nurses, experimentation and obedience to orders

In the original paper by Basil James, discussed in Chapter 1, he expressed his 'appreciation of the way in which the nursing staff co-operated so fully in the treatment'.[2] At a time when nursing was seen as subservient to the medical profession, it is arguable whether this was cooperation or obedience to his orders. One of the nurses to whom the paper refers is Gilbert Davies. He was interviewed for this book, and was asked about his thoughts on this statement:

> Erm ... I suppose it was coercion rather than cooperation really when I think about it because ... erm ... we didn't know what else to do. Our job to all intents and purposes was to follow the doctors' order ... [pause] ... I mean you have to understand the power the doctors, Nursing Officers and Matron had in those days. You stood up to attention with your thumbs down your creases, for example, when the doctor came on the ward. Likewise when the Matron or Nursing Officer came on your ward, they were checking that all beds were in line, with the wheels pointing in exactly the same direction ... erm ... the beds, well they had to be turned down from there to there [shows distance with hands] exactly – they even measured to make sure it was. No one ever told me why we had to do that. I don't suppose anyone ever thought to ask. It was the same with aversion therapy, I didn't ask why – I just did it. It was the doctor who needed to know the whys, what ifs and maybes in my day.[3]

However, an article published in the *Nursing Times* in 1965 entitled 'Aversion Therapy in Psychiatry' suggested that there was a dissonance between reality and rhetoric.[4] The quote from the article below urges nurses not to merely accept doctors' orders, but make the decision to partake in this aspect of their clinical practice only after they have reflected on their own values regarding it:

> If a nurse is asked to participate in this type of treatment it is most important that she considers her view on the matter rather than merely accepting orders. One must consider one's own motives when applying this treatment. There may be conscious or unconscious reasons for wishing to inflict pain, either on people in general or on a particular group, such as homosexuals in particular ... In its present stages the treatment is experimental, and until it has been found either to fulfil its purpose or, on the other hand, to be unsuccessful, it must remain a necessity for all concerned with its administration to look at it carefully and make their own decisions about their participation.[5]

Furthermore, in 1941 a working party was set up by the Ministry of Health, under the chairmanship of Sir Robert Wood, to review the position of the nursing profession. The working party set out to address two fundamental questions: 'What is the proper task of the nurse?' and 'What training is needed to equip her for her task?'[6] The working party reported in 1947 and it was the responsibility of the Chief Nursing Officer, Dame Elizabeth Cockayne, to set about implementing the report's recommendations.[7] Cockayne was convinced that nursing was in need of radical reform and posited that such reform had to be instigated by the nurses themselves:

> We do not want stereotyped nurses trained in a groove, but nurses capable of thinking for themselves on the wider issues of life . . . As a profession, we need to become increasingly self-analytical, to examine what we are doing and why. In these days of limited financial resources, we need to be sure that the money we have is being used in the best possible way.[8]

Interestingly, only one nurse in this study recalls reading the above article in the *Nursing Times*, and the impact this had on her clinical behaviour is discussed later. Nevertheless, what these two documents do is highlight the immense gulf between the prescriptions of theory, the intentions of policy and the realities of practice. The way nurses worked on the wards appeared to rest on the preference of the supervising doctors, sister or charge nurse. The nursing literature promoted the notion that competent nurse obeyed their superiors:

> No matter how gifted she may be, she will never be a reliable nurse until she can obey without question. The first and most helpful criticism I ever received from a doctor was when he told me I was supposed to be an intelligent machine for the purpose of carrying out his orders.[9]

This was reinforced by the medical literature, which argued that doctors have 'exclusive theoretical knowledge' affording them a certain level of control over nurses, who have 'subordinate statuses'.[10] Nevertheless, rationales to particular orders or, as to why things were done in a certain way, or even done at all were never provided:

> They would tell us what had to be done but never why. I can't ever remember being given an explanation for what I was doing or why I was doing it. In the same vein, I was never really thanked for what I did; therefore, I was never really sure if I had done something right. I just thought: 'if no one is complaining then it must be right' so I just carried on with it.[11]

Some nurses interviewed for this book felt completely unskilled to nurse the homosexuals or transvestites when they were admitted to their wards. However, despite this, they did not appear to accept the limitations of their skill set and carried on administering the treatments regardless:

I remember **** ***** [name of nurse] coming on shift the day he [male homosexual patient] was admitted. **** [name of nurse] was reporting for night duty. Well he was getting on – was too old for it really. He had never seen this treatment before, just like me. I explained it all to him in the office at handover, and I said: 'Are you alright with this?' and he said: 'Yes. Clear as mud.' The patient was still there in the morning so he must have got on with it alright. [Laughs] I mean a good nurse then was one who kept their head down, didn't ask questions, did as they were told and just got on with their work. . . . There were also some nurses who you could tell enjoyed administering these aversion treatments. There were others, myself included, who never enjoyed this aspect of their role and considered it barbaric. But, a lot of psychiatric treatments were barbaric, and the doctors had such enthusiasm for them. I suppose we just went along with it and allowed the doctors to do all the thinking.[12]

When nurses did ask questions they were often regarded as, 'audacious and impudent'.[13] Benedict Henry muses on the reasons for this:

I mean to think back, the treatments were so contrived! I mean to see a doctor coming in with a slide projector and a handful of slides, and setting it up, and then putting a couple of electrodes on this lad's body, and plugging him to this machine – it was even crueller than ECT. I remember the first time I saw it [aversion therapy for transvestism] I thought it was barbaric. And I remember asking the Charge Nurse: 'By administering the shock where is the treatment?' And of course this was regarded as an insolent and impertinent question at the time. Because it went outside the training and the training was set pieces of knowledge you regurgitated in exams, and if you were able to do that you were a competent nurse and not awkward. So it was in fact an education and training in avoiding awkwardness, because that is how you ran a very stable institution. So I just got on with it. I think the nurses and patients blinded themselves to the doctors' treatment.[14]

In many cases information was not made available to nurses working on the wards. They were often kept unaware about the patients and the reasons they had been admitted. Case notes were kept off the wards in the central office and only doctors had access to them.[15]

Staff discipline was inconsiderately managed so nurses often obeyed their superiors' orders to avoid being publicly humiliated in front of colleagues and patients:

> I remember seeing a colleague of mine severely reprimanded for not doing as he was told. He was supposed to take the patients out to the airing-court, but he hadn't, as he argued that it wasn't fair on them, as it was freezing cold outside. Firstly the Charge Nurse 'bollocked' him in front of everyone including the patients. He was then seen by the Senior Nurse and then the Superintendent. His card was marked from then on as a trouble maker and they made his life pretty bad. He didn't last much longer at the hospital and left about six months later. I was pretty sure I didn't want to go through that, so I just kept my head down and did as I was told.[16]

Nurses and obedience: a comparison
with nurses in Nazi Germany

Nurses' involvement in aversion therapy is not the only example of their adoption of arguably unethical practices and behaviours attributable to obedience to authority. This justification has been used as an explanation by nurses in support of their unethical practices in a number of historical contexts, not least nurses in Nazi Germany.[17] While it is, of course, critical to emphasise the different context and that none of the nurses in this study knowingly murdered patients in their care as the nurses under Nazi rule did, both sets of nurses did, nevertheless, administer what could now be deemed brutal treatments.[18] Indeed, some patients who received aversion therapy made this connection and used the Gestapo in Nazi Germany as a metaphor to describe the treatment they received. Furthermore, nurses in this study commented: 'I was just doing what the doctor told me to do.'[19] Given that many nurses under Nazi rule offered the same reason for their behaviour during World War II, there could be something to be learnt from a comparison.[20]

As head of the National Socialist Party, Adolf Hitler was elected as leader or 'Reichskanzler' of Germany on 30 January 1933. On appointment, he almost immediately implemented a series of extreme measures to endorse National Socialist health policy based on the concept of social hygiene and racial purity (eugenics).[21] This included the opening of the first concentration camp in Dachau and, in July 1933, the passing of a law to prevent hereditary diseases ('Gesetz zur

Verhutung erbkranken Nachwuches' or GVeN).[22] These drastic measures resulted in the forced sterilisation of 400,000 people between 1934 and 1939 in an attempt to eugenically prevent illnesses such as 'feeble-mindedness, schizophrenia, manic-depressive illness, epilepsy, Huntington's chorea, hereditary blindness, deafness and physical deformity'.[23]

On the day that German troops invaded Poland, 1 September 1939, Hitler signed the Euthanasia Decree (the 'Euthanasie-Erlaa'), and patients in Polish asylums began to be murdered. The following month, 'Aktion T4' was introduced with the founding of a central organisation in Berlin, which received reports on all psychiatric patients and where judgements were made on whether or not they would be put to death, described in official documentation as being granted a 'mercy killing'.[24] Nurses helped to collect together those who met the criteria to be killed and transport them to nominated extermination institutions in groups of 40–120. They were undressed, photographed and led naked to their death into specially constructed carbon monoxide gas chambers.[25]

This genocide went on for the next two years until 1941, when the T4 programme was officially halted; by then 70,273 psychiatric patients had been killed in this way.[26] In 1941, it was replaced with the 'Hungerkost', or starvation programme, which resulted in an estimated 90,000 deaths and the development of the 'Ostarbeiter-Sammelstellen' forced labour plan. This led to further murder, this time of the unproductive forced labours. It also marked the start of the 'Wilde Euthanasie' or wild euthanasia programme. The choice of patients to be executed then became decentralised and they were taken to one of fifteen specially created killing wards in hospitals.[27] Maria Berghs and her colleagues argue that the clandestine euthanasia programmes involved more than 296 mental, nursing and medical institutions in Poland, Germany, Russia, Austria and the Czech Republic and included healthcare professionals in those countries at all levels.[28]

Nurses were involved in differing phases of the euthanasia programmes. In the children's programmes they actively abetted in exterminating children through injections of morphine and scopolamine, by starvation, or by overdoses of other medications. Nurses assisted in the selection and elimination of concentration camp prisoners in the later 'Operation 14 f 13'; they also participated in the implementation of the 'Final Solution' and in the mass sterilisation programme.[29] They assisted with compulsory medical experiments on people, generally refused to admit and treat Jewish and homosexual people, and were, overall, 'involved in all phases of the systematic annihilation of masses of people'.[30]

This brief depiction of some of the events of the Holocaust cannot do justice to the extent of the suffering that was experienced. However, it does begin to draw some similarities with the nurses and patients in this study. Percival Thatcher, who received treatments for homosexuality, reflected on his treatment as being like 'a barbaric torture scene by the Gestapo in Nazi Germany trying to extract information from me'.[31] When we revisit the descriptions of some of the treatments administered for sexual deviations it is not surprising to see why Percival might have made this connection. There are definite parallels, as Juliette Pattinson states that, among other torturous interventions, the Gestapo deprived their prisoners of sleep and made them stay awake, subjected them to electric currents surging through their bodies, denied them light, food and medical treatment, and kept them in solitary confinement.[32] The treatment of sexual deviations with aversion therapy used a combination of all of the above.

In order to achieve participation in the practices detailed above for both the nurses in Nazi Germany and the nurses in this study who participated in aversion therapy, their clinical practice had to be acceptable to them and their moralities. The role of morality had to be limited, and in some cases, this was done by diffusing the individual responsibility that the nurses could accept for their actions.[33] Similar to the nurses in Nazi Germany, some of the nurses in this study also attempted to limit their culpability by ensuring that they were not responsible for individual patients.[34] This was done by dehumanising and objectifying the affiliation between patients and caregivers through language and administrative tasks.[35] Meanwhile, other nurses discussed the distribution of specific tasks involved in nursing homosexuals and transvestites. As with the nurses in Nazi Germany, nurses administering aversion therapies were also encouraged not to build up strong therapeutic relationships with their patients.[36] They had little difficultly in recollecting the displeasing aspects of their work caring for patients receiving treatments for sexual deviations. Zella Mullins and Ursula Vaughan remember how challenging the patient receiving chemical aversion therapy was to nurse:

> It was damned hard work looking after those homosexuals, you were on the go all night, you had to keep on at this bloke to keep taking this that and the other – observations – I mean blood pressure and testing his water, you know that went round the clock. I didn't give him the injections, we shared the jobs, my colleague gave the injections and I took his observations.[37]

> Nursing the sexual deviant was exhausting. We knew we had to 'sort them out' but it wasn't easy. The smell amongst other things was probably the worst thing; imagine a few days of 'sick', 'shit' and 'piss' in one room. . . . It must have been awful for the other patients on the ward.[38]

The terminology that Zella Mullins and Ursula Vaughan used could suggest that nurses were practising in a very task-orientated manner. Zella Mullins also mentioned the distribution of the tasks involved in nursing the patient receiving aversion therapy. Gilbert Davies casts further light on this:

> Nursing was very regimented and task orientated in those days – not least the care of patients receiving aversion therapy – particularly those receiving chemical aversion therapy. We seemed to have it pretty boxed off, and took in turns to either do and have responsibility for is [sic] obs or give the injections.[39]

The Nazi euthanasia projects had to be a furtive collective endeavour, with each individual nurse following orders, and doing specialised administration or technical intervention.[40] Berghs and her colleagues suggest that these nurses then began to focus on the performance of interventions and measuring their own responsibilities 'in narrow terms of efficiency, productivity or competence'.[41] Andrew McKie suggests that a focus on the detached nature of an intervention allows an emphasis to be shifted from victims (patients) to perpetrators (nurses) and thus the responsibilities for interventions and not those towards patients.[42] Arguably, these were also ways in which some nurses in this study limited their morality regarding the treatments they administered for sexual deviation; in order to make the situation more tolerable and acceptable to them. This too could offer a possible interpretation for their acceptance and participation in aversion therapy.

Nurses' participation in medical experiments: a comparison with the Tuskegee syphilis study

Although there had been some success treating alcoholics using aversion therapy,[43] the use of this therapy to treat sexual deviations was very experimental.[44] Besides the compulsory medical experiments conducted in Nazi Germany, arguably one of the most infamous medical experiments in the twentieth century was the case of the Tuskegee Syphilis Experiment. In 1932 the USA Public Health Service (USPHS) commenced an experiment in Macon Country, Alabama, to determine the natural course of untreated, latent syphilis in black males.[45] Investigators in the study enrolled a total of 600 disadvantaged African-American sharecroppers from Macon County, Alabama: 400 who had previously contracted syphilis before the study began and 200 without the disease who would serve as controls.[46] In exchange for participating in the study, the men were given free medical care, meals and free burial insurance. However, they were never told they had syphilis. The men were told they were being treated for 'bad blood', a local term used to describe several illnesses, including fatigue, syphilis and anaemia.[47] When penicillin became widely available in the early 1950s as the preferred treatment for syphilis, the men did not receive the drug. Indeed, on several occasions, the USPHS actually sought to prevent treatment.[48] Furthermore, in 1969, a committee at the federally operated Center for Disease Control decided that the study should be continued.[49]

The first published report of the study appeared in the medical press in 1936, and papers were published about the study every four to six years.[50] However, it was only in 1972, when accounts of the study first appeared in the national press, that the Department of Health, Education and Welfare (DHEW) curtailed the experiment.[51] At that time, seventy-four of the test subjects were still alive; at least twenty-eight, but possibly more than a hundred, had died directly from advanced syphilitic lesions.[52] In August 1972, the DHEW appointed an investigatory panel, which issued a report the following year. The panel identified the study as having been 'ethically unjustified', and argued that penicillin should have been provided to the men.[53] Moreover, it was a nurse – Eunice Rivers – who played an instrumental role in perpetuating the experiment.[54]

It was Nurse Rivers' job to serve as a liaison between the doctors who designed and ran the Tuskegee Study and the black men who were its subjects. She kept track of the men in the study, visited them and developed a trusting relationship with them and their families.[55] James Jones argues that it was the men's trust in Nurse Rivers that kept them in the study.[56] Nevertheless, while Rivers was supportive of the men in the study and provided care to them and their families, she also knew that they were being denied treatment for syphilis, yet in spite of this, she continued with her influential role in the study.[57] Jones argues that her continued participation in the study was driven by obedience to authority, namely doctors.[58] However, another interpretation proposed rested on the notion of beneficence.[59]

Evelyn Hammonds argues that Nurse Rivers 'straddled two worlds'.[60] First, being a black woman from Alabama, she knew firsthand the world of poor black people living in this state, and how segregation was very oppressive for black people in the South. She knew she had to be mindful that her job put her in close contact with white people who were threatened by her professional status. Second, she had to consider and attend to the feelings of black people who might have been disdainful towards her because of her close working relationship with white people.[61]

Rivers always maintained that she was told by doctors that the purpose of the study was to make a comparison with a similar study that was being conducted on white men in order to determine if syphilis manifested itself differently in black people.[62] The distressing symptoms of the late stages of syphilis were obvious and apparent to all, and included tumours, ulcers on the skin, bone deterioration and often severe damage to the cardiovascular and central nervous system.[63] Therefore, there was a definite need for further research in this area. Jones goes on to argue that her acceptance in this study was also compounded by the fact that three doctors, two of whom were black men, approved and participated in the study.[64]

Rivers perceived the study and its impact by maintaining that while the men did not get treated for syphilis, they did receive 'good medical care' – care they would not otherwise have received on account of their socioeconomic status.[65] As Nurse Rivers saw it, the fact that the men were given cardiograms and other expensive tests over the course of the study meant that they had access to quality care that few in their position ever received.[66] Arguably, she believed that she was at least acting beneficently by trying to do something for individuals whom others had abandoned.

There are similarities with the dynamic of Rivers' participation in the Tuskegee Study, in the sense that she was a black woman who believed she was helping other black people, and the nurses in this book who administered treatments for homosexuality, but were also themselves homosexual. As discussed in Chapter 2, some of these nurses also believed that they were acting beneficently. This could offer another possible interpretation for these nurses' acceptance of, and participation in, aversion therapy. Looking again at the nurses in Nazi Germany, some believed in the moral correctness of the euthanasia killings, and argued that for humanitarian reasons, it was better for the patients to be put out of their misery.[67] In these cases, Bronwyn McFarland-Icke posits that perceiving euthanasia as 'mercy-killing' or 'death as deliverance' enabled nurses to combine their conventional morality with involvement in euthanasia practices.[68]

Beneficence versus non-maleficence

The crux of a mental health nurse's role is to display unconditional positive regard and empathy to the patients in their care.[69] This was also argued by Richard Hunter in 1956 to be 'the very function to which mental nursing owes its inception – that is, to counter alienation by sustained, kindly human understanding and contact'.[70] Therefore, the concept of nurses displaying such interpersonal characteristics is not a contemporary notion. However, some nurses in this study, for whatever reason, were not displaying empathy to the patients in their care; indeed, it could be argued that they were displaying the opposite – antipathy. The emphasis on antipathy by the health care professional is displayed in the paper by Daniel Clarke describing a patient who received treatment for transvestism. Clarke noted: 'At one session, by a particularly happy chance, one of his [the patient's] favourite pictures fell into the vomit in the basin so that the patient had to see it every time he puked.'[71] Elliot Whitman substantiates the above:

We didn't have to talk to 'em [*sic*]. If he was emotionally distressed it still went on. As long as his body was alright. . . . I mean as long as you were shaking 'em [*sic*] up you know? Well, you were doing the work. The work's being done if he was shook up. I suppose we were being cruel to be kind.[72]

Meanwhile, Myrtle Pauncefoot recalls the instructions she was given by her superior regarding the treatment, 'The Charge Nurse said: 'Now you're to make this [chemical aversion therapy] as unpleasant as possible for him – don't be cleaning his room or giving him a sick bowl!'[73] Leith Cavill agrees and recalls the lack of empathy this patient group received:

I don't ever recall any meetings or ward rounds to discuss these [homosexual and transvestite] patients. There was a distinct lack of empathy and sensitivity to this patient group. They were seen as trouble-makers and deviants, who were put on this earth to annoy and cause trouble for everyone around them. There was a belief that they were fully responsible for entering into the culture in which they drifted.[74]

The testimonies of both the patients and nurses concur, suggesting that the nurses' role was to make the treatment as unpleasant as possible for the patient, and in parallel with the nurses in Nazi Germany, not to 'build up a strong relationship between patients and caregivers'.[75]

It was always quite furtive. They were kept in a side room and not given any real 'care' you could say. [. . .] It wasn't so much the hard work, but the unpleasantness of it. Put it this way, the cleaner didn't go into his room. You were not allowed to clean his 'sick' up, and he had to go to the toilet in his room, by that I mean he had to go in a bowl in the corner. So you get the picture, after a couple of days, the smell was nauseating. I remember retching every time I opened the door to his room, all the other patients on the ward started to complain too. [. . .] Now I know we can look back on this as barbaric, but this is what we were told the cure was for these people. We were just trying to make them better and help them in the only way we knew possible at the time. All the patients consented too, even if they were sent from court, they were given a choice of coming to us or going to prison.[76]

Some nurses accepted and participated in aversion therapy because they believed they were acting beneficently. However, by relying on the notion that they were doing well by administering aversion therapy, the nurses were not upholding the principle of non-maleficence, as the treatments were very traumatic and painful for the patients receiving them.[77] Furthermore, no former patients featured in this book reported any efficacy having received the treatments; and all stated that these treatments have had a negative long-term impact on them. Albert Holliday reflects on the treatment he received to 'cure' him of his homosexuality:

> I've never got over it. I never have. I have never come to terms with it. A guilt, a guilt, a guilt, guilt. You can live with it, but how can you forget it? I desperately wanted the treatments to work, but they didn't. [. . .] I can still have terrible flashbacks of my time in hospital and the barbaric treatments I received.[78]

Oscar Mangle remains 'troubled by the treatment'[79] he received and Herbert Bliss does not 'know how something so tortuous could have been concealed under the term "health care"'.[80] Meanwhile, Pete Price stated: 'I think three days has destroyed 25 years',[81] when he reflected on his time in hospital receiving chemical aversion therapy for homosexuality.

Negative effects from the treatment were fairly common. In a paper describing ten homosexual men treated by the psychiatrist John Bancroft, one developed phobic anxiety to attractive men and attempted suicide; one became aggressive, attempted suicide and was anorgasmic in homosexual relationships; one developed serious depression after rejection by women; one became psychotically depressed and wandered into the streets removing his clothes and one became disillusioned by the homosexual world and could no longer sustain emotionally rewarding relationships.[82]

Consent

It was not only nurses who were potentially being coerced into administering these treatments: the patients themselves also appear to have been pressured into receiving them. An example is demonstrated in the Introduction, when Percival Thatcher was given the option of imprisonment or being remanded (provided he was willing to undergo psychological treatment). In addition, the negative messages homosexuals and transvestites were receiving about themselves could have implicitly coerced men into receiving these treatments. All of these issues raise important questions regarding the validity of the patients' consent to treatment.

It has already been established that the use of aversion therapy to treat sexual deviations was highly experimental and arbitrary.[83] Bridget Dimond argues that there are two types of medical experiment: 'therapeutic' and 'non-therapeutic'. Therapeutic experiments are those designed to benefit the subject, to find a cure for their illness or alleviate their suffering. Non-therapeutic experiments are designed not to help the research subject directly but to benefit others suffering from the same disease.[84] Graham Rumbold proposes that the judgement as to whether an experiment is therapeutic or non-therapeutic has to be based on the original intention. If the intention is to benefit the subject directly then the experiment is therapeutic. If the intention is not so, then the experiment is non-therapeutic.[85] Arguably, the medical experiments carried out in Nazi Germany and the Tuskegee Syphilis Experiment were non-therapeutic experiments.

Whether aversion therapy to treat sexual deviations was a therapeutic or a non-therapeutic experiment is a contentious issue. The aim of aversion therapy was always maintained to be that it would directly benefit the patient by 'curing' them of their deviant behaviours. However, the patients who received these therapies were also experimental subjects being used to establish the efficacy of such treatments; as there were no robust evidence-based successful outcomes of using this particular therapy for people suffering from sexual deviations. In the study by King and his colleagues, they concur with the findings in this book in that the treatment did not appear to be successful in its intent to cure patients of their same sex desires, and actually had long-term detrimental effects for many.[86] Rumbold proposes that if any experiment may cause harm or inflict pain, discomfort, loss of freedom or loss of dignity in an individual (arguably aversion therapy to treat sexual deviations did all of these), then the experiment cannot be justified. This is because to do something deliberately which will cause harm to a patient is wrong.[87]

Crucial to any medical experiment or research is participant consent. That consent has to be freely given and fully informed. All the former patients interviewed for this book had consented to the treatment they received. However, there appears to be some debate as to whether this was fully informed and uncoerced and whether the patients' autonomy was respected. Barrington Crowther-Lobley recalls the information he received regarding the aversion therapy he consented to:

> The psychiatrist told me what was going to happen. But in no way was it descriptive of what I was actually subjected to. I don't recall them using the words 'aversion therapy' and they made it sound like it was a definite solution to my problem. They made it sound like I had nothing to worry about, so I agreed to it. I don't ever recall signing a consent form or anything like that, though.[88]

Furthermore, Leith Cavill reflects on the legal issue of consent to treatment:

> I think we must remember that these patients all consented to treatment, and because of this we were within our rights to administer the treatment. We never pinned anyone down and shocked them. Most were so desperate that they would have done anything.[89]

Benedict Henry recalls the kind of information the patient would receive regarding aversion therapy and what could be argued to be coercion tactics some consultants would use:

> I can recall patients being 'talked to'; invariably this would be by the consultant. There were two consultants who seemed to ... erm ... have an interest in homosexuality. I do think that the form of all discussions took the form of an assessment that was essentially pointing out to the patients that their condition was in fact an illness. And ... erm ... even if patients didn't accept that it was an illness, there was a treatment that would rectify them. And the rectification was that they would become heterosexual. So the preparation was essentially talking, informing, and getting people to agree. Erm ... I think the medical staff were not averse to saying: 'Well of course if you do not have the treatment the alternative is imponderable, in the sense that you will be back out on the street and you will be very vulnerable.' It was a case of trying to convince the patient that it was much easier to be here [hospital], as outside they would be had by the police. And of course this was very frightening to the young homosexuals at the time because ending up in prison they would get very badly treated. Patients often stated: 'If I had known what this treatment really was, I would never have agreed to it.'[90]

Some nurses believed that because the patients had consented to aversion therapy it offered them both a rationalisation to administer it and a legal safeguard. The above testimonies could suggest, however, that patients were not fully informed regarding the treatment they opted for. Therefore, in these cases the patients did not give fully informed consent. In essence, health care professionals, the media and the courts all held a paternalistic attitude towards sexual deviants, and employed implicit and explicit tactics that coerced them into receiving treatment by reducing their autonomy. Autonomy can be defined as 'the capacity to think, decide, and act on the basis of such thought and decision freely and independently and without let or hindrance'.[91] Moreover, an autonomous decision is, 'one which is undertaken voluntarily, and not under coercion, however covert that coercion may be'.[92] The strategies discussed above were an affront to the patient's autonomy because they reduced the degree of voluntariness on the part of the patient.

Initiation

Nursing patients receiving chemical aversion therapy was particularly unpleasant. Therefore, requiring participation was sometimes used by senior nurses as an opportunity to test a new recruit's suitability for mental nursing. Some nurses recounted anecdotes of how they were exposed to shocking sights or placed in an impossible position by their superiors. Elspeth Whitbread recalls such a situation when her Charge Nurse delegated a task to her:

> It was my first day as a student nurse on a new ward and the Charge Nurse said he had a 'special patient' for me. He said it would be a good opportunity for me to craft my injection technique, and we went to the clinic and drew up some apormorphine. We then walked down to the side-room and he gave me a rather pejorative description of the patient I was going to administer the injection to. I remember feeling uncomfortable about this, but I didn't want to oppose his views, as I didn't want to create a bad impression on my first day. As we got closer to the side-room the smell became apparent, and I could feel myself beginning to feel nauseous. As I opened the door to the side-room I can only describe it as comparable to a zoo: there was faeces, vomit and urine everywhere. My emotions were all over the place, I felt so sorry for the poor lad in there, but I knew I had to keep them to myself . . . [Wipes tears from her eyes] . . . The Charge Nurse said: 'Right on the bed ***** [patient's surname], time for your jab!' The patient just pulled down his trousers and lay on the bed. I had no time to object: the Charge Nurse just said: 'Off you go, then!' I gave him the injection and we

left, there was no communication with him. Nor was there any de-briefing or rationale offered to me regarding the treatment. However, I believed that my ability to undertake this task without question and devoid of emotion meant that I could be 'accepted' onto the ward.[93]

Nolan suggests that many student nurses were exploited. Nurse-tutors addressed trainees as 'nurses', but on the wards, they were referred to merely as 'attendants'.[94] Elspeth's testimony could suggest that at times nursing students were also bullied. A similar incident was related by a female nurse in Nolan's study who commenced mental nursing after completing her general nurse training:

I wanted to make a good impression on my first day, so I wore the best clothes I had. I had a hat I was especially fond of that I wore; it had a veil which came some way down my face. I must have looked like a duchess! I asked a nurse for the person in charge of the ward. She looked long and hard at me and said: 'Oh laa-dee-daa, you must be the general nurse.' I was left for a time just standing there in the middle of the ward by myself. After ten or fifteen minutes, the Sister came to me and gave me a key and told me to open side-room 3 and let the patient out. I dutifully marched along to the side-room and when I opened the door, a tall bewildered woman picked up a bucket of stale smelly urine and poured it over my hat and clothes. When I went back to the Sister, she expressed surprise in a mocking way and suggested that I must have provoked the patient. The other staff, I remember, found it hilariously funny. It was their way of dealing with someone they thought had airs and graces and needed taking down a peg or two. Though I was furious at the time and thought of storming out, I stayed.[95]

In their eagerness to be 'accepted' and their inability to question their superiors, Elspeth Whitbread and the nurse in Nolan's study had been ready to undertake anything required of them. However, in doing this, some nurses appeared to have given up their status as moral agents and become fully passive to their superiors. Nolan argues that charge nurses often showed favouritism by holding back patients' food or tobacco and dispensing them to staff they trusted. Staff members who were friends would regularly play cards or dominoes on the wards in the evening. However, new staff members were excluded until they were considered 'safe'.[96]

Humour

Some nurses in this book commented that they used humour as a coping mechanism to deal with the incongruity they faced on a daily basis on psychiatric wards – not least when nursing patients receiving aversion therapy. Humour, as Una Drinkwater commented, kept them going: 'Without it, a lot of us would have crumbled under the pressure',[97] and Cecil Asquith remarked: 'We needed a sense of humour to deal with the illogicality of what we were doing.'[98] Meanwhile, Evander Orchard reflected that having a good sense of humour was a pertinent aspect of being a good mental nurse:

> It was always a good sign for me if someone had a sense of humour. We were dealing with some pretty distressing things on a daily basis, especially nursing the patient receiving aversion therapy. Yes – a lot of the reasons why we administered these treatments was due to us not wanting or knowing how to question our superiors. But we also used humour as a way of normalising what we did. I'm not excusing what I did by saying we had a good laugh about it, but we had to develop a way of dealing with our stress and conscience before the advent of clinical supervision and the like. They [other nurses] would take the mickey out of my accent or where I came from. I never saw it as anything callous – it was just banter.[99]

Humour has been recognised as a mechanism by which emergency workers rearranged their work, released tension and created emotional alliances within their teams.[100] Thomas Kuhlman argues that 'black' or 'gallows' humour is widespread among groups who work in acute environments, or where they experience incongruity. He also suggests that black humour is an 'illogical, even psychotic, response to irresolvable dilemmas and offers a way of being sane in an insane place'.[101] Prebble proposes that mental nurses experienced incongruity on a daily basis. They also experienced a gap between the rhetoric of therapeutic efficacy and the reality of crowded wards, limited resources and staff and the challenge of nursing chronically disabled patients.[102] The nurses in this study used humour as a way of coping with the absurdity of administering aversion therapy. Arguably, it was another way of limiting their conscience in relation to engaging in this aspect of their clinical practice.

'Subordinate' state enrolled nurses

The 'subordinate' state enrolled assistant nurse (SEAN) was introduced with the Nurses' Act 1943.[103] However, enrolled nurses were not introduced in mental nursing until 1964. There had been rhetoric to capitalise on the workforce of assistant or auxiliary nurses in mental hospitals in both the 1924 Departmental Committee and the 1926 Royal Commission, although these measures had never come to fruition. This has been considered to be due to the major opposition to this new role, not least by the Athlone Sub-Committee's report on mental nursing in 1945, which rejected this rhetoric.[104] Rosemary White proposes that the Athlone Sub-Committee was strongly against SEANs entering mental nursing because the sub-committee perceived that the standard of mental nursing was not high enough for there to be second-grade nurses in addition to the registered mental nurse.[105]

However, the notion of introducing a second grade of nurse into mental nursing was severely promoted by the Ministry of Health in 1953 when they published a memorandum entitled 'Supply of Nursing Staff for Mental Hospitals and Mental Deficiency Institutions', more universally known as RHB (53) 54. Its purpose was to suggest, 'some courses of action designed to improve the staffing situation'.[106] Claire Chatterton argues that the Ministry of Health wanted to dilute the mental nurse workforce, in a purely economic move to reduce costs, by introducing 'subordinate nursing staff', which included nursing auxiliaries and SEANs.[107] Eileen Baggott proposed that the Ministry of Health published the memorandum as an anticipatory intervention, as they believed that many mental hospitals would struggle to recruit student nurses once the minimum standard of entry into the profession was implemented in 1966.[108] Prior to this, there were no minimum entry criteria, and Baggott argued that many of the student nurses at the time would have fallen into the educational category of pupil nurses.[109]

There was strong opposition to RHB (53) 54 from the Confederation of Health Service Employees (COHSE); the main trade union for mental nurses during this period.[110] The COHSE argued that the need was for more registered nurses and feared that the introduction of the SEAN into mental nursing would overload the mental hospitals with unqualified or semi-qualified staff. They also believed that it would lead to 'unqualified staff having to bear ward responsibilities after a few lectures in first aid and home nursing'.[111] Meanwhile, the RMPA rejected this grade of nurse being introduced to mental nursing mainly for pragmatic reasons. They did not have the capacity to develop, write and implement a new nursing syllabus for these proposed nurses.[112]

Nevertheless, despite opposition, by the early 1960s the GNC had drawn up, and had approved by their 'Mental Nursing and Enrolled Nurses Committee', a draft syllabus, and a record of practical instruction and experience required to enable a pupil nurse to enrol with them. Once enrolled, these nurses would be known as the shortened state enrolled nurse (SEN) following the Amendment Act 1961.[113] The SEN was officially entered into mental nursing in the Nurses' Act 1964. There was no question of a separate roll: mental SENs would be admitted to the existing roll. However, in 1969 the roll was divided into three parts: general, mental and mental sub-normality.[114] Most interesting for this study, however, is the concept of these nurses being known as 'subordinate staff'.

The testimony of three of the SENs in this study has already been explored; these nurses were also homosexual. One of the explanations they offered for their participation in administering aversion therapies for patients in the same situation as themselves, in parallel with Nurse Rivers as discussed above, was that they believed they were acting beneficently. This was further compounded by the fact that the nurses did not always possess the medical knowledge that they perceived the doctors to have, so they believed that it was pertinent for the well-being of a patient that nurses obey orders.

Moreover, all four SENs in this study suggested that the overriding reason why they participated in this aspect of clinical practice rested on the perception of subservience to authority as Zella Mullins notes:

I think we [SENs] had a harder time than most on the wards. Although we were very skilled and experienced nurses we were never rewarded monetarily or with much respect at all. We were seen as subordinate and had to take orders from the doctors and from the registered nurses. We were even seen as subordinate to third year student nurses and subsequently had to take orders from them too. I found that really difficult sometimes. Some of them were OK and valued our opinion, others thought they were a cut above the rest and went on to develop what I called 'staff nurse-itus'. By that I mean the day they qualified and donned their blue uniform they conducted them-selves in a haughty manner, thinking they knew it all. They invariably soon fell from grace and I would sometimes have to pick up the pieces. [. . .] Our training was very practical and it was more around skills than underpinning knowledge. So even if I had had the professional status to question practice, my lack of knowledge gave me little information to be able to put forward a valid argument. It was easier to just get on with the task I had been given.[115]

Indeed, the *Report of the Committee of Inquiry into Whittingham Hospital* found it particularly noteworthy that the pupil nurses (who trained for the grade of SEN) 'seem not to have expressed the same discontent' to ill-treatment of patients, fraud and maladministration at the hospital as the student nurses who were training to be RNs.[116] Dorothy Baker found that SENs gave precedence to providing atten-tion to the doctors; for example a doctor would not be kept waiting while an SEN gave attention to a patient. In one case, an SEN aban-doned the medicine round in order to write the doctor's laboratory forms. Baker also noted that SENs strove to give the 'right' answers to the doctor's questions, whether or not such answers were always factually based. This was in contrast to the ward sister who was likely to admit that she did not know the answer or had not yet had time to find out.[117] Baker went on to posit that the SENs approach to nursing care had much in common with that of nursing auxiliaries. She identified that SENs tended to be task orientated and their main focus was on easing the burden of these tasks. For example, one SEN criticised the ward sister's style of management in relation to its lack of method, the consequent waste of resources and the untoward implica-tions for the staff:

Sister's got no routine. I'm concerned about the waste of manpower [*sic*]. There's no method on here; for instance – Sister makes them take out the breakfasts one at a time from the oven, when they could have been feeding two or three patients at once and could have saved journeys and save time.[118]

Meanwhile, Elliot Whitman recalls how he felt SENs were often exploited:

We [SENs] were often left in charge of wards at night. It 'took the piss' really as even though we were seen to be subordinate and not competent to make clinical decisions we were often left in charge and had to do the job of a staff nurse for the money and status of an SEN. [...] I suppose subservience was drummed into me from day one as I started off as a nursing auxiliary. I was also in the first cohort of SENs to qualify in mental nursing following a long debate about whether we were needed in mental hospitals. There was initially some hostility to us as we were an unknown quantity and I think some staff nurses felt we were going to take their jobs so they were keen to keep us in our place I suppose. We were seen as inferior to higher ranking staff and given that there was a big emphasis on the hierarchical structure in mental hospitals, I identified myself as being quite low down this structure and, therefore, never really thought I could say 'no' to a superior.[119]

Baggott published a paper in the *Nursing Times,* in 1965, regarding the decision the previous year to introduce SENs into mental nursing. She argued that this decision was essentially positive, but only if handled appropriately. She proposed that she would like to see pupil nurses, student nurses, enrolled nurses and registered nurses all working together in 'harmony' as a team. In addition, she advocated that a pupil nurse should, 'learn at the bedside but she will know something about the patient's condition and about the nursing procedure beforehand'. She also highlights the potential risk of leaving enrolled nurses in charge of wards.[120] There was an immense gulf between the prescriptions of theory, the intentions of policy and the realities of practice.

It seems that SENs were often exploited and gained little respect from some staff in higher-ranking positions. Furthermore, they appear to have received a very pragmatic training, which placed little emphasis on underpinning theories, and this led them to feel unable to question practice. Referring to these nurses as 'subordinate' was a self-fulfilling prophecy and it was inevitable that some would take on such an obedient role. This and the notion of beneficence, could offer a possible interpretation for why the SENs in this book participated in aversion therapy for sexual deviations.

Militarisation of nursing

Many mental nurses in the early 1940s were called up and assigned to the Royal Army Medical Corps, and many ex-service personnel who had not previously worked in mental health entered mental nursing after World War II, owing to limited employment opportunities.[121] Some nurses' experiences during the war also had a positive impact on their attitude towards homosexuals and transvestites in their care (discussed in Chapter 4). Nevertheless, there were also, arguably, some negative influences that 'leaked' into civilian nursing from mental nurses' military service during the World War II.

Nolan argues that mental nursing had much in common with military service, as it offered a regimented life, where nurses had to do little thinking for themselves and where plenty of company was always available, particularly ex-servicemen.[122] Indeed, Julian Wills remarked:

> I was amazed at the number of other ex-military personnel there were at the hospital when I started my nurse training. I suppose it could have been due to the parallels: like the military, the only real thinking we had to do was to make sure we followed the rules and orders.[123]

Other individuals appeared to enter the profession after the war as a form of self-prescribed therapy to help them deal with the atrocities that they had experienced during the war:

> I suppose I needed it. I left the army all confused and totally unprepared for 'civvy' street. I suppose you could say I used nursing as a form of rehabilitation.[124]

Joanna Bourke argues that many health care professionals witnessed the war as an immense laboratory for experimentation and the testing of theories. The techniques of fear management learnt within the military context were applied, essentially unaltered, to entire populations. She proposes that the 'total environment of control' which was accepted as inevitable within the armed forces was overlain onto civilian society.[125] A doctor publishing in the *British Medical Journal* in 1940 stated that, 'the civilian population must be treated as if they were combatant troops; they must be under authority'.[126] The idea that individuals were experimental beings was thus rendered familiar and respectable through the experience of war, and could provide a possible interpretation for some nurses' acceptance of the experimental nature of aversion therapy to treat sexual deviations.

Penny Starns argues that militarisation became a distinct and deliberate feature of nursing policy during the 1940s. This was pioneered by Dame Katherine Jones, a military nurse since 1916. She was mobilised on 11 September 1939 as Senior Principle Matron on the staff of general headquarters of the British Expeditionary Force. As Matron-in-Chief of the Army, she proposed explicitly that militarisation provided an opportunity to resolve nurse status issues once and for all.[127] Jones instigated a full-blown militarisation programme for army nurses, including drill and route marching three miles into the desert and back to improve their fitness. Starns notes that while some nurses viewed the introduction of such activities as 'fun and games', others took the military procedures very seriously. In some cases these nurses would allocate beds and examine patients according to their rank – the lowest rank was last to receive medical attention – irrespective of the severity of their medical need. There was a huge emphasis placed on discipline and obedience to orders from higher-ranking officers.[128]

Hopton argues that this model of militarisation extended to civilian nursing and nurse discipline became more severe and stressed the importance of class distinction, duty and self-sacrifice.[129] Indeed, Prebble argues that the language and routines of mental nurses had similarities with military life. For example, staff rooms were called 'staff quarters' and staff dining rooms were called 'mess rooms'.[130] Furthermore, civilian nurses' uniforms were increasingly regimented: stripes on sleeves were adopted to distinguish rank. Nurses were also noted to become obsessed with punctuality in ward routines and a military attitude toward personal appearance. Their shoes were expected to be shined, shoulder epaulettes had to align with creases on sleeves, and stiffly starched aprons had to be worn.[131]

Although the nurses in the picture in Figure 9 look fairly jolly, it attests to the regimentation discussed above, as the nurses all seem to have black shoes, their stiffly starched aprons are all calf length and they all appear to be wearing caps that are attached with 'strings' and 'bows'.[132] In addition, they seem to be strategically arranged alternately with either their cape straps criss-crossing their chest or their cape straps not on show. This picture also seems to illustrate a sense of camaraderie between these nurses.

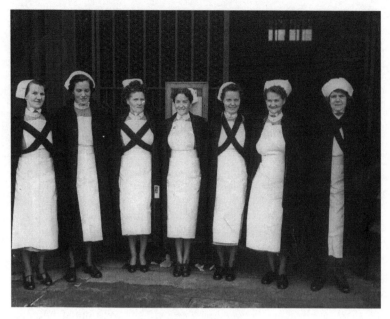

9 Mental nurses *c.*1950s

'Jack', who was interviewed in Nolan's study, took part in the 1940 campaign in France during World War II and was taken prisoner after a matter of weeks. He spent the rest of the war in PoW camps in Poland and Germany. However, he entered mental nursing after the war when his old army friend who was working as a mental nurse persuaded him to enter the profession. Jack's testimony demonstrates how daily inspections of the nurses by the superintendent meant that they were considered akin to soldiers being assessed on a parade:

> There were times when I thought I was still in the army. I must admit there were times when it was all that I had hoped army life would be. I felt very proud of my uniform and it meant a great deal to me when the Superintendent used to remark how smart I looked.[133]

Ida Ashley, who was interviewed for this book recalled a sister who had gained military experience during World War II:

> One Sister I worked under had served in the army during the war; she ruled her ward with an iron fist and with military precision. No one ever dared

169

to question her. I will never forget her daily inspections. She was very nit-picky, and my heart used to be going ten to the dozen as she examined me from head to toe.[134]

Many nurses who had served during the war returned to clinical practice in a civilian role once it had ended. Therefore, it was inevitable that they might also bring with them some of the military ideologies discussed above. This could offer a further context within which to explain the subservient role that some nurses in this book adopted.

Psychological insights into the subordinate nurses' actions

Daniel Goldhagen proposes that in some instances obedience to authority is pursued on account of an individual's self-interest, which is 'conceptualised as career advancement or personal enrichment' in total disregard of other considerations.[135] However, this explanation is untenable for the majority of nurses in this study – not least the SENs – and those who remained staff nurses for their whole careers. These nurses had no organisational or career interests to advance by their involvement in aversion therapy. They were not striving for promotion, especially the SENs, as this would have meant retraining as a registered nurse, and all expressed their unease with that prospect. Therefore, as an interpretation to participate in aversion therapy, this 'self-interest' argument fails to accord with the majority of nurses' testimonies in this book. These nurses had no career or material incentives to make them want to say 'no' to their superiors with regard to their participation in aversion therapy.

Stanley Milgram proposes that humans in general are blindly obedient to authority, and that in some cases they reflexively obey any order, regardless of its content.[136] However, Herbert Kelman and Lee Hamilton argue that this interpretation is indefensible, and claim that all obedience depends upon the existence of a favourable social and political context, in which individuals deem the commands that have been issued not to be a gross transgression of their intrinsic values and their central morality.[137] Indeed, Goldhagen suggests that if favourable social and political contexts are not in place, people will seek ways, 'granted with differential success, not to violate their deepest moral beliefs and not to undertake such grievous acts'.[138]

Arguably, the political rhetoric and media headlines regarding sexual deviations were broadly in favour of treatment with aversion therapy. There was, therefore, a favourable social and political context to these treatments. This could corroborate the influential impact that the media and political rhetoric had on the nurses' morality in relation to their participation in this therapy, and can offer further a context on which to explain their subservient behaviour in regard to this aspect of their clinical practice. Indeed, Ursula Vaughan remarked: 'I remember the press discussing "how a doctor had cured a homosexual" . . . I suppose the fact it was printed for all to see was confirmation of the good work we were doing.'[139]

Conclusion

Despite literature at the time warning nurses not to merely accept orders in relation to administering aversion therapy there appears to be some dissonance between reality and rhetoric. Some nurses in this book appeared to have behaved in a subservient, unenquiring and unquestioning manner that resulted in – or at least contributed to – behaviour, and participation in activities, that could now be perceived as professionally incongruent. There appear to be several interpretations that could help to explain why some of these nurses developed a passive obedience to authority. The passivity referred to here is around the nurses accepting orders from a superior.

Because orders to the nurses were given from a doctor, sister, nursing officer or charge nurse, or in the case of SENs from a registered nurse, this stood as a kind of guarantee of medical quality and ethical correctness of those orders. Owing to the media sanguinely reporting cases of doctors 'curing' homosexuals, this also affirmed the appropriateness of the treatment for some nurses. The combination of the media, the culture of mental hospitals during this period, the effect of militarisation in nursing and fear of harsh discipline created a fertile and receptive environment where nurses understood their ethical responsibilities in terms of a strong commitment to obedience.

There were similarities between some nurses in this study and Nurse Rivers in the Tuskegee study. This was due to some nurses believing that they were acting beneficently: the patients had consented to the treatment and they perceived that aversion therapy was the most effective intervention to cure sexual deviance at the time. However, by acting upon their notions of beneficence, they were not upholding the principle of non-maleficence.

Patients were implicitly coerced into receiving aversion therapy by the law – when they were given an option of prison or hospital – the media, and the paternalistic attitudes of nurses and doctors. The reasons for such paternalistic attitudes could have been as a result of the broadening definitions and conceptions of mental illness, and the psychiatrists' – and nurses' – endeavour to bring 'new' patients into the hospital at a time when numbers were generally being reduced. These could all have led to the health care professionals not upholding the patients' autonomy in relation to their decision to consent to the treatment.

While the different historical context was noted, and none of the nurses in this study knowingly murdered patients, unlike nurses under Nazi rule, there was an issue here of a replaying, in a minor key, of some of the dynamics between Nazi nurses and their role in the euthanasia projects, and the nurses in this study and their role in aversion therapy. As with the Nazi nurses, there is evidence to suggest that some nurses in this study overcame any reservations they may have had in relation to administering aversion therapy by focusing on specific tasks and using dehumanising language. This could offer a strand of analysis to help explain some nurses' participation in aversion therapy.

Finally, the predominant theme among the nurses in this book was that they appeared to develop a passive obedience to authority, and this chapter gives us clues as to the negative ways in which obedience to authority can work. There were others, however, who were able to covertly undermine their superiors by engaging in some fascinating subversive behaviours. Chapter 4 introduces the 'subversive nurses' in this book, and seeks to explore their testimonies, to discover how some nurses appeared to resist the powerful influences discussed above.

Notes

1 Ursula Vaughan, interviewed 12 February 2010. Parts of this chapter have been recycled from Tommy Dickinson, Matt Cook, John Playle and Christine Hallett, 'Nurses and Subordination: A Historical Study of

Mental Nurses Perceptions on Administering Aversion Therapy for 'Sexual Deviations', *Nursing Inquiry*, pp. 1–11. DOI: 10.1111/nin.12044.

2 James, 'Case of Homosexuality Treated by Aversion Therapy', p. 770.

3 Gilbert Davies, interviewed 10 February 2010; Dickinson, Cook, Playle and Hallett, 'Nurses and Subordination', p. 5.

4 Charles P. Seager, 'Aversion Therapy in Psychiatry', *Nursing Times* 26 (1965), pp. 421–424.

5 Seager, 'Aversion Therapy in Psychiatry', p. 424.

6 Nolan, *Psychiatric Nursing Past and Present*, p. 201.

7 Nolan, *Psychiatric Nursing Past and Present*, p. 202.

8 'A Brief History of the Society of Mental Nurses, 1943–1972', in Nolan, *Psychiatric Nursing Past and Present*, p. 202.

9 Sarah Dock, 'The Relation of the Nurse to the Doctor and the Doctor to the Nurse', *American Journal of Nursing* 17 (1917), p. 394.

10 Eliot Feidson, *Profession of Medicine: A Study of the Sociology of Applied Knowledge* (Chicago, 1970), p. 54.

11 Claudine de Valois, interviewed 30 December 2009.

12 Julian Wills, interviewed 4 January 2010.

13 Elizabeth Granger, interviewed 3 May 2010.

14 Benedict Henry, interviewed 23 June 2010.

15 Nolan, *Psychiatric Nursing Past and Present*, p. 227.

16 Evander Orchard, interviewed 10 August 2010.

17 For a detailed exploration of the nurses' role in Nazi Germany, see, e.g., McFarland-Icke, *Nurses in Nazi Germany*; Alison J. O'Donnell, 'A New Order of Duty: A Critical Genealogy of the Emergence of the Modern Nurse in National Socialist Germany' (unpublished PhD thesis, The University of Dundee, 2009). Hilde Steppe has also published some seminal work in this area. See, e.g., Hilde Steppe, *Krankenpflege im Nationalsozialismus* (Frankfurt, 1989). However, to mitigate any potential problems with translation, her work is not referred to unless it has been published in English.

18 While it is important to note that the aim was never to murder patients who were receiving treatments for their sexual deviations, there is at least one reported case where a patient died as a result of the chemical aversion therapy he received to 'cure' him of his homosexuality. Gerald William Clegg-Hill was a 29-year-old captain in the British army who died as result of chemical aversion therapy, which was administered to him in a military hospital on 12 July 1962: *Dark Secret: Sexual Aversion*, British Broadcasting Corporation (1996).

19 Zella Mullins interviewed, 14 July 2010.

20 See, e.g., McFarland-Icke, *Nurses in Nazi Germany*.

21 Steppe, 'Nursing in Nazi Germany', p. 745.

22 Biley, 'Psychiatric Nursing', p. 365.

23 McFarland-Icke, *Nurses in Nazi Germany*, p. 130.

24 Biley, 'Psychiatric Nursing', p. 365; McFarland-Icke, *Nurses in Nazi Germany*, p. 219.

25 Biley, 'Psychiatric Nursing', p. 365.

26 Biley, 'Psychiatric Nursing', p. 365.

27 Biley, 'Psychiatric Nursing', p. 366.

28 Maria Berghs, Bernadette Dierckx de Casterle and Chris Gastmans, 'Practices of Responsibility and Nurses During the Euthanasia Programs of Nazi Germany: A Discussion Paper', *International Journal of Nursing Studies* 44 (2007), p. 846.

29 See, e.g., McFarland-Icke, *Nurses in Nazi Germany*; Berghs, Dierckx de Casterle and Gastmans, 'Practices of Responsibility'; Susan Benedict and Jochen Kuhla, 'Nurses' Participation in the "Euthanasia" Programmes of Nazi Germany', *Western Journal of Nursing Research* 21 (1999), pp. 246–263; Henry Friedlander, *The Origins of Nazi Genocide: From Euthanasia to Final Solution* (Chapel Hill, 1995).

30 Steppe, 'Nursing in Nazi Germany', p. 748.

31 Percival Thatcher, interviewed 29 April 2010.

32 Pattinson, *Behind Enemy Lines*, p. 163.

33 Berghs, Dierckx de Casterle and Gastmans, 'Practices of Responsibility', p. 849.

34 Berghs, Dierckx de Casterle and Gastmans, 'Practices of Responsibility', p. 850.

35 It is important to note that dehumanisation of patients was used as a method of managing patients until the mid-1970s. Indeed, George Brown argues that 'One can, without exaggeration, talk of a tendency to dehumanise the patient in the welter of routine': George Brown, 'The Mental Hospital as an Institution', *Social Science and Medicine* 7 (1973), p. 409.

36 Biley, 'Psychiatric Nursing', p. 366.

37 Zella Mullins, interviewed 14 July 2010; Dickinson, Cook, Playle and Hallett, 'Nurses and Subordination', p. 5.

38 Ursula Vaughan, interviewed 12 February 2010.

39 Gilbert Davies, interviewed 10 February 2010; Dickinson, Cook, Playle and Hallett, 'Nurses and Subordination', p. 5.

40 Berghs, Dierckx de Casterle and Gastmans, 'Practices of Responsibility', p. 850.

41 Berghs, Dierckx de Casterle and Gastmans, 'Practices of Responsibility', p. 846.

42 Andrew McKie, '"The Demolition of a Man": Lessons Learnt from Holocaust Literature for the Teaching of Nursing Ethics', *Nursing Ethics* 11 (2004), p. 141.

43 Kantrovich, 'An Attempt at Associate Reflex Therapy in Alcoholism', p. 26.

44 King and Bartlett, 'Treatments of Homosexuality in Britain since the 1950s', p. 188.

45 Allan M. Brandt, 'Racism and Research: The Case of the Tuskegee Syphilis Experiment', in Susan M. Reverby (ed.), *Tuskegee's Truths: Rethinking the Tuskegee Syphilis Study* (London. 2000), p. 15.

46 James H. Jones, *Bad Blood: The Tuskegee Syphilis Experiment* (New York, 1981), p. 21.

47 'The 40-year Death Watch', *Medical World News* (18 August 1972).

48 Jones, *Bad Blood*, p. 7.

49 'The 40-year Death Watch', *Medical World News* (18 August 1972).

50 Brandt, 'Racism and Research', p. 26.

51 'Why 420 Blacks with Syphilis Went Uncured for 40 Years', *Detroit Free Press* (5 November 1972).

52 The mortality figure is based on a published report of the study which appeared in 1955. See, e.g., Jess J. Peters, Sidney Olansky, John C. Cutler and Geraldine Gleeson, 'Untreated Syphilis in the Male Negro: Pathologic Findings in Syphilitic and Non-syphilitic Patients', *Journal of Chronic Disease* 1 (1955), pp. 127–148. The article estimated that 30.4 per cent of the untreated men would die from syphilitic lesions.

53 *Final Report of the Tuskegee Syphilis Study Ad Hoc Advisory Panel* (Washington: Department of Health, Education and Welfare, 1973).

54 See, e.g., Evelyn M. Hammonds, 'Your Silence Will Not Protect You: Nurse Rivers and the Tuskegee Syphilis Study', in Susan M. Reverby (ed.), *Tuskegee's Truths: Rethinking the Tuskegee Syphilis Study* (London. 2000), pp. 340–347; Susan L. Smith, 'Neither Victim nor Villain: Eunice Rivers and Public Health Work', in Susan M. Reverby (ed.), *Tuskegee's Truths: Rethinking the Tuskegee Syphilis Study* (London, 2000), pp. 348–364; Susan M. Reverby, 'Rethinking the Tuskegee Syphilis Study: Nurse Rivers, Silence, and the Meaning of Treatment', in Susan M. Reverby (ed.), *Tuskegee's Truths: Rethinking the Tuskegee Syphilis Study* (London, 2000), pp. 365–387; Darlene Clark Hine, 'Reflections on Nurse Rivers', in Susan M. Reverby (ed.), *Tuskegee's Truths: Rethinking the Tuskegee Syphilis Study* (London, 2000), pp. 386–398.

55 Hammonds, 'Your Silence Will Not Protect You', p. 341.

56 See, e.g., Jones, *Bad Blood*.

57 Jones, *Bad Blood*, p. 24.

58 Smith, 'Neither Victim nor Villain', p. 348; Jones, *Bad Blood*.

59 Hammonds, 'Your Silence Will Not Protect You', p. 341.

60 Hammonds, 'Your Silence Will Not Protect You', p. 344.

61 Hammonds, 'Your Silence Will Not Protect You', p. 341.

62 Reverby, 'Rethinking the Tuskegee Syphilis Study', p. 370

63 Hammonds, 'Your Silence Will Not Protect You', p. 344.

64 Jones, *Bad Blood*, p. 45.

65 Neither the Tuskegee Institute nor other local hospitals had provided adequate care for the poor black people in Macon County: Hammonds, 'Your Silence Will Not Protect You', p. 345.

66 Hammonds, 'Your Silence Will Not Protect You', p. 345.

67 Berghs, Dierckx de Casterle and Gastmans, 'Practices of Responsibility and Nurses During the Euthanasia Programs of Nazi Germany', p. 849.

68 McFarland-Icke, *Nurses in Nazi Germany*, p. 227.

69 Michael Cooper, Christine Cooper and Margaret Thompson, *Child and Adolescent Mental Health Nursing Theory and Practice* (Oxford, 2005), p. 17; see also Carl Rogers, *Becoming a Person: A Therapist's View on Psychotherapy* (New York, 1995), p. 12.

70 Hunter, 'The Rise and Fall of Mental Nursing', p. 99.

71 Daniel F. Clarke, 'Fetishism Treated by Negative Conditioning', *British Journal of Psychiatry* 109 (1963), pp. 404–408.

72 Elliot Whitman interviewed 20 March 2010; Dickinson, Cook, Playle and Hallett, 'Nurses and Subordination', p. 5.

73 Myrtle Pauncefoot, interviewed 20 February 2013.

74 Leith Cavill interviewed 25 March 2010; Dickinson, Cook, Playle and Hallett, 'Nurses and Subordination', p. 5.

75 Berghs, Dierckx de Casterle and Gastmans, 'Practices of Responsibility', p. 850.

76 Elliot Whitman, interviewed 20 March 2010.

77 See Chapter 2 for the reflections regarding the treatments of the patients in this study; see also Smith, King and Bartlett, 'Treatments of Homosexuality in Britain Since the 1950s – an Oral History: the Experience of Patients', pp. 1–4; Dickinson, Cook, Playle and Hallett, '"Queer" Treatments', p. 1349.

78 Albert Holliday, interviewed 27 January 2010.

79 Oscar Mangle, interviewed 21 June 2010.

80 Herbert Bliss, interviewed 2 January 2010.

81 Pete Price interview on *Dark Secret: Sexual Aversion*, British Broadcasting Corporation (1996).

82 Bancroft, 'Aversion Therapy of Homosexuality', pp. 1417–1431.

83 King and Bartlett, 'Treatments of Homosexuality in Britain since the 1950s', p. 188.

84 Bridget Dimond, *Legal Aspects of Nursing* (London, 2004), p. 78.

85 Rumbold, *Ethics in Nursing Practice*, pp. 134–135.

86 King, Smith and Bartlett, 'Treatments of Homosexuality in Britain since the 1950s', p. 189.

87 Rumbold, *Ethics in Nursing Practice*, p. 135.

88 Barrington Crowther-Lobley, interviewed 28 April 2010.

89 Leith Cavill, interviewed 25 March 2010.

90 Benedict Henry, interviewed 23 June 2010.

91 Gillon, *Philosophical Medical Ethics*, p. 57.

92   Rumbold, *Ethics in Nursing Practice*, p. 226.
93   Elspeth Whitbread, interviewed 7 January 2010.
94   Nolan, *Psychiatric Nursing Past and Present*, p. 227.
95   Testimony of a female nurse in Nolan, *Psychiatric Nursing Past and Present*, p. 178.
96   Nolan, *Psychiatric Nursing Past and Present*, p. 178.
97   Una Drinkwater, interviewed 29 December 2009.
98   Cecil Asquith, interviewed 5 December 2010.
99   Evander Orchard, interviewed 10 August 2010.
100 Carmen Moran and Margaret Massam, 'An Evaluation of Humour in Emergency Work', *The Australian Journal of Disaster and Trauma Studies* 3 (1997), pp. 176–179.
101 Thomas L. Khulman, 'Gallows Humour for a Scaffold Setting: Managing Aggressive Patients on a Maximum Security Forensic Ward', *Hospital and Community Psychiatry* 39 (10) (1988), p. 1085.
102 Prebble, 'Ordinary Men and Uncommon Women', p. 201.
103 Eileen Baggott, 'The SEN in Psychiatric Hospitals', *Nursing Times* 29 (1965), p. 1478; Chatterton, 'The Weakest Link in the Chain of Nursing?', p. 129.
104 Chatterton, 'The Weakest Link in the Chain of Nursing?', p. 133.
105 Rosemary White, *The Effects of the NHS on the Nursing Profession* (London, 1985), p. 25.
106 Chatterton, 'The Weakest Link in the Chain of Nursing?', p. 128.
107 Chatterton, 'The Weakest Link in the Chain of Nursing?', p. 128; Nolan and Hopper, 'Mental Health Nursing in the 1950s and 1960s Revisited', p. 334.
108 Baggott, 'The SEN in Psychiatric Hospitals', p. 1478.
109 Baggott, 'The SEN in Psychiatric Hospitals', p. 1478.
110 Chatterton, 'The Weakest Link in the Chain of Nursing?', p. 138.
111 Chatterton, 'The Weakest Link in the Chain of Nursing?', pp. 138–139.
112 Chatterton, 'The Weakest Link in the Chain of Nursing?', pp. 140–141.
113 An interesting perception of the GNC's views regarding mental nursing and mental sub-normality nursing was that both the EN Mental Nurses' and EN Mental Sub-Normality Nurses' syllabuses were the same, as they determined that a different syllabus was not required: Chatterton, 'The Weakest Link in the Chain of Nursing?', pp. 142–143.
114 Chatterton, 'The Weakest Link in the Chain of Nursing?', p. 143.
115 Zella Mullins, interviewed 14 July 2010.
116 National Health Service, *Report of the Committee of Inquiry into Whittingham Hospital* (London, 1972), p. 7.
117 Dorothy Baker, 'Attitudes of Nurses to the care of the Elderly' (unpublished PhD thesis University Manchester, Manchester, 1978), p. 121.
118 Baker, 'Attitudes of Nurses to the Care of the Elderly', p. 122.
119 Elliot Whitman, interviewed 20 March 2010.
120 Baggott, 'The SEN in Psychiatric Hospitals', pp. 1478–1480.

121 See, e.g., Nolan, 'Jack's Story'; Peter Nolan, 'Attendant Dangers', *Nursing Times* 85 (12) (1989), pp. 56–59; Nolan, *Psychiatric Nursing Past and Present*; Chatterton, 'The Weakest Link in the Chain of Nursing?'

122 Nolan, 'Jack's Story', p. 25.

123 Julian Wills, interviewed 4 January 2010.

124 Nolan, 'Jack's Story', p. 27.

125 Bourke, 'Disciplining the Emotions', p. 226.

126 Maurice B. Wright, 'Psychological Emergencies in War Time', *British Medical Journal* 9 (1940), p. 576.

127 Starns, 'Fighting Militarism?', p. 194.

128 Starns, 'Fighting Militarism?', p. 196.

129 Hopton, 'Prestwich Hospital in the Twentieth Century', p. 355.

130 Prebble, 'Ordinary Men Uncommon Women', p. 52.

131 Starns, 'Fighting Militarism?', p. 197.

132 The caps were usually made of lace net (the frillier and longer the higher the authority and status). The 'strings' went either side of the ears and connected the caps with the 'bows' under the chin.

133 Nolan, 'Jack's Story', p. 25.

134 Ida Ashley, interviewed 17 July 2010.

135 Daniel J. Goldhagen, *Hitler's Willing Executioners: Ordinary Germans and the Holocaust* (London, 1996), p. 384.

136 Stanley Milgram, *Obedience to Authority: An Experimental View* (New York, 1969), p. 76.

137 Herbert C. Kelman and Lee Hamilton, *Crimes of Obedience: Toward a Social Psychology of Authority and Responsibility* (New Haven, 1989), 78.

138 Goldhagen, *Hitler's Willing Executioners*, p. 385.

139 Ursula Vaughan, interviewed 12 February 2010.

4

'Subversive nurses'

Thinking critically does not mean simple criticism. It means not simply accepting information at face value in a non-critical or non-evaluating way. The essence of critical thinking centres *not* on answering questions but on questioning answers, so it involves questioning, probing, analyzing and evaluating. The most subversive people are those that ask questions.[1]

Introduction

Some nurses in this study appeared to have adopted a predominantly subservient, unenquiring and unquestioning relationship with those in authority. While none of them steadfastly objected or refused to administer treatments for sexual deviations, some nurses, nevertheless, took huge professional risks, and did covertly question the orders they were given for the sake of their patients. They did this by engaging in what can be described as furtive and subversive behaviours to avoid administering treatments for sexual deviations. This chapter seeks to explore and describe these nurses' experiences when bending the rules in regard to administering aversion therapy, and the meaning they attached to these rule-bending behaviours. The chapter also analyses how some of these behaviours can be seen as being gendered in nature: nurses were not simply passing as nurses, they enacted particular types of masculinity and femininity which they deemed to be appropriate to evade being caught or suspected of disobeying those in authority.

Subversion and nursing

Subversive practice on the part of nurses is not a new phenomenon. While it was established in Chapter 3 that many nurses under Nazi rule engaged in some barbaric and unethical practices by obeying orders from higher authority, there are accounts of at least one nurse and two social workers who engaged in subversive activities while working under this regime. Maria Stromberger was Oberschwester (head nurse) for the SS infirmary of Auschwitz, one of Nazi Germany's most infamous concentration camps. During her work at the infirmary, she risked her life on numerous occasions to save Polish inmates from torture and death.[2] Stromberger was able to gain the inmates' trust and furtively brought food and medicine into the camp for them. She also performed an astonishing act on Christmas Day 1943 by smuggling wine, champagne and good food into the infirmary. She created a makeshift table in the attic and covered it with a clean white bed sheet. She then prepared and served a Christmas dinner to the Polish prisoners who worked in the infirmary – an act that would certainly have put her life at risk. Stromberger evaded being caught and reprimanded for her subversive behaviour because she was easily identifiable as a nurse in her white coat and able to move around Auschwitz freely without suspicion.[3]

Irena Sendler was a social worker in Warsaw, Poland. In December 1942, she was made head of Zegota's (the code name for the Council for Aid to Jews) children's department. Irena and a colleague, Irena Schultz, were sent into the Warsaw ghetto with food, clothes and medicine, including a vaccine against typhoid. However, it soon became apparent that the ultimate destination of many of the Jews was to be the Treblinka death camp. Therefore, Sendler and Schultz disguised themselves as nurses (as social workers were later banned from entering the ghetto) and orchestrated an escape network to try to save as many children as possible from this deadly fate. Some children were transported in coffins, suitcases and sacks; others escaped through the sewer system beneath the city.[4] Sendler and Schultz also appeared to take advantage of the perceived innocence and compliance of the nursing profession as a cover for their resistive work.

Debby Gould describes how, in the 1970s, labour and delivery nurses were castigated if they did not give every woman in labour an episiotomy.[5] Therefore, these nurses evaded 'orders' by deliberately dropping the episiotomy scissors at the last minute, rather than administering an intervention they deemed to be unnecessary.[6] Dorris Tinker and Jeanette Ramer discuss how nurses working with patients suffering from anorexia nervosa undermined their patients' treatment, as they did not perceive these patients to be 'sick' in its traditional sense.[7] Meanwhile, novels such as *One Flew Over the Cuckoo's Nest* (1962), *The House of God* (1978), and *The Nurse's Story* (1982) portray subversion in hospitals. Of most importance to this book, however, is Sally Hutchinson's work on 'Responsible Subversion' among nurses.[8]

Hutchinson describes how nurses bent the rules for the sake of their patients. Responsible subversion is the construct that she uses to describe such behaviours. She found nurses engaged in different degrees of responsible subversion. For example, a minor subversion was that of permitting visitors in during non-visitor hours; a major subversion included giving a medication without a medical prescription. Hutchinson found that by bending the rules, nurses were better able to work towards their identified professional goal of caring for patients. However, while these nurses viewed themselves as responsible, their means were subversive because they violated hospital policies or medical orders. There appear to be some similarities among the nurses in Hutchinson's study; Stromberger, Sendler and Schultz; and some of the nurses featured in this book.

Questioning orders

Only two female nurses in this study engaged in furtive resistive practices to avoid participating in aversion therapy for sexual deviations, and both these nurses took huge professional risks in undertaking these actions. Una Drinkwater recalls her subterfuge when she nursed a homosexual patient who had been admitted to her ward on a court order:

> I was working nights in my last year before retirement when I nursed *****
> [name of patient receiving chemical aversion therapy for homosexuality]. I can still remember his name. Now I had always prided myself for showing the utmost of respect, courtesy and empathy for the patients in my care and it sickened me knowing what we had to do to him in the futile hope

of making him heterosexual. I just thought: 'Where is the treatment in that?' I just couldn't see any benefit to it – it was punishment and torture. Especially because this particular patient was on a court order, and so he hadn't really consented to the treatment. They were given a choice: prison or hospital? Many chose hospital as no one wants to go to prison do they? So I was desperate not to get involved with it, but I knew it would be more hassle than it was worth if I refused. Not only would my life have been made hard work, because I would have been seen as a troublemaker. I also thought it will only end up being someone else doing the dirty work and they probably wouldn't have been as compassionate as me [. . .] So what I did, every two hours when I was supposed to give him the injections was this. [Pause. Takes deep breath] I went into his room and sat down on the bed next to him and asked him how he was feeling. He said he was feeling awful and burst into tears and said: 'I just want to get out.' I gave him a hug and told him I was going to help him. I told him that I was not going to give him the injections, but that I would come into his room every two hours as prescribed with the injection and pretend to give him it . . . Every two hours I drew up the apomorphine went to his room, squirted it onto the floor, and told him to pretend to be sick in a couple of minutes, once I had left [. . .] I reported to the Charge Nurse that I had given the medication. I nursed him for two nights and I spent some time with him when the other nurses were on their break. I told him that if he wanted to get out he needed to start saying that he was feeling more attracted to women and that he felt the treatment was working. [. . .] I got a thank you card and letter from him a few months after he was discharged. He thanked me for all the support I had given him, and said he was living happily with 'T'. He had confided in me that he was in love with a chap called Terrence, so I presumed it must have been him. It ended by saying he would never forget me . . . [Pause] . . . I don't think I needed any special thanks. I just questioned things that a lot of nurses didn't . . . I'm a living, thinking human being.[9]

Una's testimony corroborates the finding that nurses who did not conform to the rules and orders they were given were often labelled as 'troublemakers'. Her behaviour could be viewed in two ways: as a case of unprofessional conduct or as compassionate autonomous intervention. While Una did not overtly question practice, she did covertly question and undermine her superiors. Arguably, she conscientiously objected to this treatment owing to her intrinsic values and morals, which in turn reversed her 'conditioning' as a nurse to obey the orders of higher authority. Una recalled reading Rodney Garland's *The Heart in Exile* (1952), and she stated that this gave her 'an understanding of the challenges homosexual men faced'.[10] Therefore, her empathy towards this patient group may have been enhanced by her reading. Her behaviour could bring her trustworthiness as a nurse into question, because she reported that she had administered a prescribed treatment when she had not. Yet, the card that her patient sent her demonstrates the positive impact that her subversive behaviour had on his sense of self-efficacy.

Elizabeth Granger, a state registered nurse (SRN) who had undertaken a degree-level nurse education, recounts her resistive nursing practice as a student nurse on a conversion course to become an RMN when she was ordered to take a homosexual patient on a 'date' as part of his treatment:

I suppose being a university nurse I was more inured to questioning practice and I also enjoyed reading ... erm ... Now I remember reading an article in the *Nursing Times* about aversion therapy ... [Pause] ... I was a general nurse at the time but was due to start my conversion course in mental nursing shortly. I would have done that training first, but at the time they only did the degree in general nursing and my parents wanted me to do the degree, so I did that first. Anyway, going back to the article. I recall it saying that if a nurse is asked to administer aversion therapy, and they didn't really want to for ethical reasons, then she should say 'no'. Now I distinctly remember thinking that that's what I would do if I had to do it [administer aversion therapy] when I started my conversion course, as I thought it was barbaric, and I really had no faith in the treatment and the science it was based on was very weak if not non-existent. However, it wasn't as easy as that. The article failed to make reference to the complex hierarchical organisation of nursing and the covert and underhand bullying tactics that were used in mental hospitals to manage and get rid of oppositional people. So it was not as simple as just saying 'no'. [. . .] Luckily I only moved onto the ward once ***** [Name of patient receiving chemical aversion therapy] had finished the actual aversion therapy and he was undergoing 'social skills training'. Now this meant that the patient would have to go on a pretend 'date' with a female nurse to practice this ready for when they would do it for real – ridiculous! [Laughs]. Now they were not officially known as 'dates', this is just what we jokingly referred to them as. It was essentially about building the patient's confidence around females. We certainly weren't supposed to have any intimacy with each other or anything like that. Nevertheless, being a pretty young girl I was considered the obvious choice. I went on several 'dates' with the patient in the hospital grounds. I had a ball! He would do sarcastic impressions of the Matron and the doctor and be very effeminate – I would be in fits of laughter. He had told the doctor the treatment had worked and he was now attracted to women; but he confided to me that he had lied. I knew it hadn't worked, and he was still gay before he even told me. I wasn't bothered; I thought people should be who they are and want to be. I went back to the ward and reported that the 'date' had gone well and that the treatment appeared to have had a good effect and there was no obvious homosexual behaviour.[11]

As with Una's testimony, Elizabeth makes reference to the underhand bullying tactics that were used to 'manage and get rid of oppositional people'; and when recalling her narrative, Elizabeth was noted to laugh. This could support the finding that nurses used humour to deal with the incongruent interventions they were expected to implement when nursing patients receiving treatments for their sexual deviations. Furthermore, in contrast to the other nurses in this study, particularly the SENs, it could be argued that Elizabeth felt that her ability to question practice could be attributed to her university-based nurse education. This is an important finding and will be explored later in the chapter.

Interpreting the 'subversive' nurses' actions

The behaviours of Una Drinkwater and Elizabeth Granger could be perceived as unprofessional, given that both nurses reported that they had implemented a prescribed 'therapeutic' intervention, even though they had not. Nevertheless, their testimonies suggest that they reflected on, and covertly questioned, the orders they had been given. Una Drinkwater and Elizabeth Granger believed that they were acting in their patients' best interests when they chose to behave subversively. In 1973 the International Code of Nursing Ethics stated: 'The fundamental responsibility of a nurse is to promote health, prevent illness, restore health and alleviate suffering . . . The nurse takes appropriate action to safeguard the rights of the individual.'[12] An essential part of a nurse's role is to ensure that their patients' rights are met.[13] These include the right to autonomy; the ability to make decisions about treatment following receipt of full information; safe and considered care; and to expect whatever is done to them to be in their best interests.[14] In the majority of cases, it seems testimony proves that these rights were not upheld for patients receiving aversion therapy for sexual deviations.

Virginia Beardshaw maintains that not ensuring that nurses act in their patients' best interests is a fundamental failure for a system designed to care for vulnerable individuals.[15] Una Drinkwater and Elizabeth Granger identified that their patients' rights were not being upheld and each acted according to her own conscience. Martin Benjamin and Joy Curtis suggest 'that an appeal to conscience is based on a desire to preserve one's integrity or wholeness as a person.'[16]

Rumbold argues that such conscientious objections should be reported to a person or authority at the earliest possible opportunity.[17] However, both testimonies allude to the multifaceted negative influences that were at play in mental hospitals. Una Drinkwater 'knew it would be more hassle than it was worth' if she refused to administer the treatment.[18] Meanwhile, Elizabeth Granger reflected on 'the covert and underhand bullying tactics that were used in mental hospitals to get rid of oppositional people.'[19] This could help explain why these nurses, and others in this study, did not overtly question these practices or refuse to participate in them. Indeed, the Principal Tutor at Whittingham Hospital noted in the *Report of the Committee of Inquiry into Whittingham Hospital* that: 'There was a persistent feeling through all the staff [that] if you brought anything to light, if you dared to step out of line by doing things, then you stood on your own feet and took the consequences.' This was supported by several other witnesses, one of whom said, 'If you complained about anything you got classed as a trouble-maker . . . People could be funny with you.' Another stated: 'The atmosphere of the hospital at that time [1967] was such that you did not criticise anything.'[20]

Beardshaw found similar behaviours and noted that nurses working in mental hospitals frequently did not make complaints about ill-treatment of patients for fear of victimisation, fear of 'cover-ups', and the perception that those complaints would achieve nothing.[21] Furthermore, many of the nurses featured in the present book alluded to fears of constructive dismissal and reprisals if they made complaints or questioned the orders of higher authority. A senior trade union officer and former psychiatric Charge Nurse reported in, Beardshaw's study, what could happen when a complaint was made within a mental hospital:

> The managers make the right kind of noises . . . the veil of respectability. Then the word will get around the institution, and then the normal thing is to make the complainant see the error of his ways . . . start the process of

denying his reality. That's done in a number of subtle ways, over a drink in the social club, on the wards, little chats: 'You didn't really mean to do this . . . ' It starts off normally friendly – then, if the nurse refuses to budge, it's a case of discredit the complainant. You will find commonly, people who have complained in mental hospitals – there will have been very strenuous attempts to find weaknesses in their own character, and use those weaknesses against them . . . And then I've known extremes, like anonymous telephone calls to the person telling them to shut their mouth or else – their car interfered with – and that's the process . . . You'll get personal physical abuse, verbal abuse, ridicule. I've seen every trick in the book used against nurses who have blown the whistle.[22]

The message was clear: opposition of any kind would not be tolerated in mental hospitals. Therefore, it is not surprising that most nurses did not act on any concerns they may have had about untoward practices in such institutions. The fundamental difference between Una Drinkwater and Elizabeth Granger and other nurses in this book is that they *did* act on their concerns. While one could argue that the way they acted was unprofessional, a counter-argument might be that they acted in the best way they believed they could. Indeed, Rumbold proposes that while one has a 'prima facie obligation' to obey the law and codes of conduct, 'that obligation can be overridden in order to comply with a higher, more stringent moral obligation'.[23] Patricia Munhall described principled moral reasoning as that which depends on 'principles of justice, reciprocity, equality of human rights and of respect for the dignity of others as individuals'. A principled nurse is not a conformist, but he or she questions rules that do not serve human values.

The principled level nurse may well be the patient advocate, the change agent, the risk taker, the staunch supporter of individualistic values and, ultimately the purveyor of humanistic nursing.[24]

Like other subordinate nurses in this book, Una Drinkwater and Elizabeth Granger believed that they were acting beneficently, but in contrast to those nurses, they were behaving as principled nurses by also upholding the principle of non-maleficence.

Interestingly and coincidentally, Percival Thatcher recounted a testimony which concurs with that of Elizabeth Granger regarding the social skills training he received in hospital:

Once they stopped the aversion therapy, because I lied, and told them that it had worked, I had to do the most preposterous thing ever. I had to go on a 'date' with one of the nurses! I mean can you imagine how contrived this whole thing was . . . I thought it was going to be with the nurse who had been giving me the injections for the past few days. So I thought: 'Great. I'm going on a date with "Nurse Ratched". You're meant to be reinforcing my "heterosexuality", not turning me gay again!' Anyway, as it happens, it was a young student nurse who had just started on the ward who took me on my dates. I will NEVER forget her. She was fantastic; we had such a laugh together . . . I used to do impressions of the Matron, and we would be rolling about laughing. I trusted her so much that I actually told her that I had lied to the consultant and that I was still homosexual. Although from the way I behaved around her, which I have just described, it wouldn't have taken a genius to work that out! [Laughs] Anyway, she mustn't have said anything, as I was discharged a few weeks later.[25]

The testimonies of Percival Thatcher and Elizabeth Granger match, as both recalled the same hospital, time frame and names; however, unfortunately ethical implications dictated that I was unable to inform the individuals of this. Nevertheless, it reinforces the positive impact that Elizabeth Granger's subversive behaviour had on her patient.

Interestingly, Percival Thatcher framed his narrative around cultural constructions of psychiatry, namely the 1975 film, *One Flew Over the Cuckoo's Nest*, when he made reference to Nurse Ratched. Penny Summerfield argues that people do not simply remember what happened to them, but make sense of the subject matter by interpreting it through contemporary language and concepts available to them. Therefore, the historian needs to understand not only the narrative offered, but also the meanings invested in it and their discursive origins.[26] Nurse Mildred Ratched is portrayed as a cold, psychopathic bully in the film. She has become a popular metaphor for the corrupting influence of power and authority in establishments such as the mental hospital in which the film is set. This public representation may have shaped Percival Thatcher's memory of his time in hospital.

In these cases, Summerfield argues that such formulations are inevitably selective and can make constructions of subjectivities problematic.[27] However, the analogy that Percival Thatcher makes between the nurse who administered his aversion therapy and Nurse Mildred Ratched can be seen as a positive aspect of his testimony;

as it serves to reinforce the notion that the nurse's role in aversion therapy was to make the treatment as unpleasant as possible for the patient.

Percival Thatcher and Elizabeth Granger both highlighted the incongruity of the situation they found themselves in, when they were expected to go on a date with each other. However, even though this was a peculiar task to be assigned, it is not unique. During the World War II, women in the British First Aid Nursing Yeomanry[28] (FANY) were expected to take trainee male Special Operation Executive[29] (SOE) agents on dates and encourage them to drink alcohol. While on these dates, intoxicated trainees were then encouraged by FANYs to reveal personal details about themselves: if they did, they would be removed from the course as they were considered a 'security risk'.[30] Nolan argues that such therapeutic practices as 'habit training' and 'social rehabilitation programmes' (which the prescribed date between Elizabeth Granger and Percival Thatcher can be categorised as) were widespread in the 1960s.[31] Indeed, nurse therapist Peter Lindley stated that he taught the homosexual patient he was treating 'heterosexual social skills', which included 'advice about dating girls and petting'.[32]

Eluding suspicion

Anxiety seems a reasonable response to Una Drinkwater's and Elizabeth Granger's subversive behaviours. My assumptions regarding the possible grave repercussions of being caught engaging in such behaviours prompted me to ask questions about whether their resistive activities caused them anxiety. Rather unexpectedly, both the participants claimed in their testimonies that they were not unduly worried and managed to undertake these activities without fear. Indeed, when Una Drinkwater reflected on her subversive behaviour, she remarked, 'I have no regrets. I'm not bothered what others think about me. I did what I felt I had to do. I would do it again tomorrow if I had to!'[33] This short, insistent 'I would do it again tomorrow if I had to!' complemented by a conclusive nod of the head, gave closure to the topic of conversation. She appeared to have no professional repentance about her actions and states that other people's perceptions of her behaviour did not perturb her.

It appears that Elizabeth Granger relied on a feminine performance to enable her to evade being caught or suspected of disobeying those in authority. When Elizabeth Granger was asked how the date with the patient had gone by her charge nurse, she remarked:

> I just put on my most innocent voice, gave him a big smile, fluttered my eyelashes and said: 'It went fine. How could he possibly resist my charms?' I must have pulled it off, as I never got caught, and he [the charge nurse] just laughed flirtatiously.[34]

This interaction between Elizabeth and her superior demonstrates the powerful and effective use of conventionally feminine appearance and behaviours. By formulating her testimony in terms of 'put on' and 'pulled it off', she reveals her ingenuity and the performative way she utilised her femininity. Elizabeth found it productive to accentuate her physical appearance, and her sexual attractiveness to the opposite sex, as a way of flirting with her superior in a bid to divert his attention on to her as a sexual object rather than as a subordinate who should have carried out his orders. Beverley Skeggs argues that flirtation is behaviour intended to arouse sexual feelings or advances without emotional commitment. It involves a combination of conventional femininity (in particular passivity, powerlessness and dependence on others), the stretching of traditional femininity (typified by directly engaging in dialogue), and the reproduction of heterosexuality.[35]

Conversely, Una Drinkwater used a less glamorous performance to elude suspicion of her subversive behaviours. When recalling how she orchestrated her resistive behaviour, she remarked:

> Now you have to remember, I was in my final year before retirement, so I was getting on it bit. [Laughs] I was on shift with two other, much younger male nurses, one of whom was the Charge Nurse. So I said to the other two nurses: 'I'll look after the homosexual chap. I'll leave you strapping lads to look after the others. I don't want to be grappling we [sic] any o [sic] them lot at my age!' So they just left me to it. In their eyes I was an old woman who came in with her knitting and homemade cakes for them; they were more interested in 'protecting' me than anything else.[36]

Una utilised her mundane appearance to coordinate her subversive work. By resting on, and exploiting, her perceived frailty (which may have been emphasised by bringing in her knitting and cakes), she constructed an identity of someone who should be protected rather than suspected of any rule-bending practices. Interestingly, there is a paradox between her performance of fragility and the psychological strength that her performance required. Outwardly, Una wanted to be perceived as frail, but intrinsically she was actually a very strong character who was able to manipulate a very controlled environment for the sake of her patient.

Furthermore, her testimony suggests that there were some potentially violent patients on the ward, and by suggesting that the male nurses tend to these patients, she reinforced her fragility by her comment, 'I don't want to be grappling we [*sic*] any o [sic] them lot at my age!'[37] She also incited and appealed to traditionally masculine behaviours by implying that the two male nurses were the most appropriate to deal with aggressive patients. Ironically, Una inverted traditional gender norms, despite apparently strengthening them. In addition, the homosexual patient may have been perceived to present no physical threat – reinforcing stereotypes of weakness and effeminacy, but to subversive effect.

The testimonies of Elizabeth Granger and Una Drinkwater also highlight some similarities with Maria Stromberger's subversive behaviour. She was successful in her ability to smuggle food into Auschwitz because she drew upon the perceived innocence of the nursing profession. She wore her white nurse's coat at all times, as it had a dual purpose: it allowed her to pass unnoticed around the camp and neighbouring village of Oswiecim, and it also enabled her to conceal matchboxes, pens and food containers.[38]

While the most subversive nurses in this book appear to be Una Drinkwater and Elizabeth Granger, there were also two male nurses who engaged in rule-bending activities while nursing patients receiving treatments for sexual deviation. Although their subterfuge did not have the same professional implications as for the female nurses, something can be learned from a comparison. Benedict Henry recalls, 'Even though we were not really supposed to, I tried to sit down with the patient and offer them support.'[39] Meanwhile, Julian Wills, who served alongside a homosexual man during World War II, recalls nursing patients receiving aversion therapy:

I have already told you about the chap I served with in the war who was homosexual, and we got on really well. So this made me really question the appropriateness of the treatments these men were given just because they were homosexual. Now we weren't supposed to talk to them [the patients receiving aversion therapy], but I always made time to talk to em [sic]. A lot were in because they believed that everybody thought that they were some dirty, predatory deviant, so I thought it was my job to let em [sic] know that was not the views of everyone. I would sit down with them and have a cigarette, but only when no one was looking. I didn't want to get into trouble you see. A Charge Nurse saw me doing this once, and quizzed me about it. He said: 'You looked a bit friendly with that homosexual in the day room before?' . . . I'm not proud of what I said next, but I did the best thing I could think of at the time. I just laughed and said: 'What do you mean? As if I would want to talk to a dirty queer!' He [the Charge Nurse] just laughed and said: 'You had me worried for a minute there.' He must have believed me, as he never said nowt [sic] no more about it.[40]

Julian's exposure to homosexuals during World War II had a positive effect on his attitude towards these individuals in his care. His testimony also attests that there were significant implications if you were caught disobeying those in higher authority. However, in contrast to the female nurses' tactics to avoid suspicion of engaging in subversive behaviours, Julian's defence was less resourceful and inventive. Nevertheless, his strategy was successful, as the charge nurse did not continue to question him about his behaviour. Julian's testimony was appropriate to his gender: he made a 'macho' retort, which was aimed at reinforcing his masculinity and demonstrating that he fitted into the (possibly homophobic) culture of the ward. This distanced him in the eyes of colleagues from any sympathy or collusion with the homosexual patient.

University-based nursing education

Elizabeth Granger's testimony highlights that she attributed her subversive behaviour to the fact that she was a 'university nurse'. Indeed, she was one of the first nurses to graduate from the integrated Arts degree and SRN training at the University of Edinburgh. This course was one of the first attempts to educate nurses in university and ran between 1960 and 1965. Thereafter, it was changed to the BSc Social Sciences (Nursing) degree.[41] Other experimental courses combining degrees with nurse training were developed during the 1960s, notably Sheffield University, St George's Hospital in cooperation with the

University of Surrey, and the Brighton Hospitals Group with Sussex University. Christine Hallett argues that none treated nursing itself as an academic subject. The Victoria University of Manchester was the first to offer a degree in Nursing.[42]

A key driver in the development of university-based nurse education was Colin Fraser Brockington, Professor of Social and Preventative Medicine at the University of Manchester.[43] Brockington believed that the benefit of establishing a degree programme for nurses would be twofold. Initially, it would improve the status and formalise the training of nurses and health visitors. Second, it would allow individuals who were of 'superior intellect' to make use of their capacity for analysis and creativity. His perception was that, historically, if such individuals had wanted to pursue a nursing career, then they had felt obliged to suppress their 'capacity for intellectual and creative work, in order to become conventional, passive and compliant'.[44] Moreover, concurring with Elizabeth Granger's testimony, one of the central functions of the university nurse was to question practice.[45] Indeed, Mrs Comber-Higgs, Matron of Crumpsall Hospital, Manchester (where the students on the University of Manchester 'Manchester Scheme' undertook their clinical experience), was noted to remark:

> Oddly enough, the presence of the diploma students seems to stimulate our own nurses to ask more questions. It has been stressed to the girls on the university course that they are students and that it is their job to ask more questions, while our own students [undertaking traditional nurse training] are often diffident about taking up the ward sister's time, or feel that they themselves are too busy to ask questions.[46]

Despite the fact that these were pioneering courses, these nursing students often met challenges, which included 'stress in the face of resentment'[47] and the 'burden of being different'.[48] Some of them felt that they did not fit on the wards and others believed that nurses undertaking the traditional nurse training were better prepared for a career in nursing.[49] Moreover, despite the aim of the university-based nurse education programmes being to create nurses who questioned practice, in a study which explored the experiences of nursing students who undertook the same nurse education programme as Elizabeth Granger at the University of Edinburgh, the majority of participants in this study noted that their questioning minds were not well received by the ward sisters.[50]

Karen Luker argues that the university nurse was in some sense assigned to a category of 'deviance' because they challenged the essence of what most conventionally trained nurses had learnt to accept.[51] It seems that parallels can be made here with Elizabeth and her patient Percival Thatcher, as both may have been perceived as 'deviant'. For one because Elizabeth had become a nurse through an unorthodox route and Percival was homosexual. When students elected to read nursing at university, they did so without realising that they were about to become members of a stigmatised group, therefore, in this sense they did not choose to be different.[52] This could offer a context to explain Elizabeth's subversive behaviour, she may have easily empathised with Percival, as she identified what it was like to have an all-embracing feeling of being different through no fault of your own, thus strengthening the resolve to support the 'underdog'.

In an occupation such as nursing, with its tradition of a hierarchical style of administration where experience in terms of years of service counts, and the quest of knowledge for its own sake is given a low priority, university nurses may have been seen to defy a moral order which formed the basis for the ranking system. Therefore, Elizabeth may have been perceived with suspicion by the mental nurses she was working alongside. First, she was already an SRN, and such nurses were often viewed by mental nurses as predominately middle class and female – in contrast to themselves, who they identified as principally working class and male.[53] Furthermore, mental nurses were deeply suspicious of SRNs, as senior positions in mental hospitals were often denied to nurses unless they were dual qualified as a SRN and RMN.[54] Even worse Elizabeth was a university-educated nurse, which was unusual within a mental hospital, as the first university-based mental nurse education programmes were not implemented until the late 1970s.[55]

It appears that many university nursing students developed dynamic ways to present themselves as acceptable and to gain favour with the ward staff. This tactic involved information control concerning what they did or did not know and self-denigration, which they thought would undermine the preconceived expectations of the ward staff in relation to university nurses.[56] Luker proposes that the nursing students had to be particularly vigilant in controlling information about the university side of their life. Knowledge of the theoretical underpinnings of nursing practice may have been seen by conventionally trained nurses as threatening.[57] This could offer a further context within which to explain Elizabeth's behaviour. By virtue of her educational background, Elizabeth may have been viewed as a double threat to the mental nurses. Therefore, it could be reasoned that she may have subversively bent the rules. Even though she made an appeal to her own conscience, she also managed to fit in with the compliant culture of the mental hospital. Elizabeth would have had a lot to lose; being a student nurse, her qualified colleagues could potentially have failed her. She may not have wanted to draw attention to herself or to be perceived as oppositional by her colleagues, nor, to be seen as overtly questioning practice.

Responsible subversion

Hutchinson argues that responsible subversion occurs when nurses bend the rules for the sake of their patients. She posits that there are four phases that characterise the process of responsible subversion: evaluating, predicting, rule bending and covering. Although they are written in a linear fashion, in reality they occur almost simultaneously over a period of only a few minutes. During the evaluating phase, the nurse analyses the patient/context, the rule itself, and his or her own motives. They evaluate the rule or order they have been issued – its sources, purpose and possible effects. It is assessed as to whether it makes rational sense.[58] It seems Elizabeth and Una could not make rational sense of the orders they had been issued, which moved them into the next phase of predicting.

During the predicting phase the nurse anticipates the consequences of the planned behaviour for the patient, the self (the nurse bending the rule), and the rule maker (the doctor or nursing superior). Generally, this process happens quickly because it is the patient's situation that inspires the rule bending. The nurses' awareness of the need for self-preservation is strong. This is the stage where Una Drinkwater and Elizabeth Granger both believed that voicing their conscientious objections to these treatments would have caused them problems.

Rule bending is the third phase of responsible subversion. Hutchinson argues that there are three kinds of circumstances where nurses may bend the rules:

1 when nurses have tried and been unsuccessful in getting a rule changed or they expect they would be unsuccessful;
2 when they have no immediate access to doctors or have determined that the doctor should not be interrupted at this time; and
3 when they believe their behaviour is indicative of good nursing judgement.[59]

Rule bending may occur publicly, making others aware of the responsible subversion, or privately. Elizabeth and Una both bent the rules privately. The circumstances that possibly led to this behaviour were that they expected that their attempts to change or question the medical orders would have been unsuccessful; and they believed their planned rule bending was 'indicative of good nursing judgement'.

The strategies chosen for rule bending depend upon many variables, including the context, the rule makers, the patient, the rule and the nurse. One strategy involves stalling, which enables nurses to avoid following through a doctor's order. Some nurses in Hutchinson's study referred to a 'code slow'. This meant that nurses and others walked slowly to a patient who had coded (experienced a respiratory or cardiac arrest). They participated in a slow code by calling the code slowly, walking to it slowly and moving slowly once in the patient's room. One nurses described doing slow codes 'when the patient wanted to be allowed to die peacefully and when he is in terrible shape and there is no hope and he has suffered so'.[60] Hutchison also found that critically evaluating the right time for rule bending often ensured success. Arguably, some nurses in this study used this strategy. As Una Drinkwater commented: 'I spent some time with him when the other nurses were on their break.'[61] Meanwhile, Julian Wills remarked, 'I would sit down with them [homosexual patients] and have a cigarette, but only when no one was looking.'[62] Finally, Hutchinson argues that other strategies nurses use for rule bending include: exaggerating or even lying about clinical symptoms. Elizabeth Granger, Julian Wills and Una Drinkwater would have used a combination of these strategies to orchestrate their rule-bending behaviours.

The final stage of responsible subversion is covering. This is a self-protective process that nurses rely on when they bend the rules. As the nurses are consciously and willingly bending the rules, they clearly recognise the potential for negative consequences. The aim of these protective manoeuvres is to prevent these consequences. Nurses select a covering strategy that aids them in not getting caught or provides an explanation if they are caught bending the rules. In the majority of cases nurses keep their rule-bending behaviours secret. One nurse in Hutchinson's study described the responsible subversion process as 'invisible practice', 'We don't admit to people that we do it. We don't have conversations about it.'[63] Indeed, Elizabeth Granger, Julian Wills and Una Drinkwater disclosed that this was the first time they had revealed their rule-bending behaviours to another person since they happened.

Arguably, the subversive nurses in this study were aware of the potential personal consequences of their behaviours, which is why they so carefully evaluated, predicted and covered their activities. Many of the actions taken by these nurses reveal caring behaviours. Moreover, their subversive actions exhibit their belief in the autonomy (self-determination) of the patient and in the concept of beneficence.

Conclusion

There are some possible interpretations for why the nurses in this study may have bent the rules. It seems that one of the main reasons was that they conscientiously objected to the treatments. However, owing to the way oppositional people appear to have been managed within mental hospitals, these nurses did not feel that they could overtly question the appropriateness of aversion therapy to cure sexual deviations. In the case of Elizabeth Granger, her university-based nurse education may also have encouraged her to behave in this way in order to be accepted into the culture of the mental hospital.

An examination of the above testimonies also demonstrates that femininities and masculinities were sometimes used by the subversive nurses in this study to avert the suspicion of their engaging in resistive activities. In essence, these gendered performances were the best cover for their subversive behaviour. While these enactments appeared to be successful for the participants in this study, there may have been other nurses who also engaged in subversive activities but were caught. Therefore, such performances may not have been foolproof for all nurses. There may also have been – yet unrevealed – nurses who steadfastly refused to participate in this aspect of clinical practice. However, the testimonies throughout this study concur in so far as many nurses did not voice their concerns or question practice. Mental nurses had good reasons to keep quiet about any conscientious objections they may have had. Conflict of loyalties and fears of victimisation inhibited free speech within many mental hospitals. There is no doubt that the subversive nurses who covertly questioned practice in this study were empathic and upheld the principles of beneficence and non-maleficence. Moreover, as their actions appeared to have had a positive long-term impact on their patients' sense of self-efficacy, one could argue that these nurses were 'responsibly subversive'.

Notes

1 Jostein Gaarder, *Sophie's World: A Novel about the History of Philosophy* (London, 1995), p. 128.
2 Susan Benedict, 'Maria Stromberger: A Nurse in the Resistance in Auschwitz', *Nursing History Review* 14 (2006), pp. 189–202.
3 Benedict, 'Maria Stromberger', p. 196.
4 'Irena Sendler', *Daily Telegraph* (12 May 2008); 'Irena Sendler, Lifeline to Young Jews, Is Dead at 98', *The New York Times* (13 May 2008).
5 This is a cut in a woman's perineum (the area between the vagina and anus). The cut makes the opening of the vagina a bit wider, allowing the baby to come through it more easily.
6 Debby Gould, 'Professional Dominance and Subversion in Maternity Services', *British Journal of Midwifery* 16 (2008), p. 4.
7 Dorris E. Tinker and Jeanette C. Ramer, 'Anorexia Nervosa: Staff Subversion of Therapy', *Journal of Adolescent Health Care* 4 (1983), pp. 35–39.
8 See, e.g., Sally Hutchinson, 'Responsible Subversion: A Study of Rule-Bending Among Nurses', *Scholarly Inquiry for Nursing Practice: An International Journal* 4 (1990), pp. 3–17; Sally Hutchinson, 'Nurses and Bending the Rules', *Creative Nursing* 4 (2004), pp. 4–8.
9 Una Drinkwater, interviewed 29 December 2009.
10 Una Drinkwater, interviewed 29 December 2009.

11 Elizabeth Granger, interviewed 3 May 2010.
12 International Code of Nursing Ethics (1973) in Virginia Beardshaw, *Conscientious Objectors at Work* (London, 1981), p. 45.
13 Dimond, *Legal Aspects of Nursing*, p. 65.
14 Martin Benjamin and Joy Curtis, *Ethics in Nursing* (New York, 1992), p. 34.
15 Beardshaw, *Conscientious Objectors*, p. 45.
16 Benjamin and Curtis, *Ethics in Nursing*, p. 29.
17 Rumbold, *Ethics in Nursing Practice*, p. 249.
18 Una Drinkwater, interviewed 29 December 2009.
19 Elizabeth Granger, interviewed 3 May 2010.
20 National Health Service, Report of the Committee of Inquiry into Whittingham Hospital (London, 1972), p. 30.
21 Beardshaw, *Conscientious Objectors*, p. 45.
22 'Testimony of Male Trade Union Officer and former Charge Nurse', in Beardshaw, *Conscientious Objectors*, p. 36.
23 Rumbold, *Ethics in Nursing Practice*, p. 258.
24 Patricia Munhall, 'Moral Reasoning Levels in Nursing Students and Faculty in a Baccalaureate Nursing Programme', *Image* 12 (1980), pp. 57–61.
25 Percival Thatcher, interviewed 29 April 2010.
26 Summerfield, 'Culture and Composure', p. 67.
27 Summerfield, 'Culture and Composure', p. 69.
28 The FANY was a voluntary civilian women's organisation established in 1907 to bridge the divide between the front line and medical stations. During World War I about 400 FANYs drove ambulances and other vehicles in England, France and Belgium: Marcus Binney, *The Women who Lived for Danger* (London, 2002), p. xiii.
29 In 1938, the British Secret Intelligence Service (SIS, also known as MI6) established Section D, which gained its name on account of the 'destruction' caused by sabotage and subversion undertaken in the Balkans. Military Intelligence Research established that insurgent warfare could assist in diverting the enemy troops if used in juxtaposition with the regular armed forces. Following the Nazi 'blitzkrieg' of the Low Countries, the withdrawal of the British Expeditionary Force from Dunkirk and the surrender of France, the new British War Cabinet under Winston Churchill sanctioned a higher priority for acts of sabotage and subversion. On 27 May 1940, they agreed to a reorganisation of bodies concerned with subversive activities; this led to the establishment of the SOE on 1 July 1940.
30 Pattinson, *Behind Enemy Lines*, p. 53.
31 Nolan, *A History of Mental Health Nursing*, p. 124; see also Allyon and Michael, 'The Psychiatric Nurse as Behavioral Engineer', pp. 323–334.
32 Peter Lindley, 'Sexual Deviation in a Young Man', *Nursing Mirror* 8 (1977), p. 64.
33 Una Drinkwater, interviewed 29 December 2009.

34 Elizabeth Granger, interviewed 3 May 2010.
35 Beverley Skeggs, *Formations of Class and Gender: Becoming Respectable* (London, 1997), p. 128.
36 Una Drinkwater, interviewed 29 December 2009.
37 Una Drinkwater, interviewed 29 December 2009.
38 Benedict, 'Maria Stromberger', p. 197.
39 Benedict Henry, interviewed 23 June 2010.
40 Julian Wills, interviewed 4 January 2010.
41 Jane Brooks, 'The First Undergraduate Nursing Students: A Quantitative Historical Study of the Edinburgh Degrees, 1960–1985', *Nurse Education Today* 31 (2011), p. 634.
42 Christine Hallett, 'The 'Manchester Scheme': A Study of the Diploma in Community Nursing, the First Pre-Registration Nursing Programme in a British University', *Nursing Inquiry* 12 (4) (2005), p. 292.
43 Christine Hallett, 'Colin Fraser Brockington (1903–2004) and the Revolution in Nurse-Education', *Journal of Medical Biography* 16 (2008), p. 89.
44 Hallett, 'The 'Manchester Scheme', p. 289.
45 Joanne Howard and Julia I. Brooking, 'The Career Paths of Nursing Graduates from Chelsea College, University of London', *International Journal of Nursing Studies* 24 (3) (1987), p. 183.
46 Comber-Higgs (1960) cited in Hallett, 'The 'Manchester Scheme', p. 291.
47 Hallett, 'The 'Manchester Scheme', p. 288.
48 Karen A. Luker, 'Reading Nursing: The Burden of Being Different', *International Journal of Nursing Studies* 21 (1984), pp. 1–17.
49 Jo Brand, *Look Back in Hunger* (London, 2009), p. 228.
50 Brooks, 'The First Undergraduate Nursing Students', p. 635.
51 Luker, 'Reading Nursing', p. 2.
52 Luker, 'Reading Nursing', p. 3.
53 Harrington, *Voices Beyond the Asylum*, p. 8.
54 Claire Chatterton, '"A Thorn in its Flesh?" Maud Wiese and the General Nursing Council', *The Bulletin of the UK Association for the History of Nursing* 1 (1) (2012), p. 41.
55 Brand, *Look Back in Hunger*, p. 228.
56 Luker, 'Reading Nursing', p. 4.
57 Luker, 'Reading Nursing', p. 5.
58 Hutchinson, 'Responsible Subversion', p. 8.
59 Hutchinson, 'Responsible Subversion', p. 10.
60 Hutchinson, 'Responsible Subversion', p. 11.
61 Una Drinkwater, interviewed 29 December 2009.
62 Julian Wills, interviewed 4 January 2010.
63 Hutchinson, 'Responsible Subversion', p. 14.

5

Liberation, 1957–1974

Many members of the GLF [Gay Liberation Front] can testify to the ineffectiveness of aversion therapy in reorientation of their sexual desires and to the totally destructive effect [this] has had on their personality and adjustment. Our plan, therefore, is for homosexuals seeking advice from you to be given reassurances from you that they are fully capable of living a full, worthwhile and happy life and that many other men and women are doing just that. This positive attitude substituted for attempts to provide treatment and cure will spare many from intense and undue suffering.[1]

Introduction

The Sexual Offences Act became law in 1967, decriminalizing sex between two consenting male adults over the age of 21 in private in England and Wales.[2] However, for many gay[3] men who were not considered 'respectable homosexuals', this new legal climate provided little benefit to them because of where they were meeting men for sex and how they were conducting themselves in public. These 'other' men remained socially excluded, subject to legal proceedings and medical treatments. Many gay men were unhappy with the conservative imperative of the 1967 Act and its exclusion and condemnation of gay men who did not express their sexuality through coupledom and domesticity. Through a fresh gay liberation movement, these aggrieved men created an attitudinal shift that led to a better understanding of sexual identity and community. They advocated for greater acceptance of sexual variance, for the removal of homosexuality from psychiatric diagnostic manuals and, as demonstrated in the letter above, the curtailment of medical treatments for homosexuality.

The period also witnessed a fresh women's liberation movement and a new stress on individual freedoms, which was, in part, inspired by the civil rights movement in the USA and other general 'counter-cultural' shifts. This period also witnessed a shift in the media representations of sexually deviant individuals; and the press were beginning to question the treatments used to 'cure' these individuals. This chapter explores the consequences of these piecemeal cultural and representational shifts as nurses came to see the treatments they were administering for sexual deviation as inappropriate as ideas of deviance shifted.

In parallel to this fresh gay visibility and radicalism, the nursing profession was also undergoing changes. The advent of 'nurse therapists' witnessed nurses being trained in advanced clinical practice roles, enabling them to be more autonomous practitioners. This period also marked the era of public inquiries into the care of the mentally ill, and the plight of these individuals was moved up the political agenda. This chapter also examines the implications of these changes.

Reform, 1957–1967

Jivani argues that the Conservative government refused to act on the Wolfenden report in 1957 because they believed its recommendations were 'in advance of public opinion'.[4] The lack of action by the government in response to the report appeared to confirm to the police that homosexuality was still not to be tolerated in any form – the police frequently raided the meeting places of homosexual men and employed secret surveillance tactics and agent provocateurs throughout the late 1950s and early 1960s.[5] Indeed, Jivani argues that the report had a paradoxical effect and things actually became worse for homosexuals between 1957, when the report was published, and 1964 when the Director of Public Prosecutions intervened, and requested that the police 'ease off' these individuals.[6]

Resistance to homosexual law reform was observed in a number of ways and many reformers were ironically using the same language of illness, sin and despair as those opposing legal change.[7] However, British society was undergoing a rapid if uneven transformation by the mid-1960s. The homosexual may have been considered unusual, but the unusual was in vogue, and gay men were at the forefront of 'Swinging London'.[8] Dominic Sandbrook argues, however, that the Swinging Sixties did not create the extensive social and 'cultural revolution' that has sometimes been supposed and was actually a decade of 'caution, conservatism and convention' marred by unemployment and recession.[9] Nevertheless, Cook argues that there was a change in attitudes which came with economic expansion and affluence, and a mounting frustration with puritanical moral codes.[10] These attitudinal shifts were being influenced by international notions of individual liberty. In the western world, individuals were beginning to question the definitions of 'difference'.

The civil rights movement in the USA during the 1960s, which put the onus on individual freedoms as well as the rights of certain groups, was filtering through into the UK. On both sides of the Atlantic, women's liberation advocated for equality and sexual, cultural and social independence. Harold Wilson's Labour government of 1964 embarked on a series of social reforms on abortion, divorce and the death penalty. There were student protests at the London School of Economics in 1967 and student riots in Paris in 1968, which suggested that groups that were not traditionally in the political mainstream were claiming the power and ability to express their specific concerns. Meanwhile, the 'summer of love'[11] and the professed sexual revolution led to deliberation around issues of sexual pleasure and monogamy.[12]

By 1965, arguably Britain's most daring playwright, its most commended avant-garde artist and its most esteemed composer – Joe Orton, Francis Bacon and Benjamin Britten – were all openly homosexual.[13] Television documentaries in 1965 and 1967 included homosexual men speaking on their own behalf.[14] Radio became more irreverent, and in the comedy *Round the Horne*, Kenneth Williams and Hugh Paddick traded in homosexual stereotypes and were sharp and self-confident.[15] More broadly, along with the film *Victim* (1961), a tragic tale of homosexuality, blackmail and suicide, all the above covertly pushed the case for reform. Visibility may have made homosexual men easier targets after Wolfenden, but as the years went by, knowledge also decreased public fear, which had been prompted by ignorance.

This change in climate – and government – brought Wolfenden's recommendations back into the political mainstream. In April 1966,

Lord Arran reintroduced his Bill to the Lords decriminalising homosexuality along the lines recommended by Wolfenden. Leo Abse guided the Bill through the Commons, where it passed by 244 votes to 100 on its first reading. The Sexual Offences Act became law on 27 July 1967, decriminalising sex between two consenting male adults over the age of 21 in private.[16] The distinction between public and private was pertinent: for purposes of the law 'public' was anywhere where a third party was likely to be present; and it remained illegal for more than two men to have sex together.[17] Indeed, Lord Arran accentuated the conservative import of the act when he asked homosexual men 'to show their thanks by comporting themselves quietly and with dignity'.[18] He went on to argue: 'Homosexuals must continue to remember that, while there may be nothing bad in being homosexual, there is certainly nothing good'.[19]

The contentious Labouchère Amendment of 1885 had been annulled. However, for many homosexual men this change in the law was simply not substantial enough. The only beneficiary of the law reform was the middle-class 'respectable' homosexual who expressed his sexuality through coupledom and domesticity. Many homosexual men did not fall into this category and refused to 'comport themselves quietly'. These 'other' men remained beyond the law because of where they were having sex, where they were picking up men and how they were conducting themselves in public.[20] Houlbrook maintains that homosexual men who could not, or would not, fit into the confines of the new Act remained the subject of 'social opprobrium and regulatory intervention'.[21]

It is important to note that the 1967 Sexual Offences Act and the new legal climate it supposedly opened up did not appear to have a radical effect on reducing the numbers of patients being referred for treatment of their sexual deviations. One rationale for this is because the recorded incidence of indecency between men in public actually doubled between 1967 and 1977.[22] This offers a context to explain why the treatments continued despite the new legal climate.

Gay liberation

In the years after law reform, the gay voice was largely ineffective.[23] However, the Stonewall riots[24] in New York in July 1969 appeared to invoke a fresh gay liberation movement in both the USA and the UK. The gay activists in the USA eventually went on to disrupt several annual meetings of the American Psychiatric Association (APA) in the early 1970s, which provided the impetus for the eventual removal of homosexuality from its diagnostic manual (explored later in the chapter).

In the UK, the riots across the Atlantic enthused student activists Aubrey Walker and Bob Mellors to hold meetings in the London School of Economics in October 1970. These weekly meetings subsequently led to the development of the Gay Liberation Front (GLF), which was governed by a philosophy of pride and publicised sexual and subcultural variance as positive and life enhancing.[25] Their policy included a number of immediate demands around issues of equality under the law, the end to workplace discrimination, the reform of sex education in schools and the right for gay people to 'be free and hold hands and kiss in public'.[26]

Although homosexual men had been individually defiant in the past, the existence of the GLF gave a united support to homosexuals, some of whom were very angry in relation to the exclusivity of the law reform.[27] Oscar Mangle recalls, 'The GLF voiced what we had all been thinking and feeling for so many years. It was an exciting time for us, there was a real feeling that things were changing for the better.'[28] However, there were other gay men who were not so in favour of the GLF. They believed that the radical members of the GLF made demands on all gay men and many felt underrepresented as despite the GLF's open-door policy, owing to their other responsibilities, many men had too little time to dedicate to GLF activities. Some men simply disliked the disruption to the status quo and the challenge to an established scene.[29]

The GLF was behind the first Gay Pride event of July 1972, which saw 1,000 people march from Trafalgar Square to Hyde Park for a picnic and party.[30] Lisa Power argues, however, that despite this event being a success, the GLF had already started to falter because of internal conflicts, and by 1972, it had disbanded with considerable bitterness.[31] Nevertheless, by the time the GLF disintegrated in 1972, it had already made a huge impact.

There seemed to be shifts and changes on the part of the public, and many homosexual men were beginning to embrace the term 'gay' as a form of self-definition.[32] Papers such as the *Guardian*, the *Observer* and even the conservative *Daily Telegraph* began using the word to describe homosexuals and increasingly the word was used without quotation marks around it.[33] However, Cook argues that even this new terminology 'raised heckles'.[34] Peter Dennis believed that the 'queer' world 'had lost its charm [. . .] now you're either gay or you're straight, you're one or the other. It's lost a certain amount of its colour for the fact that it's no longer underground.'[35]

In the 1970s, gay men and transvestites began to appear in the arts and the media in a way in which they had never been portrayed before.[36] In 1975, Hollywood obtained the rights to the play *The Rocky Horror Show* and made it into a movie. In the same year, Thames produced *The Naked Civil Servant* – after the BBC turned it down – adapted from Quentin Crisp's autobiography of the same title. The film was a huge success and went on to win a number of awards. Jeffrey Weeks mentions that there was minimal hostility to this film. A survey conducted by the Independent Broadcasting Authority revealed that, while 3 per cent of viewers had switched off, 85 per cent stated that they did not find the film shocking.[37]

Nevertheless, in spite of the gay liberation movement creating a new visibility of gay lives which helped to challenge antagonism towards homosexuality, British culture remained broadly hostile and grudging in its liberalism.[38] In an opinion poll for *Gay Times* in 1975, most participants supported the 1967 legislation. However, 45 per cent believed that there should be curbs on gay men working in teaching and medicine, and the notion of gay men being a danger to young people persisted.[39] Many men were still noted to struggle with isolation and rejection, and despite some parents working hard to 'come to terms with having a gay son, many still viewed their "choice" as tragic and/or abhorrent'.[40] This could offer a further context to explain the reason for the continuation of treatments for homosexuality into the mid-1970s despite legal reform, gay liberation and the removal of 'homosexuality' from the APA's diagnostic manual. Men continued to seek treatment because of the shame that continued to be placed on them by society and their families. Indeed, Ida Ashley remarked:

> I breathed a sigh of relief when they changed the law, but it would take a lot more than a new law and a gay rights movement to wipe away people's

entrenched prejudices. I was treating homosexuals well into the 1970s, because they were still very troubled by their sexual desires.[41]

The fresh attitude and pride embraced by some gay men also had its roots in other new cultural, social and political movements. Within this period, some individuals were beginning to live counter-cultural lifestyles, and the way people lived their lives in the UK were changing in a very visible, and for some, disturbing way. Protests against the Vietnam War and anti-racism grew in size and enthusiasm. Recreational drugs such as LSD and marijuana became more readily accessible and used. Superficial changes, such as colourful clothes, the mini-skirt and bikini for women and long hair for men, defied conventional norms of behaviour and appearance. Popular music was changing as the glam rock era emerged and David Bowie appeared as the flamboyant, androgynous alter ego Ziggy Stardust. Peter Ackroyd argues that Bowie challenged traditional gender roles and made transvestism more broadly acceptable.[42] There was also the emergence of anti-establishment thinking, including challenges to the institution of psychiatry with the emergence of the 'counter-psychiatry' movement.[43]

The 'counter-psychiatry' movement

Nick Crossley argues that counter-psychiatry[44] was essentially a movement which criticised psychiatry. It questioned its very basis, its purpose, its fundamental conception of mental illness and the very distinction between 'madness' and sanity.[45] The movement challenged and criticised psychiatry and consequently influenced attitudes towards institutional psychiatric care. Crossley proposes that it was under the impact of counter-culture that the counter-psychiatry movement emerged.[46]

The movement was essentially pioneered through the seminal investigation by Erving Goffman into American psychiatric hospitals in the 1960s, which proved to be very critical of the mental health system. Goffman had personal experience of institutionalisation as a patient suffering from tuberculosis. He also had an interest in other people's experiences of this phenomenon. He found that the social structure of mental hospitals resembled that of a 'total institution'. Here the primary concern of staff was to ensure that patients conformed; this was achieved by forcing patients to enact their lives within a confined and observable space. This corroborates the finding in Chapter 3, which identified that many staff in mental hospitals held paternalistic attitudes to those in their care. Moreover, Goffman's book *Asylums*,[47] published in 1961, along with the work of Thomas Szasz,[48] brought about a radical rethinking of care for the mentally ill in the USA and both had a considerable influence in Britain.[49]

A key figure in the counter-psychiatry movement in the UK was Ronald David Laing.[50] According to Crossley, Laing was a 'charismatic counter-cultural guru and formed a nucleus of "movement individuals" around which the anti-psychiatry movement was formed in the UK and abroad'.[51] He challenged the fundamental assumptions and practices of psychiatry. He argued that the specific definitions of, or criteria for, hundreds of psychiatric diagnoses or disorders were vague and arbitrary, and left too much room for opinions and interpretations to meet basic scientific standards.[52] Laing was also noted to develop and experiment with alternative treatments for mental health problems, such as 'therapeutic communities'.[53]

The psychiatric and medical profession were being more broadly criticised by the likes of the playwright Joe Orton in his play *What the Butler Saw* in 1969.[54] In 1976, Ivan Illich argued in his book *Medical Nemesis: The Expropriation of Health* that the medical establishment had become a major and disabling threat to health and that this had 'reached the proportions of an epidemic'. He named this new epidemic 'iatrogenesis'. The name came from 'iatros', the Greek word for 'physician', and 'genesis', meaning 'origin'.[55] He went on to argue that deviance was now 'legitimate' only because it merits and justifies medical interpretation and treatment.[56] In essence, medical treatments had become a new form of punishment and social control.

'Psychiatrists in a shift. Declare homosexuality no mental illness'

A pioneer in the eventual removal of homosexuality from psychiatric diagnostic manuals was Evelyn Hooker, a psychology professor.

She presented an important challenge to the sickness model in her 1957 article reporting that there was no difference in the psychological adjustment of groups of homosexual and heterosexual men.[57] Nevertheless, David Eisenbach argues that the medical profession perceived her methodology as weak and her research sample to be too small, and largely discounted her work.[58] However, with the advent of the US gay liberation movement in the early 1970s, assertive gay activists began using this work to challenge the 'sickness' label that had been ascribed to homosexuality. During this time, activists began appearing on television talk shows to criticise the psychiatric establishment's beliefs on homosexuality.[59] Indeed, one New York psychologist told *The New York Times* that 'the Gay liberation movement is the best therapy the homosexual has had in years'.[60]

The most effective political tactic that the gay liberation movement used on both sides of the Atlantic was the 'zap'.[61] Just as these activists had zapped political offices and fund-raisers, psychiatrists were also vulnerable to this. The Student Homophile League at Columbia University, USA, launched the first public demonstration against the psychiatric establishment in 1968; gay and lesbian revolutionaries from around the USA targeted meetings of mental health professionals. In the same year, these individuals held a press conference to condemn the US government's plans to build a centre for the cure of 'sexual deviants', a plan that the activists compared to 'the [Nazi] final solution'.[62]

The US GLF was noted to be very confrontational in its campaign against the sickness model, and in 1970, the GLF interrupted an APA convention. During this zap, a prominent psychiatrist remarked: 'I never said homosexuals were sick – what I said was that they had displaced sexual adjustment.' The GLF activists were not happy with this and one member was noted to bellow, 'That's the same thing "motherfucker"!'[63] Furthermore, when an Australian expert described his use of electric aversion therapy to make 'unhappy homosexuals' responsive to women, a protester remarked, 'Where did you do your residency? Auschwitz?'[64] Eisenbach argues that the GLF were not satisfied with shouting from the gallery during this zap and the demonstrators called for an official voice at the conference: 'We've listened to you, now listen to us.'[65] The majority of the psychiatrists in the audience were annoyed and demanded their money back from the APA. One asked the police to shoot the protesters.[66]

At the end of the demonstration, a liberal psychiatrist, Kent Robinson, approached one of the activists, Larry Littlejohn. Robinson agreed to lead an effort from within the APA to organise a panel of homosexuals to speak at the next convention. Robinson was successful in his effort, and he managed to convince the APA to include a panel of gay men and women who rejected the sickness diagnosis in its 1971 annual convention in Washington DC.[67] A key GLF member in their campaign to challenge the sickness diagnosis was Frank Kameny. Although he was invited to this convention, the GLF decided to zap it anyway to attract media attention. At the opening ceremony, Kameny sat in the audience as an honoured guest while dozens of GLF demonstrators burst into the hall from the door behind the stage. In the confusion Kameny seized the microphone and declared: 'Psychiatry is the enemy incarnate. Psychiatry has waged a relentless war of extermination against us. You may take this as a declaration against you!'[68] The activists also demanded that a stall marketing aversion therapy equipment be immediately removed or they would tear it down. To avoid further disruption, it was dismantled. This event marked the alliance of Kameny and Robinson to persuade sympathetic psychiatrists to support a resolution to remove homosexuality from the APA's Diagnostic Statistical Manual (DSM).

The following year, at its Dallas convention, Robinson was able to influence the APA to hold a discussion called 'Psychiatry, Friend or Foe to Homosexuals? A Dialogue'. People were only invited to the discussion if they were sympathetic to the removal of the sickness designation. Frank Kameny and Barbara Gittings (another prominent member of the GLF) were joined on the panel by Robert Seidenberg and Judd Marmor, who represented sympathetic psychiatrists.[69] Furthermore, Gittings managed to convince Marmor that a homosexual psychiatrist should be included on the panel. However, it proved very difficult to find someone who was willing to discuss his homosexuality in front of his colleagues, as the APA officially barred homosexuals from careers in psychiatry.[70] Nevertheless, Gittings managed to find Dr John Fryer. However, Fryer only agreed to do this on the condition that he could use the pseudonym Dr H. Anonymous, and that he could wear a wig and mask and use a voice-distorting microphone.[71]

Dr H. Anonymous was smuggled into the convention through back corridors into a packed lecture hall. During his address, he highlighted the fact that there were more than 200 homosexual psychiatrists attending the convention:

> As psychiatrists who are homosexual, we must know our place and what we must do to be successful. If our goal is high academic achievement, a level of earning capacity equal to our fellows, or admission to a psychoanalytical institute, we must make sure that we behave ourselves, and that no one in a position of power is aware of our sexual preference.[72]

When Dr H. Anonymous finished, the audience honoured his brave presentation with a standing ovation. Frank Kameny noted that the Dallas convention was the first convention in which only positive views on homosexuality were voiced in the public forums.[73] Moreover, Eisenbach argues that whether or not the APA's new consideration for homosexuals resulted from education, sympathy or intimidation, it marked a turning point in the relationship between psychiatry and the gay community.[74] The intellectual tide seemed to be turning against the sickness model by 1972. The APA's leadership was also changing during the early 1970s and a group of young psychiatrists formed the Committee for Concerned Psychiatry, which worked to get liberals elected to APA offices in order to alter the profession's positions on social issues such as feminism and homosexuality. This included John Spiegel, a closet homosexual, being elected president of the APA in 1973. Furthermore, Charles Silverstein from the Gay Activist Alliance (GAA) had also joined forces with the GLF against the sickness diagnosis.[75]

While the GLF in the USA appeared to be the most influential in tackling homophobic rhetoric in psychiatry, there were also protests to these treatments in the UK. The GLF in the UK had a subgroup entitled 'The Anti-Psychiatry Group' who critically challenged the notion that homosexuality was a mental illness.[76] The Albany Trust[77] began using questionnaires to survey patients who had received treatment in psychiatric facilities to cure them of their sexual deviations. The results were fairly damning and the Trust started offering gay men counselling to come to terms with their sexuality.[78]

In an article entitled 'Aversion Therapy is Like a Visit to The Dentist' in *Gay News* in 1972, Peter Tatchell, a member of the GLF, recalls his protest against two of Britain's leading psychiatrists' advocacy of aversion therapy as a 'cure' for homosexuality. On 2 November 1972, the London Medical Group held a symposium on aversion therapy. Peter Tatchell attended to challenge what he believed to be the psychiatric abuse of gay men by psychiatrists Professor Hans Eysenck and Dr Isaac Marks. When Dr Marks, a senior lecturer and consultant psychiatrist at the Maudsley Hospital, tried to reassure his audience that the pain and discomfort experienced by the patient receiving aversion therapy was greatly exaggerated and, in fact 'it is just like a visit to the dentist ... It is no different from any other form of therapy', Tatchell challenged his statement by citing patients who had undergone aversion therapy and were now chronically depressed. This led to a verbal altercation between Tatchell and the psychiatrists, which resulted in Tatchell being 'violently assaulted' as 'ten heavies ... dragged' him from the symposium.[79]

In 1973, the APA Committee on Nomenclature (the committee responsible for editing the DSM) held a meeting, to which they invited GAA members Ron Gold and Charles Silverstein. Gold had a long history of undergoing torturous psychiatric treatment in a bid to cure him of his homosexuality, and he talked openly about the negative effects this had on him. There had been no plans to revise the DSM until 1978. However, Gold implored the committee to revise it immediately and thereby bring 'to pass a more enlightened medical and social climate'.[80] Silverstein was a PhD student in psychology and knew that if he was going to convince the APA to revise the diagnosis of homosexuality he needed to make an articulate argument that displayed an understanding of systems and classifications. He read the committee a long statement that surveyed the work of Kinsey and Hooker and quoted Freud's sympathetic letter to an American mother regarding her son's homosexuality.[81] Byer argues that while the committee was moved by Gold's narrative, it was Silverstein's calm and professional appeal that impressed them most. They agreed to hold a debate at the APA convention in Hawaii later that year.[82]

The debate, entitled 'Should Homosexuality be in the APA Nomenclature?' found that the panel members were broadly in favour that homosexuality should be included on the agenda for discussion in the nomenclature. Indeed, the debate inspired Robert

Spitzer, a Columbia University psychoanalyst, to join the fight against the sickness diagnosis.[83] Spitzer analysed the DSM to uncover something common to pathologies that did not apply to homosexuality. He found that people who suffered from most disorders listed in the DSM usually experienced serious distress or their conditions interfered with their overall functioning. He submitted a report to the Nomenclature Committee arguing that while homosexuality might not fall within the 'normal' range of sexual behaviour, it did not impair social effectiveness. He argued that for behaviour to be listed as a psychiatric disorder, it had to be accompanied by subjective distress and/or 'some generalized impairment in social effectiveness or functioning'. He also made reference to Hooker's study comparing functioning levels of homosexuals and heterosexuals and concluded that since general functioning was not necessarily impaired, homosexuals could not be diagnosed as having a disorder.[84]

Nevertheless, the Nomenclature Committee was divided on Spitzer's report and the proposed revision of the DSM to remove homosexuality. To avoid further debate, the committee passed the issue to the Council on Research and Development, who advised the APA on matters of policy. The Council approved Spitzer's proposal, as its policy was to accept the advice of the experts on the sub-committees. However, Eisenbach argues that it is possible that the council failed to notice that Spitzer was not an 'expert' on homosexuality.[85] The debate regarding the removal of homosexuality as a diagnosis was then moved to the Assembly of District Branches, and then to the Reference Committee, and finally it reached the APA board of trustees.

On 15 December 1973, the APA board of trustees voted unanimously to remove homosexuality from the DSM, and the following year, the seventh printing of the DSM version II excluded homosexuality as a diagnosable illness.[86] Homosexuals were no longer considered mentally ill by the APA, and their DSM was widely used in the UK. Ron Gold summed up their decision, simply saying, 'We've won!'[87] The media were keen to report this decision and ran front-page headlines such as The New York Times' 'Psychiatrists in a Shift. Declare Homosexuality no Mental Illness.'[88] Meanwhile, in mock relief, the Gay Community News announced: 'It's Official Now: We're Not Sick.'[89]

Eisenbach argues that the removal of homosexuality from the DSM was based on science and politics. He notes that Spitzer wanted to help fight the social problem of homosexual discrimination by finding a scientific argument for the revision. However, his argument that a condition had to impair general functioning was flawed. Eisenbach posits that if, as Spitzer argued, a condition had to impair general functioning or cause great distress to be considered a disorder, then paedophilia, for example, would have not been considered a mental illness.[90] Nevertheless, Bayer argues that while the revision of the DSM did not 'launch an unrestrained march toward social acceptance of homosexuality; it did move the power of "the experts" to the side of the gay rights movement.'[91]

Nurse therapists

Not only were there changes and developments in the ways that homosexuals were viewed by society, psychiatry and the law during this period: the profession of mental nursing was also experiencing changes and developments. Younger nurses starting out in the late 1960s and early 1970s were exposed to the social changes discussed above, and Nolan argues that this prepared them to challenge older nurses about their attitudes towards patients and staff.[92]

In parallel with the wider society, nurses were beginning to question a culture which required them and patients to conform to institutional norms. Nevertheless, these nurses found that there was an enormous resistance to change and senior nurses were reluctant to disrupt the 'status quo' by backing younger staff against more experienced staff, even when cruelty to patients was an issue.[93] Indeed, Hopton argues that many of the asylum type practices were present in mental hospitals until well into the 1970s.[94] The tide was beginning to turn, however.

The 1960s witnessed the era of public inquiries into mental health care. Most of these inquiries were instigated by nurses writing letters to various prominent figures regarding patient care.[95] One of these letters, which was published in *The Times* on 10 November 1963, was of significant importance and it was signed by ten individuals:

We, the undersigned, have been shocked by the treatment of geriatric patients in certain mental hospitals, one of the evils being the practice of stripping them of their personal possessions. We have now sufficient evidence to suggest that this is widespread . . . We shall be grateful if those who have encountered malpractices in this sphere will supply us with detailed information, which would of course be treated as confidential.[96]

The contents of the letters received by ten signatories became the basis of a book entitled *Sans Everything: A Case to Answer*.[97] The book noted the degrading misery of the older adult in hospitals and demonstrated that, with only minimal effort, their circumstances could be positively changed. Nolan argues that many claimed that the book was exaggerated. However, it was highly persuasive and prompted closer scrutiny of the treatment of other vulnerable groups in care, including the mentally ill.[98] It also broke the tradition of secrecy in mental hospitals, as other nursing staff started to come forward condemning the treatment of patients in mental hospitals.

The 1969 Ely Hospital Inquiry report[99] was instigated by a letter sent to the *News of the World* from a nursing auxiliary, which was subsequently forwarded to the Health Minister.[100] The Ely Report delineated cruelty to patients, pilfering of food and the unresponsiveness of senior nursing management, medical staff and the Physician Superintendent to reports of malpractice, at Ely Hospital, Cardiff.[101] More findings, some more severe, were also made during inquiries at other hospitals.[102] Moreover, many of the subsequent reports that were published from these inquiries revealed that nurses in mental hospitals were unable to either recognise, or act on, gross deficiencies in the care of their patients.

In a possible response to this escalating crisis, The Department of Health and Social Security published its paper entitled *Psychiatric Nursing Today and Tomorrow* in 1968. The paper posited that the patient is 'an active participant and not a passive object for the exercise of medical skill' and went on to advocate that 'the nurse is the key therapeutic figure'.[103] Chatterton argues that this document instigated a cultural change within mental nursing, and the title of 'mental nurse' was replaced by the term 'psychiatric nurse'.[104]

During the 1970s, psychiatric nurses started to analyse their skills by undertaking their own studies into psychiatric nursing.[105] Key researchers during this period were Annie Altschul and David Towell, who proposed that nurses were not skilled in establishing and maintaining therapeutic interpersonal relationships with patients, and argued that they had no theoretical basis on which to stand when caring for mental patients.[106] They suggested that the root cause was a problem with nurse education, which they found to still be institutionalised, with minimal opportunities for innovation. Moreover, according to Nolan, the work of these researchers stimulated wide-ranging discussions and closer examination of nursing practices.[107]

A pioneering development during the 1970s was the introduction of the nurse therapist. These nurses autonomously practised adult behavioural psychotherapy for a range of clinical problems likely to respond to brief behavioural psychotherapy: one such problem was sexual deviation. Charlie Brooker argues that nurse therapists were agents to effect lasting change in patients, and allowed psychiatrists to fulfil other roles for which they were trained, including being consultants, researchers and teachers.[108]

This dynamic new role was initiated for several reasons, including pressure of demand for services, which according to Geoff Russell had far outstripped supply. Russell went on to argue that the bulk of psychiatric patients could no longer expect to have a psychiatrist as their main therapist.[109] There were also pressures to economise, as medical training up to finals, according to the *Observer* on the 24 July 1977, cost approximately £40,000, which was fifteen times the average national per capita income. Nurse training was £4,400, which was less than twice the average national per capita income.[110] Coupled with salary differences on graduation, the government was naturally interested in using non-medical staff to satisfy the demand for therapists. Finally, there was pressure from dissatisfied nurses, who felt that many traditional nursing roles had been taken over by social workers, occupational therapists and domestic supervisors.[111] Junior nurses often perceived their role as little more than issuing medicines and being vaguely supportive, while senior nurses, since the Salmon Report,[112] felt generally confined to administration or teaching and many felt as frustrated as their juniors.[113]

Selection for nurse therapy courses was rigorous. All potential trainees had to have as a minimum qualification the RMN certificate. Applicants also had to attend an interview and had to demonstrate:

A desire to work in behavioural therapy, initiative, capability of working increasingly independently with adult neurotic patients and an ability to earn the respect of colleagues in other health care professions.[114]

It is arguable, from the last requisite, 'an ability to earn the respect of colleagues in other health care professions', that people involved in developing the role foresaw that this new position might cause conflict with other health care professions. They were right. The main opposition came from clinical psychologists, who preferred to restrict behavioural work to their own discipline. The nurse therapist was unwelcome to them, as they viewed these nurses as medically orientated, academically naive and a block towards clinical psychologists working autonomously.[115] Ida Ashley reflects on this strained working relationship:

> We had to have a fairly thick skin at times, particularly in relation to psychologists' attitude towards us. Many were not happy about our new role and some had a distinct lack of respect for us. I believe they did not perceive us to be 'level' with themselves in relation to educational status. Nevertheless, without 'bigging' ourselves up, we were a very intelligent, resilient and tenacious group of nurses. The selection and training we underwent was rigorous and I feel that the innovators of our role were aware of the challenges we were likely to face and selected and trained us with this in mind.[116]

The training course was eighteen months in duration, of which twelve months were given to intensive training at the training centre and six months to placement at a general practice, a health centre or another hospital. The teacher–trainee ratio was approximately 1:3. The syllabus included interview skills, with emphasis on the behavioural analysis of patients' problems and subsequent negotiation of appropriate treatment goals. According to Brooker, the importance of clinical documentation was reiterated throughout the course, especially where communication with other professionals was necessary.[117] Again, this could be interpreted as a tacit apprehension the nurses had towards other members of the health care team. Trainees were also taught how to apply a wide range of specific behavioural techniques and essentially to recognise the limits of their own competence. The training methods were wide ranging and included the use of closed circuit television monitoring and feedback, clinical demonstrations, seminars, lectures and reviews.

The nurse therapists' worth was demonstrated in the treatment of sexually deviant patients. Peter Lindley discussed his practice as a nurse therapist treating 'sexual deviation in a young man' in the *Nursing Mirror* in 1975, stating that he was responsible for prescribing and administering electrical aversion therapy for a young man with homosexual desires. Lindley summarised that the patient had improved, as his 'homosexual desires had diminished'.[118] In 1977, Isaac Marks, Julian Bird and Peter Lindley found that for the ten patients who completed treatment for their sexual deviation with a nurse therapist, the frequency of the patients' sexually deviant behaviour diminished, and they concluded that nurse therapists thus produced useful improvement in patients with sexual disorders. The paper, however, fails to comment on the small sample size and the self-reported nature of the findings: as shown in Chapter 1, many patients were able to subvert their health care professionals by feigning heterosexuality or repulsion with their transvestism. Furthermore, there are no follow-up findings on these patients.[119] Moreover, Neil McConaghy, a psychiatrist, concluded in 1976 in *The British Journal of Psychiatry* that aversion therapies would appear not to have altered the patients' pre-existing sexual orientation and the practitioners involved did not consider the significant damage wrought by these treatments.[120] The nurse therapists were claiming to be successful in an already discredited area of care.

The nurse therapists, who worked in the latter part of the study period, considered themselves autonomous practitioners: 'We had a lot of autonomy and could make decisions about and prescribe treatment of our own accord.'[121] Furthermore, it appears that these nurses were also following the 'nursing process'[122] and were responsible for assessing, planning, implementing and evaluating the treatment for patients in their care. This can be demonstrated in a number of primary manuscript sources, available in *Nursing in Behavioural Psychotherapy: An Advanced Clinical Role for Nurses* (1977), a book published by the Royal College of Nursing, which traces the development of this advanced practice role.[123] This book contains an assessment tool entitled 'The Guide to Sexual History', which the nurse therapists used to assess their patients' sexual history.[124] In a 'Treatment Plan and Progress Summary' the nurse therapist has developed a care plan with treatment formulations and aims for a patient with a diagnosis of 'homosexuality'.[125] Finally, it also appears that the nurses evaluated the efficacy of the treatment they were implementing. In the 'Nurse-Therapist's Letter to the General Practitioner at One Month Follow Up', the nurse states:

> Throughout the course of the treatment he [the patient] was able to report a lessening in intensity and frequency of urges to indulge in homosexual activity, until he was no longer troubled by these thoughts or desires ... When seen recently at a one-month follow-up interview his progress had been maintained.[126]

The training the nurse therapists received equipped them with a theoretical basis on which to stand when treating their patients, which was in broad contrast to other nurses in this book, especially the SENs. The nurse therapists also identified the importance of developing a therapeutic relationship with patients in their care. Indeed, nurse therapist Peter Lindley considered:

> It essential to establish a very good working relationship with 'John'. Our first three sessions were spent chatting about his problem in order to arrive at a clear picture of his situation.[127]

Once again this is in contrast to other nurses in this study, as Gilbert Davies, who nursed patients receiving chemical aversion therapy in the early 1960s, remarked: 'We didn't have to talk to 'em [sic]. If he was emotionally distressed it still went on.'[128] However, despite this new found education, the evidence base for aversion therapy to treat sexual deviation was still very limited. The nurse therapists were still doing something quite spurious, as the efficacy of the treatments they were implementing still relied on self-reported outcomes from the patient and had already been discredited by a psychiatrist in *The British Journal of Psychiatry*.[129]

It is impossible to measure whether the nurse therapists treated patients with any more humanity than psychiatrists had done. One psychiatrist from Michael King's study gave an interesting reflection regarding nurse therapists' attitudes towards electrical aversion therapy:

> It was the nurses who actually gave the aversion therapy ... The nurse would sit in another room when the treatment was taking place. I can't

remember now whether they had a one-way mirror or something like that. I was surprised that the nursing staff didn't feel more strongly because one hears of nursing staff having conscientious objections to termination of pregnancy or even sometimes giving ECT. It surprises me that they didn't say: 'I don't want to do this treatment'. There was some sort of physical barrier between the nurse and the patient.[130]

Interestingly, this psychiatrist is directing the responsibility for administering aversion therapy on to the nurses, as they were the ones 'who actually gave' it.[131] In fact, one could argue that she perceived herself as working within a higher moralistic framework than the nurses, which is ironic given that she did not appear to voice any objections to these treatments at the time either. Moreover, Greta Gold gives an interesting reflection of a nurse therapist's attitude towards her when the nurse administered electrical aversion therapy to her: 'Tears began running down my face and the nurse said: "What are you crying for? We have only just started!" . . . [Chokes] . . . I was speechless.'[132] Therefore, some of these nurses may have been equally as antipathetic to their patients as the doctors. However, Ida Ashley remarked, 'The nurse therapists role was to provide support and reassurance. We would talk to them about their homosexuality and not just shock them as people often think.'[133]

During this period, community care had returned to the political agenda, and in 1975, the report entitled *Better Services for the Mentally Ill* was published.[134] The report evaluated the current state of psychiatric services and outlined a plan for future services. These included reducing overcrowding in hospitals by increasing the number of patients being treated in the community. The report also noted that staffing levels and community facilities at present were inadequate to properly support patients in the community. As it became increasingly apparent that community services were the way forward for mental health care, it was evident that nurses needed training to support them in making the transition from hospital to the community. This led to the development of the first course for Community Psychiatry Nurses (CPNs) at Chiswick College in the early 1970s and, analogous to the nurse therapists, CPNs were soon to gain recognition as autonomous practitioners. Moreover, by the 1970s nurses were acquiring specialist skills dealing with specialist groups, which was very much in contrast to their generalist work in mental hospitals.[135]

It is important to note that the majority of the papers discussing the work of nurse therapists with sexually deviant patients were published in the mid- to late 1970s. Interestingly, this was also after the APA removed homosexuality as a diagnosis in 1974. There are a number of explanations for this. Many of the patients discussed in these papers had a paedophilic or cross-dressing element to their sexual desires.[136] Owing to the obvious risk paedophiles may pose, such sexual desires remain classifiable as a mental disorder and, albeit not with aversion therapy in the majority of cases, treatments are still administered for these individuals.[137] In addition, despite education and liberalism regarding transvestism and transsexuals,[138] transvestism remains classifiable as a mental disorder.[139] Furthermore, before an individual can undergo gender reassignment surgery, he or she has to be diagnosed with the psychiatric diagnosis of Gender Dysphoria.[140] This could offer a context to explain why treatments for transvestism continued.

It is difficult to quantify the impact of the APA's decision to remove homosexuality from its DSM on homosexual men and nurses in the UK. King argues that the decision did have some impact in the UK, and highlights that the treatments appeared to peter out in parallel with the growing profile of gay liberation.[141] Furthermore, ironically, just as the media appears to have had a positive impact in promoting these treatments, they also appear to have supported their curtailment.

In 1970, former nurse Claire Rayner wrote an article in the *Daily Mail* entitled: 'Should Shame be the Cure?' She argued that doctors were unjust in their use of chemical aversion therapy as it stripped patients of their dignity and inflicted pain and shame on them.[142] The *Glasgow Daily Record* ran an article entitled: 'Doctors are the "Problem" Men.'[143] The article stated that homosexuals are more at risk from medicine than from the law. In 1971 *The Sunday Times* ran an article entitled: 'Fears Over Aversion Therapy Grow: Using Shock Tactics to Bend the Mind.'[144] The article by Peter Pringle describes a homosexual patient who suffered a heart attack while receiving electrical aversion therapy. It also includes excerpts from Dr Reginald Beech, Consultant Psychologist at Nerthern Hospital, UK. In 1968,

PSYCHOLOGY

Fears over aversion therapy grow:

Using shock tactics to bend the mind

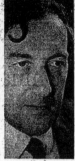

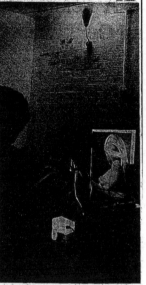

ROBERT JOHN used to drink two bottles of whisky a day to give him enough courage to pick up men in pubs and live as a homosexual in a sleepy London suburb. But alcohol began slowing down his reactions and affecting his memory. Mr John desperately wanted help.

A London psychiatrist said he could treat him. The medicine was aversion therapy—a highly controversial method of punishing the patient to change his behaviour. Alcoholics are made to vomit violently while sipping their favourite drink; homosexuals are given electric shocks while looking at pictures of male nudes, and tobacco addicts have smoke blown in their faces for hours at a time.

The efficacy of this somewhat crude therapy has always been questioned and now an increasing number of doctors will not use it. But Mr John was apparently thought to be a suitable case for treatment. His psychiatrist never imagined that his efforts to salvage his life would very nearly kill him.

First the alcoholism. At each of 15 sessions Mr John was given an injection to make him feel nauseous, then a pint of salt water followed by his favourite drink whisky. He could then have any other drinks he fancied from beer to a liqueur. When the vomiting started it was prolonged and painful.

At the end of three weeks his craving for alcohol ceased. But his homosexual feelings were not affected and Mr John feared that if he did nothing about them he would take to the bottle again.

He asked the psychiatrist if aversion therapy could make him a heterosexual. At home there was considerable pressure on him to get married and have children, and he well liked the idea.

There was no definite answer since aversion therapy is still only regarded as an experimental cure. Nevertheless he decided to try it.

He had five sessions in four days each lasting about half an hour. The process is simple and extremely unpleasant. The patient sits in a darkened room in front of a screen on to which are projected "homosexual" pictures of male nudes interspersed with an occasional nude female. The patient controls the projector and if he lingers too long on the male pictures he is given an electric shock in the arms and legs. He can look at the female pictures for as long as he likes.

At the end of the fifth session Mr John could not get out of his seat. His arms and legs were like lead weights. He had suffered a heart attack and spent the next

'Dr Beech: I can't imagine any Iron Curtain country has ever inflicted on captured spies the kind of treatment which may be handed out during electrical aversion. It is far too unpleasant.'

10 weeks in bed. During the treatment (at the end of last year) he lost three stones—from 11 to eight, which he still weighs. It is hard to take for a man of 6ft 1in.

It is this kind of horrific, albeit isolated, example of the unexpected side effects of aversion therapy (Mr John's heart passed all the necessary tests before the treatment) that is gradually turning doctors away from it. It is also the reason why fewer homosexuals are agreeing to undergo it as the activities of homosexual reform groups like the Albany Trust, the Committee for Homosexual Equality and the vociferous Gay Liberation Front have quickly spread the word.

But there is also an increasing amount of clinical data which shows that the treatment is more often a failure than a success.

In one experiment published in America 4,000 cases of

alcoholism were treated. Fifty per cent of the patients did not touch alcohol for up to five years but this figure dropped to 13 per cent at the end of 10 to 15 years. Some experiments have even showed an 80 per cent relapse rate after a few weeks. The success rate for sexual offenders appears to be directly dependent on the motivation. For example, those sent for treatment by the courts do not, as a rule, make good patients, because they are forced into it.

But perhaps most important are the doses of the drugs and the strength of the electric shocks used to create the aversion. It has been found that different doses and different strengths are needed for each patient and therefore there are no guidelines. Furthermore, there are two schools of thought on the electric treatment. One says that a lot of medium shocks below the "terror level" work and another advocates large shocks over a short period.

The "after-care" treatment also causes concern. One psychologist admitted that the "after care" for electric aversion, a portable self-shocker unit carried by the patient who gives himself a shock whenever he feels the urge to return to his previous behaviour, could create a masochistic tendency. "We just don't know what kind of monsters we're producing," said the doctor.

So what are the alternatives? Current research has returned to Pavlov, the classical behaviour therapist of the 1920's. He taught his dogs to salivate at the ring of a bell because they associated the bell with food. A painless experiment.

In a current experiment a group of psychologists found that after only one hour, they could get a sexual response from looking at a screened picture of an old boot when it was continually followed by a series of sexy pin-ups.

Using the same basic thesis Dr Reginald Beech, a consultant psychologist, was able to woo a paedophiliac off his desire for little girls. Put simply, a picture of a mature female body was followed by a series of immature female bodies to which, of course, the patient had an immediate sexual response. Eventually, on the Pavlovian theory, he was getting a sexual response from the mature body and at the end of the course experienced a satisfactory mature heterosexual act.

Apart from its obvious unpleasantness the use of aversion therapy for homosexuals has raised the inevitable ethical outcries of whether homosexual

behaviour can be cured. Michael De-la-Noy, director of the Albany Trust, says: "For homosexuals, the homosexual condition is basically as 'normal' and irreversible as heterosexuality is for heterosexuals.

"Homosexuals who seek aversion therapy or who are advised to undergo it would be far better served by sympathetic help to become happy, well-adjusted homosexuals."

In fact there is strong evidence that many homosexuals suffer from a condition referred to as heterophobia—or fear of the opposite sex. To treat them by electric aversion therapy would in effect be to frighten an already scared man. For these cases another technique is in use. The patient is first given a muscle relaxant and then with the help of a doctor "talked through" a heterosexual act. The prospects

for permanent removal of phobias after several such sessions are apparently promising.

But for the moment its use continues at several hospitals and clinics throughout this country. Dr Beech, in his book, Changing Man's Behaviour, says of the treatment: "The techniques of aversion therapy are likely to have considerable appeal to the more strict and authoritarian members of society who may feel such methods to be entirely suitable for application to deviant and little-understood behaviour."

He wrote that three years ago. Last week he said: "I can't imagine any Iron Curtain country has ever inflicted on captured spies the kind of treatment which may be handed out during electrical aversion. It is far too unpleasant."

Peter Pringle

Grim decor for one male patient undergoing the cure

10 *Sunday Times* 'Fears Over Aversion Therapy Grow: Using Shock Tactics to Bend the Mind'

he advocated in his book, *Changing Men's Behaviour*, that electrical aversion therapy was 'entirely suitable for application to deviant and little-understood behaviour'. Nevertheless, Beech admits in *The Sunday Times* article that, on reflection, this intervention was inappropriate: 'I can't imagine any Iron Curtain country has ever inflicted on captured spies the kind of treatment which may be handed out during electrical aversion. It is far too unpleasant'.

Claudine de Valois recalls the influence the press had on her perceptions of the treatments she had administered for sexual deviations:

> I remember in the 1970s that the press started to change direction in regard to their views on these treatments. Historically they had promoted them now they were condemning them. I had already started to feel guilty about the treatments I had given in the 1960s, but reading these articles in the media really confirmed to me that the treatments were wrong.[145]

Meanwhile, Ida Ashley recalls the influence that gay liberation appeared to have on these treatments:

> On reflection, I think the greater acceptance and understanding that gay liberation created, in the end, had a lot more impact in decreasing the number of referrals I received. [. . .] Nurses, myself included, were beginning to see homosexuals as no different from any other individual.[146]

Arguably, the new found radicalism of gay liberation and shifts and changes within the media were a lot more influential in curtailing these treatments than the APA's decision. They also appeared to influence the nurses' views that using aversion therapy to cure homosexuality was inappropriate. Nevertheless, despite liberalism and education about transvestites and transsexuals, which allowed these individuals to be more broadly accepted by society, they did not appear to have the same medical liberalism as homosexuals. These individuals still remain open to psychiatric diagnosis and evaluation.

In spite of the APA's decision to drop the term homosexuality as a diagnosis, it is important to note that the World Health Organization (WHO) did not follow suit until 1990. The term was eventually removed from their diagnostic manual in 1992 with the introduction of the *International Classification of Diseases Edition 10 Classification of Mental and Behavioural Disorders* (ICD-10).[147] Nevertheless, none of the participants in this study stated that they received treatments after 1974. There is a dearth of literature describing these treatments for purely homosexual desires after 1974, and the treatments appeared to peter out in the mid- to late 1970s.[148]

Conclusion

This chapter has explored the assertive journey to gay liberation. While the new 1967 Act essentially legalised homosexual sex between consenting men, the many restrictions within the new legislation meant that many homosexual men were still open to social exclusion, legal proceedings and medical treatments. For the men who did not express their sexuality through coupledom and domesticity, prosecution continued. This led to their being offered the option of imprisonment or remand provided they were willing to undergo psychological treatment, and as this book has demonstrated, many chose the latter.

During this period wider society was also beginning to change. In the western world, individuals were beginning to question the definitions of 'difference'. In parallel to these changes, gay men and women were starting to unite and promote sexual and subcultural difference as positive and life enhancing as gay liberation emerged – individuals were actively and vocally refuting the sickness label and the treatment that had come to accompany it. The media were starting to become more accepting of sexual difference during this period and ran headlines questioning the efficacy of medical treatments for homosexuality. This new found gay assertion and change in direction from the media appeared to have a positive effect on some of the nurses in this book, as they began to view the treatments they administered as inappropriate as ideas of deviance shifted. Moreover, while the APA decided to remove homosexuality from its DSM in 1973, it appears to have been the impact of gay liberation and shifts and changes on the part of the media that essentially led to the curtailment of aversion therapy to cure homosexuality.

During this period, nurses working in psychogeriatric care began to question practices, which led to a number of public investigations. These investigations were also seen to spread to the rest of mental health care as the plight of the mentally ill and their conditions of treatment and care became a public issue. Community care was now back in the political mainstream and new roles were created, including advanced practice roles such as the CPN and nurse therapist. In contrast to the nurses who cared for patients receiving treatments for sexual deviations in the earlier part of the study, these advanced practice nurses appeared to have a theoretical basis upon which to stand when treating their patients. Nevertheless, although nurse therapists believed they had a scientific foundation for their work, they were still administering a spurious intervention, as the treatment's efficacy still relied on self-reported outcomes from the patient. Furthermore, ironically, these nurses were claiming success in an area of care that had already been discredited.

Notes

1 The Hall Carpenter Archives (HCA), London School of Economics, HCA/EPHEMERA/1148, Letter from the West London Gay Liberation Front's Anti-Psychiatry Group to a local GP about treatment of homosexuality in 1972.
2 Men in Scotland, Northern Ireland, Guernsey, Jersey and the Isle of Man had to wait until 1980, 1982, 1983, 1990 and 1993 respectively.
3 As with the rest of the book, the terms 'gay' and 'homosexual' are used interchangeably throughout this chapter. However, in keeping with the terminology used during the period, the term 'gay' is used more frequently.
4 Jivani, *It's Not Unusual*, p. 141.
5 See, e.g., HCA/Grey Papers/1/2 (a) Sexual Offences: records relating to actions on homosexual law reform from the Departmental Committee on Homosexuality and Prostitution; HCA/GREY Grey Papers.
6 Jivani, *It's Not Unusual*, p. 138.
7 Cook, *A Gay History of Britain*, p. 175; See also HCA/GREY material relating to the HLRS, 1958–1984; HCA/GREY/1/2 HLRS Executive Committee: agendas and minutes.
8 Jivani, *It's Not Unusual*, p. 141.
9 Dominic Sandbrook, *White Heat: A History of Britain in the Swinging Sixties* (London, 2006).
10 Cook, *A Gay History of Britain*, p. 169.
11 The Summer of Love was a social phenomenon that occurred during the summer of 1967. Individuals began experimenting with different lifestyles, which included communal living and the sharing of resources often with total strangers. It has been seen as a defining moment of the 1960s, as the hippie movement came into public awareness.
12 Cook, *A Gay History of Britain*, p. 185.
13 Jivani, *It's Not Unusual*, p. 141.
14 Weeks, *The World We Have Won*, p. 67; Cook, *A Gay History of Britain*, p. 176.
15 See, e.g., Ryan Powell, 'Man Country: A Social History of 70s Gay Cinema' (unpublished PhD thesis University College, London, 2010).
16 Between 1958, when Parliament first debated Wolfenden's recommendations, and 1967, when the law was finally changed, the issue was raised in Parliament six times before the seventh attempt was successful and went on to its second readings.

17 For example, the definition of 'private' was such that a locked hotel room was deemed to be a public place: therefore, two men in such a situation could still be prosecuted. See, e.g., Higgins, *Heterosexual Dictatorship*.

18 Jeffery-Poulter, *Peers, Queers & Commons*, p. 94.

19 Jivani, *It's Not Unusual*, p. 153.

20 HCA/CHE/9/46 Police Harassment Working Party correspondence and papers on cottaging (seeking and engaging in sexual acts in public toilets); Cook, *A Gay History of Britain*, p. 177.

21 Houlbrook, *Queer London*, p. 254.

22 Tim Newburn, *Permission and Regulation: Law and Morals in Post-War Britain* (London, 1992), p. 62.

23 See, e.g., Lisa Power, *No Bath But Plenty of Bubbles: Stories from the London Gay Liberation Front, 1970–73* (London, 1995).

24 The Stonewall riots were a number of unprompted, violent demonstrations against a police raid that took place in the early morning hours of 28 June 1969, at the Stonewall Inn, in the Greenwich Village neighbourhood of New York City. They are often cited as the first instance in American history when people in the homosexual community retaliated against and challenged a government-backed system that discriminated against sexual minorities. Eisenbach argues that they have become the defining event that marked the start of the gay rights movement in the USA and around the world. See, e.g., David Eisenbach, *Gay Power: An American Revolution* (New York, 2006), pp. 80–115.

25 See, e.g., HCA/EPHEMERA/1148 West London Gay Liberation Front; Cook, *A Gay History of Britain*, p. 180.

26 Cook, *A Gay History of Britain*, p. 180.

27 Jivani, *It's Not Unusual*, p. 201.

28 Oscar Mangle, interviewed 21 June 2010.

29 Davidson, *And Thus Will I Freely Sing*, p 110; Cook, *A Gay History of Britain*, p. 187.

30 Jeffery-Poulter, *Peers, Queers & Commons*, p. 106; HCA/EPHEMERA/1148 West London Gay Liberation Front.

31 Power, *No Bath But Plenty of Bubbles*, p. 87.

32 Jones, *Tales from Out in the City*, p. 106.

33 Jivani, *It's Not Unusual*, p. 181.

34 Cook, *A Gay History of Britain*, p. 183.

35 Peter Dennis, *Daring Hearts: Lesbian and Gay Lives in 50s and 60s Brighton* (Brighton, 1992), p. 37.

36 See, e.g., Powell, *Man Country*.

37 Weeks, *Coming Out*, p. 228; Jivani, *It's Not Unusual*, pp. 181–182.

38 Cook, *A Gay History of Britain*, p. 191.

39 See, e.g., HCA/ALBANY TRUST/16/61 National Council for Civil Liberties

Report 8: Homosexuality and the Teaching Profession, August 1975; Cook, *A Gay History of Britain*, p. 191.

40 Cook, *A Gay History of Britain*, p. 191.

41 Ida Ashley, interviewed 17 July 2010.

42 Ackroyd, *Dressing Up*, 17.

43 Prebble, '*Ordinary Men and Uncommon Women*', p. 193.

44 'Counter-psychiatry' and 'anti-psychiatry' are used interchangeably.

45 Nick Crossley, 'R. D. Laing and The British Anti-Psychiatry Movement: A Socio-Historical Analysis', *Social Science Medical* 47 (7) (1998), p. 878.

46 Crossley, 'R. D. Laing', p. 879.

47 Erving Goffman, *Asylums* (New York, 1961).

48 See, e.g., Thomas S. Szasz, *The Myth of Mental Illness: Foundations of Theory and Personal Conduct* (New York, 1961).

49 Nolan, *A History of Mental Health Nursing*, p. 124.

50 See, e.g., Ronald David Laing, *Sanity, Madness and the Family* (London, 1964).

51 Crossley, 'R. D. Laing', p. 879.

52 See, e.g., Laing, *Sanity, Madness and the Family*.

53 Therapeutic communities aimed to establish a more self-governing, patient-led form of therapeutic milieu environment. They tried to avoid the controlling and demeaning practices of many psychiatric institutions of the time. The central philosophy was that patients were active participants in their own and each other's mental health care and that responsibility for the daily running of the community was shared among the clients and the staff. See, e.g., Maxwell Jones, *Social Psychiatry in Practice: The Idea of a Therapeutic Community* (Harmondsworth, 1968); David Cooper, *Psychiatry and Anti-Psychiatry* (London, 1967); Crossley, 'R. D. Laing', p. 885.

54 The play is a farce and revolves around an unprofessional psychiatrist – Dr Prentice – attempting to seduce his attractive prospective secretary: Alan Sinfield, *Out on Stage: Lesbian and Gay Theatre in the Twentieth Century* (New Haven, 1999), p. 271.

55 Ivan Illich, *Medical Nemesis: The Expropriation of Health* (London, 1976), p. 3.

56 Illich, *Medical Nemesis*, p. 4.

57 Evelyn Hooker, 'Male Homosexuality in the Rorschach', *Journal of Projective Techniques* 21 (1957), pp. 18–31.

58 Eisenbach, *Gay Power*, p. 229.

59 Eisenbach, *Gay Power*, p. 231.

60 'The Changing View of Homosexuality', *The New York Times* (28 February 1971).

61 Zaps were public confrontations of individuals (mainly politicians) or organisations, aimed at forcing the recipients to address the issue of homosexuality and gay rights. Eisenbach argues that they not only accomplished

the political feat of forcing individuals to address the issue of homosexuality, but they also enabled participants to feel a sense of power – 'gay power': Eisenbach, *Gay Power*, pp. 130–131.

62 Henry Minton, *Departing from Deviance* (Chicago, 2002), p. 254; John D'Emilio, *Sexual Politics, Sexual Communities* (Chicago, 1998), p. 216.

63 Dudley Clendinen and Adam Nagourney, *Out for Good: The Struggle to Build a Gay Rights Movement in America* (New York, 1999), pp. 201–203.

64 'Gays and Dolls Battle the Shrinks', *Washington Post* (15 May 1970).

65 Eisenbach, *Gay Power*, p. 232.

66 Minton, *Departing from Deviance*, p. 255; Eisenbach, *Gay Power*, p. 232.

67 Drescher and Merlino, *American Psychiatry and Homosexuality*, p. 43.

68 Bayer, *Homosexuality and American Psychiatry*, pp. 103–105.

69 Eisenbach, *Gay Power*, p. 233.

70 Drescher and Merlino, *American Psychiatry and Homosexuality*, p. xvii; Eisenbach argues, however, that gays were able to quietly enter the profession and flourish. Indeed, at the annual APA conventions, dozens of 'closeted' homosexual psychiatrists gathered together in gay bars to convene what they jokingly referred to as the GAY-PA: Eisenbach, *Gay Power*, p. 233.

71 Bayer, *Homosexuality and American Psychiatry*, pp. 57–58; Eisenbach, *Gay Power*, p. 233.

72 Drescher and Merlino, *American Psychiatry and Homosexuality*, pp. 17–18.

73 Alvarez, *Homosexuality*, p. 216; Eisenbach, *Gay Power*, p. 234.

74 Eisenbach, *Gay Power*, pp. 234–345.

75 Drescher and Merlino, *American Psychiatry and Homosexuality*, p. 121; Eisenbach, *Gay Power*, p. 235.

76 The Anti-Psychiatry Group's work is demonstrated in the letter at the beginning of this chapter. See, also HCA/EPHEMERA/1148 West London Gay Liberation Front interim statement 'the Counter Psychiatry Group of the GLF'; Cook, *A Gay History of Britain*, p. 180.

77 The Albany Trust was a UK registered charity founded in May 1958. The Trust worked in collaboration with the Homosexual Law Reform Society and eventually developed into an innovative counselling organisation for gay men, lesbians and sexual minorities: See, e.g., HCA/ALBANY TRUST/10.

78 See, e.g., HCA/ALBANY TRUST/10/4 Malik Survey on psychosexual treatment. Completed questionnaires on psychiatric facilities for homosexuals in the London area; HCA/ALBANY TRUST/10/6 Eva Bene survey regarding use of medical and psychiatry treatment.

79 'Aversion Therapy Is Like A Visit To The Dentist', *Gay News* 11 (1972).

80 Bayer, *Homosexuality and American Psychiatry*, p. 119.

81 See the Introduction of this book for a copy of Freud's letter; Eisenbach, *Gay Power*, p. 238.

82 Bayer, *Homosexuality and American Psychiatry*, p. 120.
83 Eisenbach, *Gay Power*, p. 240.
84 Clendinen and Nagourney, *Out for Good*, p. 217; Eisenbach, *Gay Power*, p. 241.
85 Eisenbach, *Gay Power*, p. 242.
86 American Psychiatric Association, *Seventh Printing Diagnostic Statistical Manual Version II* (Arlington, 1974).
87 Eisenbach, *Gay Power*, p. 247.
88 'Psychiatrists in a Shift. Declare Homosexuality no Mental Illness' *The New York Times* (16 December 1973).
89 'It's Official Now: We're Not Sick', *Gay Community News* (16 December 1973).
90 Eisenbach, *Gay Power*, pp. 241–242.
91 Bayer, *Homosexuality and American Psychiatry*, p. 157.
92 Nolan, *A History of Mental Health Nursing*, p. 133.
93 Brand, *Look Back*, p. 190.
94 Hopton, 'Prestwich Hospital in the Twentieth Century', p. 355.
95 Nolan, *A History of Mental Health Nursing*, p. 135.
96 *The Times* (10 November 1963).
97 Barbara Robb, *Sans Everything: A Case to Answer* (London, 1967). See, also Her Majesty's Stationery Office, Command 3687: *Findings and Recommendations Following Inquiries into Allegations Concerning the Care of Elderly Patients in Certain Hospitals* (London, 1968).
98 Nolan, *A History of Mental Health Nursing*, p. 135.
99 Her Majesty's Stationery Office, Command 3975: *Report of the Committee of Inquiry into Allegations of Ill-Treatment of Patients and other Irregularities at Ely Hospital Cardiff* (London, 1969).
100 Nolan, *A History of Mental Health Nursing*, p. 135.
101 Command 3975: *Report of Ely Hospital Cardiff*.
102 See, e.g., Beardshaw, *Conscientious Objectors*, pp. 84–88.
103 Department of Health and Social Security, *Psychiatric Nursing Today and Tomorrow* (London, 1968), pp. 45.
104 Chatterton, 'The Weakest Link in the Chain of Nursing?', p. 6.
105 Nolan, *A History of Mental Health Nursing*, p. 137.
106 Annie Altschul, *Patient–Nurse Interaction: A Study of Interactive Patterns in Acute Psychiatric Wards* (Edinburgh, 1972); David Towell, *Understanding Psychiatric Nursing* (London, 1975).
107 Nolan, *A History of Mental Health Nursing*, p. 137.
108 Charlie Brooker, 'Nurse Therapist Trainee Variability: The Implications for Selection and Training', *Journal of Advanced Nursing* 8 (1983), p. 322.
109 Geoff F. M. Russell, *Policy for Action* (London, 1973), p. 56.
110 'The True Cost of Training a Doctor', *Observer* (24 July 1977).
111 Royal College of Nursing, *New Horizons in Clinical Nursing* (London, 1976).

112 The Salmon Report on Nursing Management in 1966 was welcomed as a policy for psychiatric nurses. The report created a new role of 'Nursing Officer', which doubled the number of nurses in management roles. They played a key role in clinical supervision, management and personnel work. However, Nolan has posited that the role was never formally evaluated and, therefore, it is impossible to say what, if any, improvements were made to nursing practice with their introduction. They did, however, provide more opportunities for nurses to progress their careers and enter management positions: Nolan, *A History of Mental Health Nursing*, p. 134.

113 Julian Bird, Isaac Marks and Peter Lindley, 'Nurse Therapists in Psychiatry: Developments, Controversies and Implications', *British Journal of Psychiatry* 135 (1979), p. 321.

114 Brooker, 'Nurse Therapist Trainee Variability', p. 322.

115 Bird, Marks and Lindley, 'Nurse Therapists in Psychiatry', p. 328.

116 Ida Ashley, interviewed 17 July 2010.

117 Brooker, 'Nurse Therapist Trainee Variability', p. 322.

118 Lindley, 'Sexual Deviation in a Young Man', p. 63.

119 Marks, Bird & Lindley, 'Behavioral Nurse Therapists', p. 27.

120 Neil McConaghy, 'Is Homosexual Orientation Irreversible?', *British Journal of Psychiatry* 129 (1976), pp. 356–563.

121 Ida Ashley, interviewed 17 July 2010.

122 Nursing practice was first described as a four-stage (assess, plan, implement and evaluate) process: by Ida Jean Orlando in 1958.

123 Isaac M. Marks, 'Nursing in Behavioural Psychotherapy: An Advanced Clinical Role for Nurses', *Royal College of Nursing* (London, 1977).

124 Marks, 'Nursing in Behavioural Psychotherapy', Appendix A7.

125 Marks, 'Nursing in Behavioural Psychotherapy', p. 135.

126 Marks, 'Nursing in Behavioural Psychotherapy', p. 134.

127 Lindley, 'Sexual Deviation in a Young Man', p. 64.

128 Gilbert Davies, interviewed 10 February 2010.

129 McConaghy, 'Is Homosexual Orientation Irreversible?', pp. 356–563.

130 Female psychiatrist interviewed as part of a study by Michael King, *Doubts about the Treatments*, available at: www.treatmentshomosexuality.org.uk/index.php/en/narratives-en (last accessed 29 December 2011).

131 Michael King, *Doubts about the Treatments*.

132 Greta Gold, interviewed 24 March 2010.

133 Ida Ashley, interviewed 17 July 2010.

134 Department of Health and Social Security, *Better Services for the Mentally Ill*, Cmnd.6233 (London, 1975).

135 Nolan, *A History of Mental Health Nursing*, p. 137.

136 See, e.g., Lindley, 'Sexual Deviation in a Young Man', pp. 63–64; Marks, 'Nursing in Behavioural Psychotherapy', p. 133.

137 See, e.g., Ray Blanchard, 'The DSM Diagnostic Criteria for Paedophilia', *Archives of Sexual Behaviour*,16 (2009), pp. 1–11.

138 The Beaumont Society was formed in 1966. This is a support group based in the UK for transgendered people, and then as now it is important in terms of alternative configurations of support and non-medical models of explanations; see also HCA/EPHEMERA/568 Transsexual Action Organisation (TAO) 'Transsexual Information', two leaflets and one pamphlet by the TAO.

139 The current versions of the Diagnostic Statistical Manual and the International Classification of Diseases both classify transvestism as a mental disorder: 'Transvestic Fetishism' (DSM: 302.3) American Psychiatric Association, *Diagnostic Statistical Manual Version IV* (Washington, 1994) and 'Transvestism' (ICD: F64.1) World Health Organization, *The International Classification of Diseases Version 10 Classification of Mental and Behavioural Disorders* (Geneva, 1992).

140 NHS Choices available at: www.nhs.uk/Conditions/Genderdysphoria/ Pages/Introduction.aspx (last accessed 15 May 2012).

141 Michael King, 'Dropping the Diagnosis of Homosexuality: Did it Change the Lot of Gays and Lesbians in Britain?', *Australian and New Zealand Journal of Psychiatry* 37 (6) (2003), pp. 684–688.

142 'Should Shame Be The Cure?', *Daily Mail* (10 September 1970).

143 'Doctors are the "Problem" Men', *Glasgow Daily Record* (28 November 1974).

144 'Fears Over Aversion Therapy Grow: Using Shock Tactics to Bend the Mind', *The Sunday Times* (9 May 1971).

145 Claudine de Valois, interviewed 30 December 2009.

146 Ida Ashley, interviewed 17 July 2010.

147 World Health Organization, *The International Classification of Diseases version 10 Classification of Mental and Behavioural Disorders* (Geneva, 1992).

148 Smith, King and Bartlett, 'Treatments of Homosexuality in Britain Since the 1950s', p. 2.

Concluding remarks

It is fairly clear that the nurses in this study did not deliberately set out to inflict pain and distress on homosexuals and transvestites in their care. A variety of circumstantial factors provided momentum for the development and implementation of medical 'treatments' to 'cure' these individuals. The medicalisation of sexual deviation can be traced back to the late nineteenth century. However, World War II appears to have been a critical point in this medicalisation. In spite of the war exposing the British to different and more liberal sexual attitudes, this was also the period when the idea of homosexuality as a pathology was more universally adopted by psychiatrists in both Britain and the USA.

There appeared to be a cultural shift in the immediate post-war years urging the nation to return to pre-war values. This was marked by a growing emphasis on domesticity, 'traditional' family life and social order, with which it was believed that homosexual men were at odds. There was never any dedicated campaign by the police to target these individuals during the 1950s; however, arrests did increase.[1] This left homosexual men and transvestites living through this period fearful, hyper-vigilant and cautious of the police.

A crucial event during this period seems to have been the Montagu trial in 1954. This appeared to mark the nadir of the persecution of homosexual men in Britain and largely persuaded the liberal intelligentsia that something had to be done regarding the perceived 'problem' of homosexuality.[2] This led to the formation of the Wolfenden Committee in 1954. The committee reported in 1957 and recommended that homosexuality between consenting adults over the age of 21 should be decriminalised. A further recommendation was that medical treatments should be made available to homosexuals to cure them of their disorder – reinforcing the notion that homosexuality was the result of an ingrained condition, which could be cured.

Following Wolfenden there was a distinct altering of notions about homosexuality from a criminal perspective to understandings of the subject as pathology. This was coupled with what Chris Waters describes as the 'therapeutic state', based on the belief that experts, with their 'modern knowledge', could assist in the eradication of any number of social maladies.[3] In a two-pronged attempt to prove that their clinical practice was as socially useful as it was humane, psychiatrists began optimistically promoting their worth in being able to cure sexual deviation by reporting successful outcomes.[4] Indeed, for many men, discovering that there was a 'cure' for their disorder gave them a sense of hope and legitimacy.

By the late 1950s, homosexuality was brought into the public consciousness by media, literary, medical, sociological and legal discourses. These played a role in shaping public knowledge about who the sexual deviant was and what he represented. However, they were all portraying mixed messages with regard to sexual deviation, leaving the recipients very confused.[5] Moreover, along with the courts, these public, somewhat prejudicial discourses created a favourable social and political context for the treatments. They helped to shape unsympathetic family, police and social attitudes, which in turn tacitly coerced men into receiving treatment. These factors were an affront to the patient's autonomy because they reduced the degree of voluntariness on the part of the patient.

These mixed public discourses of sexual deviation also created uncertainty for the nurses in this study. The nurses were also exposed to a number of contextual factors in their clinical practice, which may have influenced their decision to administer aversion therapy to cure sexual deviations. The introduction of the Mental Treatment Act 1930 brought a wave of therapeutic optimism around the possibility of curative treatment for mental patients. This led to the introduction of new somatic treatments, which were rather brutal and distressing for those who received them.[6] Indeed, some nurses in this study also administered or witnessed these invasive somatic treatments, and their participation was influenced by psychiatrists' elementary justifications for them.

With the introduction of such treatments, some nurses took on more advanced roles. However, the vast majority had no theoretical underpinning for the interventions they were implementing. Essentially, nurses were unaware that what passed for treatment in their workplace might represent no more than the penchant of their particular medical superintendent, based on no firm evidence at all. Moreover, exposing nurses to these somatic treatments may have normalised the implementation of 'therapeutic' interventions, which caused distress to patients. This could offer a context to, at least in part, explain some nurses' acceptance that such disturbing interventions as aversion therapy were a normal, and morally acceptable, part of a larger venture that promised positive outcomes. In essence, the ends *could* justify the means.

The training the nurses received regarding sexual deviation promoted the notion that homosexuals and transvestites were deviants in need of psychiatric evaluation.[7] However, their training appears to have given little, if any, attention to equipping nursing students with the skills required to nurse these individuals, and the nurses in this book reported that they felt unprepared when they were admitted onto their wards. This was compounded by the wider debate regarding how to view the sexual deviant that was being promoted in the media and literary works. In short, nurses did not receive a training that was based on a coherent and robust knowledge regarding these individuals.

With the implementation of the Mental Health Act 1959, the emergence of rhetoric around community care, the introduction of new health and social care practitioners, and the reduction in patient numbers within mental hospitals, many nurses and psychiatrists felt their profession was under threat. In combination with the discourses concerning the lack of consensus on the optimal way to deal with the problem of sexual deviants, some psychiatrists – and nurses – may have developed and implemented treatments for the these individuals as a tacit way of bringing 'new' patients into the mental hospital. This could have been in a pragmatic and perhaps not even acknowledged attempt to protect their jobs and enhance their profile. It further marked out a specialism and a specialist discourse.

Although some nurses in this study sensed that there was something wrong in administering aversion therapy, their participation appears to have been encouraged and reinforced by specific informal, possibly deleterious, features of mental hospital life. The stresses of institutional life may have destabilised the individual initiative of mental nurses: insensitive staff discipline, fears of victimisation and the betrayal and abuse of colleagues and senior staff may have threatened the performance of even the most conscientious nurse. However, the most noteworthy feature within such institutions appears to have been the passive obedience of nurses to authority.

The nurses within this book are presented as if they were polar opposites. The reality was much more complex and it may be too simplistic to present them as either 'subordinate' or 'subversive'. It is unlikely that there was any malevolence underpinning their motivations to administer aversion therapy. Arguably, the subordinate nurses in this study who carried out the treatment fall into three categories (in so far as it is possible to categorise).

Some subordinate nurses appeared to have behaved in an unenquiring and unquestioning manner. They accepted that their role was to carry out, uncritically and without question, whatever medical staff or their nursing superiors had prescribed. Nurses may have obeyed their superiors' orders to avoid being publicly humiliated in front of colleagues and patients. This was compounded by the fact that the nurses, especially the SENs, did not always possess the medical knowledge that they perceived the doctors to have, so they believed that it was pertinent for the well-being of a patient that nurses obey orders. Nevertheless, the knowledge of the medical staff in relation to aversion therapy for sexual deviations was also poor.

These treatments had a very limited evidence base, they were extremely experimental and they lacked regulation. Furthermore, with no general protocol or ethical guidelines, the treatment of choice in aversion therapy was often the unilateral decision of the consultant psychiatrist. This highlights the power that the medical profession appeared to hold at the time. These nurses seem to have been swamped by this medical power and the influential culture of the institution, which dictated that nursing was learnt 'by watching the example of others, based on "common sense" assumptions and concern with neatness rather than on research-based theory'.[8]

Other subordinate nurses sensed that there was something wrong in what they were doing. However, they appeared to overcome any reservations they may have had regarding administering aversion therapy by limiting their culpability. They did this by ensuring that they were not responsible for individual patients, while others used humour. Furthermore, nurses were encouraged not to build up strong relationships with their patients receiving aversion therapy. They avoided relating to these patients by dehumanising and objectifying them through language, and focusing on specific tasks. By taking refuge in the technical challenges of administering the therapy, these nurses receded their patients from view as objects of moral concern.

While it was highlighted that none of the nurses in this study knowingly murdered patients, unlike nurses under Nazi rule, there was an issue here of a replaying, in a minor key, of some of the dynamics between Nazi nurses and their role in the euthanasia projects, and the nurses in this study and their role in aversion therapy, as similar strategies were used by Nazi nurses to limit their accountability in relation to the unethical acts they implemented.[9] There are also similarities with some nurses in this study and with Nurse Rivers's participation in the Tuskegee study.[10] Indeed, Rivers was a black woman believing she was helping other black people, and some nurses in this book administered treatments for homosexuality, but were themselves homosexual. Meanwhile, Thaddeus Chester sensed that there was something wrong in administering aversion therapy. However, he believed that objecting to the treatments or refusal to assist with them may have brought his own sexuality into question, which motivated him to participate in this clinical practice.

Finally, some subordinate nurses genuinely believed that they were acting beneficently. These nurses appeared to believe, at the time, that aversion therapy was the most effective intervention to cure sexual deviants. However, reliance on the principle of beneficence led the nurses to become 'beneficently paternalistic'. Essentially, the patients were being told what was good for them without regard for their own needs or interests.[11] By acting based on their notions of beneficence, these nurses were not upholding the principle of non-maleficence, as the treatments were very traumatic and painful for the patients receiving them. Indeed, no former patients in this study reported any efficacy of the treatments and all stated that they had a negative long-term impact on them.

The predominant theme among the nurses in this book was that they appeared to be engulfed by the culture of the institution, which cultivated a passive obedience to authority. Other nurses, however, albeit a small minority, were able to engage with this culture in clever ways and covertly undermine their superiors by engaging in some fascinating subversive behaviours. Essentially, these nurses were doing the opposite of some of the subordinate nurses: they were questioning the orders they had been given by those in authority. In parallel with some of the subordinate nurses, they also argued that their behaviours were based on the notion of beneficence. Nevertheless, in contrast to the subordinate nurses, the subversive nurses were upholding the principle of non-maleficence when they chose to engage in resistive practices. Indeed, one could argue that these nurses were 'responsibly subversive' and their rule-bending behaviours had a positive long-term impact on their patients' sense of self-efficacy.

Within mental nurses' clinical practice there was an immense gulf between the prescriptions of theory, the intentions of policy and the realities of practice. For example, one article published at the time urged nurses not to merely accept doctors' orders, but to make the decision to partake in aversion therapy only after they had reflected on their own values regarding it.[12] However, only Elizabeth Granger recalled reading this article and, aided by her university-based nurse education, this might have encouraged her to act on her conscientious objections to the treatments.

The later part of the period covered by this book witnessed a new stress on individual freedoms that was, in part, inspired by the civil rights movement in the USA and other general counter-cultural shifts. This period also witnessed a sympathetic shift in the media representations of sexually deviant individuals, the APA's decision to remove the term homosexuality from its DSM and the inception of nurse therapists.

In contrast to the nurses who cared for patients receiving treatments for sexual deviations in the earlier part of the study, the nurse therapists appeared to have a theoretical basis upon which to base their clinical practice. However, the testimony of a former patient who was treated by a nurse therapist indicated that this particular nurse was equally as antipathetic as the doctors. Moreover, in spite of the emphasis among nurse therapists believing they had a scientific foundation for their work, they were still administering a spurious intervention, as the treatment's efficacy still relied on self-reported outcomes from the patient. Furthermore, ironically, these nurses were claiming success in an area of care that had already been discredited. In their quest for professionalisation, nurse therapists were taking on the mantle of the controlling clinical practitioners.

The participants in this study may not be representative of all the people who underwent or administered treatment for sexual deviations, as some individuals may have been reluctant to take part, or may have died or emigrated. In respect to the former patients who participated in the study, it may have only been those most perturbed by the treatments they received who wanted to participate. There may also have been nurses who steadfastly refused to participate in this aspect of clinical practice. Meanwhile, some nurses may have had sinister – yet unrevealed – motivations underpinning their participation in this area of clinical practice.

All the former patients who participated in this study reported that the treatments they received had been ineffective in altering their sexual desires, as they either remained homosexual or eventually underwent gender reassignment surgery. It is, however, important to bear in mind that if these treatments had been effective for some individuals in so far as they were now heterosexual, these people might have been reluctant to come forward to tell their story. Therefore, this book cannot address the full reality of the issues raised by these treatments.

Nevertheless, in spite of the above possible shortcomings to a research study, this book, arguably, indicates the value of an in-depth study such as this. It shows how issues might resonate with wider histories without actually representing them. Moreover, it illustrates how experience is necessarily fragmentary and contradictory and broad sweeps of histories can sometimes miss too much – especially when the focus of the study is on how people felt and thought.[13] In essence, this book makes a case for the inclusion of local and micro history in this kind of work.

This book enhances our understanding of sexuality in relation to nursing as a profession by discovering a hitherto neglected history of gay life in mental hospitals, and sits at the nexus of memory studies, histories of subjectivities, and histories of post-war Britain. In doing so, it offers a fresh understanding of the draw of mental nursing to gay men and supplements previous work regarding gay life at sea and within the military during World War II.[14] By identifying this previously hidden and multifaceted homosexual male sub-culture within the mental hospitals and discovering that different types of gay male nurses had their own implicit rules and behaviours, which included status distinctions between the lower ranking SENs and the nursing officers in the higher ranks, it relates to Matt Houlbrook's seminal work regarding camp 'queans' and the 'respectable middle class queer' men.[15] It adds to this debate and contributes to our understanding about status, class and sexual identity among gay men.

This book offers a new insight into the role of mental nurses caring for patients receiving aversion therapy for sexual deviation. As the first focused study exploring the nurses' role in caring for sexually deviant patients, it provides a basis for further historical analysis of this subject and related issues. This book can offer insights into the way nurses may behave when a particular set of social, political and contextual factors are at play. In addition, it presents an important area of nurse ethics and socialisation by analysing how nurses make decisions about what is professionally right and wrong in a context of ambiguity, frustration and conflict. Overall, this study displays how histories of discourse do not map straightforwardly on to histories of everyday life. It exposes the tensions in relations between the two, and the equivocal way in which nurses read and listened to influential cultural outputs and acted in accordance with these.

First, the culture of many mental hospitals – and their nurses – was custodial, impersonal and ritualised. The work of nurses was largely constrained by the asylum-type conditions in which they worked, and the character and quality of patient care was largely influenced by the medical staff, who appeared to have overriding control of both the institution and the nurses working within it. In addition, owing to their limited knowledge base, some nurses believed that it was pertinent for the well-being of a patient that nurses obey orders. They took on the status offered to them of obedient followers of orders.

Furthermore, nurses were exposed to prejudicial attitudes towards homosexuals and transvestites, which were being expressed by the media and by literary, medical, sociological and legal discourses.

Indeed, Herbert Kelman and Lee Hamilton argue that all obedience depends upon the existence of a favourable social and political context, in which individuals deem the commands that have been issued not to be a gross transgression of their intrinsic values and their central morality.[16] The rhetoric regarding sexual deviants during the 1950s and 1960s created a favourable social and political context for these treatments. Without judgement, this resulted in a set of actions that, on reflection, were ethically unjustified, brutal and harmful to the patients receiving them. What was lacking at the time was a culture in which nurses possessed the knowledge base and self-efficacy to voice their concerns and to question those in authority.

It is envisaged that this book might act to reiterate the need for nurses to ensure that their interventions have a sound evidence base, and that they constantly reflect on the moral and value base of their practice; and the influence that science, societal norms and contexts can have on changing views of what is regarded as acceptable practice. We can learn much from studying aspects of our profession's past in which our actions, even if countenanced by the context in which they were situated, did not serve patients and society well.

Notes

1 Houlbrook, *Queer London*, pp. 19–43.
2 Weeks, *Coming Out*, p. 164; Jivani, *It's Not Unusual*, p. 111.
3 Waters, 'Disorders of the Mind', p. 151.
4 See, e.g., James, 'Case of Homosexuality Treated by Aversion Therapy'; 'How Doctor Cured a Homosexual', *Observer* (18 March 1962).
5 See, e.g., Rees and Usill, *They Stand Apart: A Critical Survey of the Problem of Homosexuality;* Westwood, *Society and the Homosexual;* 'Evil Men', *Sunday Pictorial* (25 May 1952).
6 See, e.g., Crossley, 'The Introduction of Leucotomy'; James, 'Insulin Treatment in Psychiatry'; Kragh, 'Shock Therapy'; Berrios, 'The Scientific Origins of Electroconvulsive Therapy: A Conceptual History'.
7 See, e.g., Ackner, *Handbook for Psychiatric Nurses*, pp. 108–116; Bachelor, *Henderson and Gillespie's Textbook of Psychiatry*, pp. 197–209.
8 Hopton, 'Prestwich Hospital in the Twentieth Century', p. 360.
9 See, e.g., Berghs, Dierckx de Casterle and Gastmans, 'Practices of Responsibility', p. 850.
10 Reverby, 'Rethinking the Tuskegee Syphilis Study'.
11 Gillon, *Philosophical Medical Ethics*, p. 87.

12 Seager, 'Aversion Therapy in Psychiatry', p. 424.
13 Ginzburg, Tedeschi and Tedeschi, 'Microhistory', pp. 10–35; Cook, 'Gay Times': Brixton Squats in 1970s London', pp. 1–26.
14 See, e.g., Baker and Stanley, *Hello Sailor!*; Vickers, *Queen and County*.
15 For a more detailed exploration of class within homosexual urban culture see, e.g., Houlbrook, *Queer London*, pp. 167–195.
16 Kelman and Hamilton, *Crimes of Obedience*, 78.

Epilogue

The APA's 1974 decision to remove homosexuality from its DSM, along with social protests and a newly emerged gay liberation movement, eventually led to the curtailment of medical treatments to cure homosexuality. A conservative turn in the 1980s, however, provided the cultural and social foundations to reclassify homosexuality as a contagious pathology, and this could offer a context to explain why the WHO took a further eighteen years before it mirrored the APA's decision to remove homosexuality from its diagnostic manual.

In 1981, the Centre of Disease Control in the USA reported that five young men had died from a rare form of pneumonia in Los Angeles. A year later, on 4 July 1982, 37-year-old Terry Higgins became the first known person in Britain to die of an AIDS-related disease at St Thomas' Hospital, London.[1] This virulent and completely unpredictable pathogen endangered homosexual men and threatened to undo the social advances that had been made for homosexuals in the previous two decades.

The social reaction to AIDS during the first few years of the epidemic was permanently marked by the unique social distribution of the disease. With more than 90 per cent of reported cases coming from intravenous drug users, gay and bisexual men, the community expressed not only its fears about contagion but also its moral judgement. Before the term 'AIDS' was first coined in 1982, it had been labelled 'Gay Cancer' or 'GRID' (Gay-related immune deficiency), and there was a strong sense that the condition was associated with sexual identity rather than sexual practice.

Just under a decade after homosexuality had been demedicalised, the power of the medical profession was being brought into intimate contact with the gay community, and once again medicine was compelling homosexual men to examine their behaviour.[2] The media were shaping a lot of public perception regarding the epidemic, and headlines such 'Gay Plague' characterised gay men as plague bearers who were highly contagious.[3] Press coverage such as this created a backlash against homosexuals in the 1980s and served to confirm all the lingering prejudices, which had lain dormant during the 1970s. 'Andy' recalls, 'It was OK to hate gay people again because we carried a plague – "The Gay Plague".'[4] There was rhetoric around compulsory testing for all gay men and even of quarantine.

In 1983, work began on revising the WHO ICD-9 (the predecessor to the ICD-10, which still classified homosexuality as a psychiatric disorder). It is interesting to note that this was just as the AIDS epidemic was coming to the fore along with its strong association with homosexual men. Indeed, in Britain, by March 1983, there were six reported cases of AIDS, and by July that year, this figure had more than doubled. By October 1985, the number of cases had risen to 241 and, while it was difficult to measure the exact number of individuals infected in Britain, the most widely held assumption at the time was that it was at least 20,000.[5] By 1986, the catastrophic worldwide implications of the AIDS epidemic were becoming ever more apparent. In June of that year, the USA Public Health Service predicted that by 1991 there would be 270,000 cases of AIDS in the USA alone.[6] This could offer a context to explain why the WHO delayed its decision to remove homosexuality from its diagnostic manual.

Nevertheless, the AIDS crisis reunited gay men in a way that had not happened since the 1970s and new protests groups, like 'Act Up' and 'Outrage', emerged employing similar tactics to the GLF.[7] Gay men were also gaining a higher profile in the arts and media by the late 1980s, with Sir Ian McKellen sensationally 'coming out' during a radio debate.[8] These all played a role in dissipating the initial panic around HIV and AIDS.

On 17 May 1990, the General Assembly of the WHO decided to remove homosexuality from their list of mental disorders.[9] The International Lesbian, Gay, Bisexual, Trans and Intersex Association argue that this action served to end more than a century of medical homophobia and constitutes a historic date and a powerful symbol for members of the GLBTIQ community. Therefore, on 17 May every year, this decision is remembered when 'The International Day Against Homophobia and Transphobia' is celebrated.[10]

Notes

1 Cook, *A Gay History of Britain*, p. 195.
2 Drescher and Merlino, *American Psychiatry and Homosexuality*, p. 127; Bayer, *Homosexuality and American Psychiatry*, p. 204.
3 Jivani, *It's not Unusual*, p. 189.
4 'Andy', whose testimony appears in Jones, *Tales from Out in the City*, p. 94.
5 Jivani, *It's not Unusual*, p. 186.
6 Bayer, *Homosexuality and American Psychiatry*, p. 204.
7 Jivani, *It's not Unusual*, pp. 198–199.
8 Cook, *A Gay History of Britain*, p. 208.
9 It was eventually removed from their diagnostic manual with the introduction of the *International Classification of Diseases Edition 10 Classification of Mental and Behavioural Disorders* (ICD-10), published in 1992.
10 International Lesbian, Gay, Bisexual, Trans and Intersex Association, *May 17th is the International Day Against Homophobia*. Available at: http://ilga.org/ilga/en/article/546 (last accessed 21 May 2012).

Appendix: biographies of the twenty-five interviewees whose testimonies have been referred to

The twenty-five participants who were interviewed for this book are described below. All names have been changed, as discussed within the Introduction. Some of the participants did not want to give a great deal of biographical information, as they wished to remain unrecognisable for their own security today.

Nurses

Gilbert Davies interviewed 10 February 2010
Born 1912. Trained as a mental nurse and qualified in 1936. Worked as a staff nurse in various mental health settings before retiring in the 1960s. Sadly, Gilbert passed away in 2010, aged 98.

Elliot Whitman interviewed 20 March 2010
Born 1935. Commenced work as a nursing auxiliary in 1953 aged 18. In 1964 he commenced as a pupil nurse and was in the first cohort of SENs in mental nursing to qualify. Worked as an enrolled nurse in various mental health settings before retiring in the 1990s. He now lives in London with his partner.

Elizabeth Granger interviewed 3 May 2010
Born 1944. Undertook a university-based SRN nurse education at Edinburgh University in the early 1960s. She worked as a staff nurse in a cottage hospital for six months once she qualified. However, she always wanted to pursue a career in mental nursing. Therefore, she

commenced a conversion course at her local psychiatric hospital and qualified as a mental nurse in 1967. She soon became a ward sister and eventually became the director of nursing for a large private group of nursing homes before she retired in the 1990s. Sadly, Elizabeth passed away in 2012, aged 68.

Una Drinkwater interviewed 29 December 2009
Born 1911 in Galway in the Republic of Ireland. Due to very poor job prospects in Ireland, she moved to England in 1929 to live with her cousin. Almost immediately she found a job at the local county asylum as a nursing student and qualified in 1933. She worked as a staff nurse there for her whole career before retiring in 1963. Una never married and she sadly passed away in 2010, aged 98.

Ursula Vaughan interviewed 12 February 2010
Born 1937. Trained as a mental nurse and qualified in 1960. Worked as a staff nurse in various mental health settings before retiring in 2005. She now lives in Cork in the Republic of Ireland.

Thaddeus Chester interviewed 8 August 2010
Born 1930. Trained as a mental nurse and qualified in 1951. He eventually became a nursing officer before he retired in 1985. He now lives in Inverness with his partner.

Evander Orchard interviewed 10 August 2010
Born 1946. Commenced as a pupil nurse in 1965, qualifying in 1967. He worked as a State Enrolled Nurse in various psychiatric hospitals around the UK before retiring in 2001. He now lives in Belfast with his partner.

Ida Ashley interviewed 17 July 2010
Born 1940 in Blackpool, Lancashire. She trained as a mental nurse, qualifying in 1961. She went on to train as a nurse therapist and went on to become a sister at a specialist behaviour therapy research and treatment unit. She is now retired and lives in Cardiff with her husband.

Cecil Asquith interviewed 5 December 2010

Born 1947 in Huddersfield. Unsure about what direction he wanted his career to follow after leaving school, his mum suggested that he consider mental nursing. He went along to his local mental hospital and was initially accepted as a cadet nurse for six months before commencing his nurse training in 1965, aged 18 years. Once qualified he embarked on a shortened general nursing programme and qualified as a general nurse, as at the time he believed this would increase his chances of promotion later in his career. Cecil returned to mental nursing and became a community psychiatric nurse. He eventually became a professor of mental health nursing. He has now retired and lives in Manchester with his wife.

Julian Wills interviewed 4 January 2010

Born 1921. Within weeks of the outbreak of World War II Julian was called up for military service, and he took part in many campaigns during the war. Feeling his life was lacking direction once the war was over, he followed up an advert in the local paper about the mental hospital in his village, which was recruiting staff. He went along and was offered a place as a student nurse, and qualified as a mental nurse in 1950. He worked as a staff nurse for the rest of his career. He retired to Bournemouth with his wife. Sadly, Julian passed away in 2012, aged 91.

Elspeth Whitbread interviewed 7 January 2010

Born 1939. Bored with her job as a secretary, she responded to an advert for mental nursing which showed a nurse assisting with 'brain surgery'. She was successful in her application and commenced her nurse training in 1957, qualifying in 1960. Elspeth eventually became a clinical nurse manager of an older adults mental health service. She retired in 1994 and now lives in Cornwall with her husband.

Claudine de Valois interviewed 30 December 2009

Born in 1933 in Calais, France. She responded to an advertisement in a French newspaper in 1951, advertising for staff for a mental hospital in England. She was successful at the interview and moved the same year, and qualified as a staff nurse in 1955. Here she met her future husband, also a nurse, and decided to stay in the UK. She eventually became a nurse tutor until her retirement in 1988. She returned to France with her husband on their retirement and currently lives in Dijon, France.

Myrtle Pauncefoot interviewed 7 November 2012

Born in 1944 in Douglas, Isle of Man. Trained as a mental nurse in London and qualified in 1965. She worked as a staff nurse in a psychiatric hospital in London for a year before she commenced her 'mental sub-normality' nurse training in 1966. She qualified as a nurse for the 'mentally subnormal' in 1968, and took a job as a 'night nurse' in a nursing home, where she worked until her retirement in 2009. On retirement, she returned to the Isle of Man with her husband, where they receive regular visits from their many grandchildren.

Benedict Henry interviewed 23 June 2010

Born in 1942 in the West of Ireland. Benedict spent eight years in a monastery studying theology, bible scriptures and teaching. However, he felt that there was not a great deal to do after this. Therefore, he moved to London in the early 1960s and commenced work in a pharmacy. However, he took an instant dislike to this. He was a keen runner, and during a meeting his running club held at the Maudsley Hospital in London one weekend, he realised that many of the hospital staff had great sporting opportunities, and that there were a lot of other people from Ireland there. This prompted him to begin his nurse training in 1963, qualifying in 1966. Benedict worked in mental health nursing for the remainder of his career and eventually became a professor of mental health nursing. He currently lives in Staffordshire with his wife.

Zella Mullins interviewed 14 July 2010

Born 1947. Commenced as a pupil nurse in 1966, qualifying in 1968. She worked as a state enrolled nurse in various psychiatric hospitals around Scotland before retiring in 1987. She now lives in Edinburgh with her husband.

Maude Griffin interviewed 20 October 2012

Born 1933 in Stepney, London. Commenced as a student nurse in 1951, qualifying in 1954. She eventually became the night sister of psychiatric hospital in London before retiring in 1988. She still lives in London with her husband.

Leith Cavill interviewed 25 March 2010

Born 1940. Commenced his pupil nurse training in 1966, qualifying in 1968. He worked as a state enrolled nurse in London and Jersey until he retired in 2002. He still lives in Jersey with his partner.

Patients

Oscar Mangle interviewed 21 June 2010

Born 1929. Grew up in a small rural farming village in Lancashire. Moved to London in 1947. Worked in retail his whole career until he retired in the 1980s. He retired to the Isle of Man. Sadly Oscar passed away in 2012, aged 85.

Albert Holliday interviewed 27 January 2010

Born 1928 in Sheffield, and then moved to London to attend art school in 1946, aged 18. Worked as a painter his whole career. Now retired and lives in Cornwall, but he still loves to paint.

Greta Gold interviewed 24 March 2010

Born 1935, in a fishing village in Cornwall. Worked as a bus driver for many years. Underwent gender reassignment surgery in 1982 and went on to train as a social worker. She is now retired and lives in London with her partner.

Barrington Crowther-Lobley interviewed 28 April 2010

Born 1940 in Kingston, Jamaica. He emigrated to the UK with his parents and brother in 1951, aged 11. He read history at university and eventually went on to teach history in a secondary school and subsequently became the head teacher. He retired in 2005, and lives in Devon with his partner.

Molly Millbury interviewed 31 December 2010

Born 1945, Liverpool. She initially worked on the docks with her father. Molly underwent gender reassignment surgery in 2000 and now owns a successful hat designing business. She lives in London with her partner.

Percival Thatcher interviewed 29 April 2010

Born 1930, in London, and lived there all his life. He trained as a butcher in the family butcher's shop and eventually inherited the business from his father. Sadly, Percival passed away in 2012, aged 82.

Herbert Bliss interviewed 2 January 2010

Born 1920 in Salisbury, Wiltshire. He served in the RAF during the war. Herbert was captured by the Japanese during the fall of Singapore and interned in a PoW camp in Osaka Japan. He went on to read English at university after the war. Worked as a university lecturer in English literature until his retirement in 1980. Sadly, Herbert passed away in 2011, aged 91.

Ughtred Lovis-Douglas interviewed 4 November 2012

Born 1941. His father was a high ranking officer in the British army, which meant that he travelled a lot in his childhood. He read Veterinary Medicine at University. Ughtred went on to set up his own veterinary practice. He retired in 2001, and moved to Buckinghamshire with his partner. However, they are often away on a cruise enjoying their retirement.

Bibliography

Archival sources

Files held at The National Archives, formerly the Public Record Office

Kew, London

B/107/1/2 – memo. By Professor John Glaister, 30 June 1955.

CAB/195/11 – minutes of a meeting with Home Secretary and Prime Minister discussing issues around prostitution and homosexuality.

HO345/2 – Adair to Roberts, 4 October 1956.

HO345/9 – Proceedings of the Wolfenden Committee on Homosexual Offences and Prostitution (PWC), Summary Record of 21st Meeting, March 1956.

HO 345 7: CHP II – memorandum submitted by Harold Sturge, metropolitan magistrate, Old Street.

HO345/10 – note on WC discussion meetings, 11 and 12 September 1956.

HO 345 12 – CHP TRANS 8, Q633, 3.

HO 345 14, CHP TRANS 32 – two witnesses called by chairman (28 July 1955).

HO345/15, CHP/TRANS/41, PWC – evidence of W. Boyd, 1 November 1955.

HO345/15, CHP/TRANS/42, PWC – evidence of TD Inch, 'Sexual Offenders: treatment in prisons'.

HO345/12 and /16 – PWC, 15 October 1954, 10 April 1956.

The Hall Carpenter Archives, London School of Economics

London

HCA/EPHEMERA/1148 – Letter from the West London Gay Liberation Front's Anti-Psychiatry Group to a local GP about treatment of homosexuality in 1972.

HCA/Grey Papers/1/2 (a) – Sexual Offences: records relating to actions on homosexual law reform from the Departmental Committee on Homosexuality and Prostitution.

HCA/GREY – Material relating to the HLRS, 1958–1984.

HCA/GREY/1/2 HLRS – Executive Committee: agendas and minutes.

HCA/CHE/9/46 – Police Harassment Working Party correspondence and papers on cottaging.

HCA/EPHEMERA/1148 – West London Gay Liberation Front.

HCA/ALBANY TRUST/16/61 – National Council for Civil Liberties Report 8: Homosexuality and the Teaching Profession, August 1975.

HCA/EPHEMERA/1148 – West London Gay Liberation Front interim statement, 'The Counter Psychiatry Group of the GLF'.

HCA/ALBANY TRUST/10/4 – Malik Survey on psychosexual treatment. Completed questionnaires on psychiatric facilities for homosexuals in the London area.

HCA/ALBANY TRUST/10/6 – Eva Bene survey regarding use of medical and psychiatry treatment.

HCA/EPHEMERA/568 – Transsexual Action Organisation (TAO) 'Transsexual Information', two leaflets and one pamphlet by the TAO.

Royal College of Nursing Archives

Edinburgh

Marks, Isaac. *Nursing in Behavioural Psychotherapy: An Advanced Clinical Role for Nurses* (London, 1977).

Seager, Charles, P. 'Aversion Therapy in Psychiatry', *Nursing Times* 26 (1965), pp. 421–424.

Oral history interviews

Conducted by author
Date of interview/Pseudonym applied to interviewee

29/12/2009 Una Drinkwater
30/12/2009 Claudine de Valois
04/01/2010 Julian Wills
07/01/2010 Elspeth Whitbread
27/01/2010 Albert Holliday
02/02/2010 Herbert Bliss
10/02/2010 Gilbert Davies
12/02/2010 Ursula Vaughan
20/03/2010 Elliot Whitman
24/03/2010 Greta Gold
25/03/2010 Leith Cavill
28/04/2010 Barrington Crowther-Lobley
29/04/2010 Percival Thatcher
03/05/2010 Elizabeth Granger

21/06/2010 Oscar Mangle
23/06/2010 Benedict Henry
14/07/2010 Zella Mullins
17/07/2010 Ida Ashley
08/08/2010 Thaddeus Chester
10/08/2010 Evander Orchard
05/12/2010 Cecil Asquith
31/12/2010 Molly Millbury
20/10/2012 Maude Griffin
04/11/2012 Ughtred Lovis-Douglas
07/11/2012 Myrtle Pauncefoot

Newspapers

'A Night in a Workhouse', *Pall Mall Gazette* (4 January 1866).

'The Lunacy Problem', *The Times* (5 April 1877).

'Porter's Punishment', *News of the World* (30 October 1932).

'If Guilty They Would be Gassed While in Court', *Reynolds* (18 December 1938).

'Sailor Cleared of Manslaughter', *News of the World* (26 October 1947).

'Evil Men', *Sunday Pictorial* (25 May 1952).

'Scotland Yard to Smash Homosexuality', *The Sydney Morning Telegraph* (25 June 1953).

'The Problem of Homosexuality: report by clergy and doctors', *The Times* (26 February 1954).

'Final Day of the Montagu Trial', *Daily Sketch* (24 March 1954).

'The Squalid Truth', *The Sunday Pictorial* (25 September 1955).

'One Million Need This New Clinic', *Express* (23 August 1957).

'What the Papers Say about the Report', *Evening News* (5 September 1957).

'Planned to Help a Million', *Mail* (6 September 1957).

'Sex Pills for Scots in Jail', *The Sunday Pictorial* (16 February 1958).

'Growing Problem of the Homosexual', *The Scotsman* (5 June 1959).

'Control Must Come Before Cure', *The Scotsman* (6 June 1959).

'"Twilight" Men Can Be Cured', *The Sunday Pictorial* (5 February 1961).

'Treatment of Homosexuals: Public Opinion Hostile', *Glasgow Herald* (28 September 1961).

'How Doctor cured a Homosexual', *Observer* (18 March 1962).

'Homosexuality Research Unit', *Birmingham Post* (25 November 1964).

'Gift to Start Homosexuality Research Unit', *Manchester Daily Telegraph* (25 November 1964).

'£6,000 Gift for Research into Homosexuality', *Guardian* (25 November 1964).

'Offer for Study of Homosexuality', *The Scotsman* (26 November 1964).

Bibliography

'Homosexuals Cured More Easily in Prison', *Guardian* (10 October 1965).

'A Neurosis Is Just A Bad Habit', *The New York Times* (4 June 1967).

'A Nursing Sister's Advice to Homosexuals', *Johannesburg Star* (25 November 1968).

'Gays and Dolls Battle the Shrinks', *Washington Post* (15 May 1970).

'Should Shame Be The Cure?', *Daily Mail* (10 September 1970).

'The Changing View of Homosexuality', *New York Times* (28 February 1971).

'Fears Over Aversion Therapy Grow: Using Shock Tactics to Bend the Mind', *The Sunday Times* (9 May 1971).

'Aversion Therapy Is Like A Visit To The Dentist', *Gay News* 11 (1972).

'The 40-year Death Watch', *Medical World News* (18 August 1972).

'Why 420 Blacks with Syphilis Went Uncured for 40 Years', *Detroit Free Press* (5 November 1972).

'Psychiatrists in a Shift. Declare Homosexuality no Mental Illness', *The New York Times* (16 December 1973).

'It's Official Now: We're Not Sick', *Gay Community News* (16 December 1973).

'Doctors are the 'Problem' Men', *Glasgow Daily Record* (28 November 1974).

'The True Cost of Training a Doctor', *Observer* (24 July 1977).

'Mistaken Identity', *The Guardian* (31 July 2004).

'Irena Sendler', *Telegraph* (12 May 2008).

'Irena Sendler, Lifeline to Young Jews, Is Dead at 98', *The New York Times* (13 May 2008).

'An Uneasy History', *Attitude Magazine* (March 2010).

Documentaries

Dark Secret: Sexual Aversion (1996), BBC 2. Dir, Hilary Clarke.

Films

Design for Living (1933), Dir. Ernst Lubitsch.

Look up and Laugh (1945), Dir. Basil Herbert Dean.

Brief Encounter (1945), Dir. Sir David Lean.

Internet sources

International Lesbian, Gay, Bisexual, Trans and Intersex Association, *May 17th is the International Day Against Homophobia*. Available at: http://ilga.org/ilga/en/article/546 (last accessed 21 May 2012).

King, Michael, 'Doubts about the Treatments', available at: www.treatmentshomosexuality.org.uk/index.php/en/narratives-en (last accessed 29 December 2011).

NHS Choices available at: www.nhs.uk/Conditions/Genderdysphoria/Pages /Introduction.aspx (last accessed 15 May 2012).

National Union of Teachers, 'Equal Pay & The Equal Pay Act 1970' available at: i.teachers.org.uk/node/12977 (last accessed 27 January 2012).

Official publications

Department of Health and Social Security, *Psychiatric Nursing Today and Tomorrow* (London, 1968).

Department of Health, Education and Welfare, *Final Report of the Tuskegee Syphilis Study Ad Hoc Advisory Panel* (Washington, 1973).

Department of Health and Social Security, *Better Services for the Mentally Ill*, Cmnd.6233 (London, 1975).

Her Majesty's Stationery Office, Command 3687: *Findings and Recommendations Following Inquiries into Allegations Concerning the Care of Elderly Patients in Certain Hospitals* (London, 1968).

Her Majesty's Stationery Office, Command 3975: *Report of the Committee of Inquiry into Allegations of Ill-Treatment of Patients and other Irregularities at Ely Hospital Cardiff* (London, 1969).

Powell, Enoch, J. Speech by the Minister of Health, the Rt Hon. Enoch Powell. *Report of the Annual Conference of the National Association for Mental Health* (London, 1961).

Royal College of Nursing, *New Horizons in Clinical Nursing* (London, 1976).

Tooth, George C. and Newton, Michael P. 'Leucotomy in England and Wales, 1942–1954', *Great Britain Ministry of Health Reports on Public Health and Medical Subjects No. 104* (London, 1961).

Autobiographies

Brand, Jo. *Look Back in Hunger* (London, 2009).

Price, Pete. '*Namesdropper*' (Liverpool, 2007).

Biographies

Fallowell, Duncan and Ashley, April. *April Ashley's Odyssey* (London, 1982).

Unpublished theses

Adams, John. 'Challenge and Change in a Cinderella Service: A History of Fulbourn Hospital, Cambridgeshire, 1953–1995) (unpublished PhD thesis, The Open University, 2009).

Arton, Michael. 'The Professionalization of Mental Nursing in Great Britain, 1850–1950' (unpublished PhD Thesis, University of London, 1998).

Carpenter, Diane. 'Above All a Patient Should Never Be Terrified: An Examination of Mental Health Care and Treatment in Hampshire' (unpublished PhD Thesis, University of Portsmouth, 2010).

Chatterton, Claire S. '"The Weakest Link in the Chain of Nursing?" Recruitment and Retention in Mental Health Nursing, 1948–1968' (unpublished PhD Thesis, University of Salford, 2007).

Church, Olga. 'That Nobel Reform: The Emergence of Psychiatric Nursing in the United States, 1882–1963' (unpublished PhD Thesis, University of Illinois, 1982).

D'Antonio, Patricia. 'Negotiated Care: A Case Study of the Friends Asylum, 1800–1850' (unpublished PhD Thesis, University of Pennsylvania, 1992).

Harrington, Valerie. 'Death of the Asylum: The Run-Down and Closure of Prestwich mental hospital' (unpublished MSc Thesis, University of Manchester, 2004).

Harrington, Valerie. 'Voices Beyond the Asylum: A Post-War History of Mental Health Services in Manchester and Salford' (unpublished MPhil/PhD Transfer Report, University of Manchester, 2005).

Martin, Angela. 'Determinants of Destiny: The Professional Development of Psychiatric Nurses in Saskatchewan' (unpublished MA Thesis, University of Regina, 2003).

Maude, Philip. 'The Development of the Community Mental Health Nursing Services in Western Australia: A history (1950 to 1995) and Population Profile' (unpublished Master of Nursing Thesis, Edith Cowan University, Perth, 1996).

Mitchell, Duncan. '"No Claim to be Called Sick Nurses at All". An Historical Study of Learning Disability Nursing' (unpublished PhD Thesis, London South Bank University, London, 2000).

Nolan, Peter. 'Psychiatric Nursing Past and Present: The Nurses' Viewpoint' (unpublished PhD Thesis, University of Bath, 1989).

O'Donnell, Alison, J. 'A New Order of Duty: A critical Genealogy of the Emergence of the Modern Nurse in National Socialist Germany' (unpublished PhD thesis, The University of Dundee, 2009).

Powell, Ryan. 'Man Country: A Social History of 70s Gay Cinema' (unpublished PhD Thesis, University College London, 2010).

Prebble, Kate. 'Ordinary Men and Uncommon Women: A History of Psychiatric Nursing in New Zealand Public Mental Hospitals' (unpublished PhD Thesis, University of Auckland, 2007).

Tipliski, Veryl. 'Parting in the Crossroads: The Development of Education in Psychiatric Nursing in Three Canadian Providences, 1909–1955' (unpublished PhD Thesis, University of Manitoba, 2003).

Published sources: primary and secondary

Abbott, Pamela and Sapsford, Robert. *Research Methods for Nursing and the Caring Professions* (London, 2007), pp. 267.

Abramson, Lyn Y. 'Relevance of Animal Learning Models to Behavioural Psychotherapy', *British Association for Behavioural and Cognitive Psychotherapies* 4 (1976), p.2.

Ackner, Brian. *Handbook for Psychiatric Nurses* (London, 1964).

Ackroyd, Peter. *Dressing Up Transvestism and Drag: The History of an Obsession* (Norwich, 1979).

Allan, Callen. 'The Treatment of Homosexuality', *Medical Press* 235 (1956), p. 141.

Altschul, Annie. Patient–Nurse Interaction: A Study of Interactive Patterns in Acute Psychiatric Wards (Edinburgh, 1972).

Allyon, Teodoro and Michael, Jack. 'The Psychiatric Nurse as Behavioral Engineer', *Journal of Experimental Analysis of Behavior* 2 (1959), pp. 323–333.

Aggleton, Peter. *Deviance* (London, 1987).

Allison, Fred, H. 'Remembering a Vietnam War Fire Fight: Changing Perspectives Over Time', in Robert Perks and Alistair Thompson (eds), *The Oral History Reader*, 2nd edn (Oxon, 2006), pp. 211–220.

Alvarez, Walter. *Homosexuality* (New York, 1974).

American Psychiatric Association. *Diagnostic Statistical Manual Version I* (Arlington, 1952).

American Psychiatric Association. *Seventh Printing Diagnostic Statistical Manual Version II* (Arlington, 1974).

American Psychiatric Association. *Diagnostic Statistical Manual Version IV* (Washington, 1994).

'Anomaly'. The Invert and His Social Adjustment (London, 1948).

Anderson, Charles. 'On Certain Conscious and Unconscious Homosexual Responses to Warfare', *British Journal of Medical Psychology* 2 (1945), pp. 157–162.

Ashforth, Blake E. and Kreiner, Glen E.'"How Can they do It?" Dirty Work and the Challenge of Constricting a Positive Identity', *Academy of Management Review* 24 (1999), pp. 413–434.

Atwood, Kathryn J. *Women Heroes of World War II* (Chicago, 2011).

Babbie, Earl R. and Benaquisto, Lucia. *Fundamentals of Social Research* (New York, 2009).

Bachelor, Ivor R. C. Henderson and Gillespie's Textbook of Psychiatry (Oxford, 1962).

Baggott, Eileen. 'The SEN in Psychiatric Hospitals', *Nursing Times* 29 (1965), p. 1478.

Baker, Dorothy. 'Attitudes of Nurses to the care of the Elderly' (unpublished PhD thesis University Manchester, Manchester, 1978), p. 121.

Baker, Paul and Stanley, Jo. *Hello Sailor! The Hidden History of Gay Life at Sea* (London, 2003).

Baly, Monica E. 'The National Health Service', in Monica E. Baly (ed.), *Nursing & Social Change* (New York, 1995).

Bancroft, John. 'Aversion Therapy of Homosexuality: a Pilot Study of 10 Cases', *The British Journal of Psychiatry* 115 (1969), p. 1418.

Bancroft, John. *Deviant Sexual Behaviour: Modification and Assessment* (Oxford, 1974).

Barker, John C. 'Behavioural Therapy for Transvestism: a Comparison of Pharmacological and Electrical Aversion Techniques', *British Journal of Psychiatry* 111 (1965), pp. 268–276.

Barlow, David H. 'Increasing Heterosexual Responsiveness in the Treatment of Sexual Deviation: a review of the Clinical and Experimental Evidence', *Behaviour Therapy* 4 (1973), p. 655.

Basu, Shbrabani. *Spy Princess the Life of Noor Inyat Khan* (Stroud, 2006).

Bayer, Ronald. *Homosexuality and American Psychiatry: The Politics of Power* (Princeton, 1987).

Beardshaw, Virginia. *Conscientious Objectors at Work* (London, 1981).

Beck, Gad. *An Underground Life: Memoirs of a Gay Jew in Nazi Berlin* (Wisconsin, 1999).

Benedict, Susan and Kuhla, Jochen. 'Nurses' Participation in the "Euthanasia" Programmes of Nazi Germany', *Western Journal of Nursing Research* 21 (1999), pp. 246–263.

Benedict, Susan. 'Maria Stromberger: a Nurse in the Resistance in Auschwitz', *Nursing History Review* 14 (2006), pp. 189–202.

Benedict, Susan and Georges, Jane M. 'Nurses and the Sterilization Experiments of Auschwitz: a Postmodernist Perspective', *Nursing Inquiry* 13 (4) (2006), pp. 227–288.

Benjamin, Martin and Curtis, Joy. *Ethics in Nursing* (New York, 1992).

Berrios, German E. 'The Scientific Origins of Electroconvulsive Therapy: a Conceptual History', *History of Psychiatry* viii (1997), p. 106.

Berghs, Maria., Dierckx de Casterle, Bernadette and Gastmans, Chris. 'Practices of Responsibility and Nurses During the Euthanasia Programs of Nazi Germany: A Discussion Paper', *International Journal of Nursing Studies* 44 (2007), p. 846.

Bieber, Irving. *Homosexuality* (New York, 1965).

Bierer, Joshua. 'Stilboestrol in Out-Patient Treatment of Sexual Offenders: A Case Report', *British Medical Journal* (1950), pp. 935–936.

Biley, Francis. 'Psychiatric nursing: living with the legacy of the Holocaust', *Journal of Psychiatric and Mental Health Nursing* 9 (2002), p. 365.

Bingham, Stella. *Ministering Angels* (Over Wallop, 1979).

Binney, Marcus. *The Women who Lived for Danger* (London, 2002).

Bird, Julian, Marks, Isaac and Lindley, Peter. 'Nurse Therapists in Psychiatry: Developments, Controversies and Implications', *British Journal of Psychiatry* 135 (1979), p. 321.

Blanchard, Ray. 'The DSM Diagnostic Criteria for Paedophilia', *Archives of Sexual Behaviour*, 16 (2009), pp. 1–11.

Bland, Jed. *Transvestism and Cross-Dressing: Current Views* (London, 2004).

Bland, Lucy and Doan, Laura. *Sexology Uncensored The Documents of Sexual Science* (Cambridge, 1998).

Blatz, Perry. 'Craftsmanship and Flexibility in Oral History: a Pluralistic Approach to Methodology and Theory', *The Public Historian* 12 (4) (1990), p. 12.

Borland, Katherine. "That is not what I said". Interpretative Conflict in Oral Narrative Research', in Robert Perks and Alistair Thompson (eds), *The Oral History Reader*, 2nd edn (Oxon, 2006), p. 319.

Boschma, Geertje. *The Rise of Mental Health Nursing: A History of Psychiatric Care in Dutch Asylums, 1890-1929* (Amsterdam, 2003).

Boschma, Geertje., Scaia, Margaret., Bonifacio, Nerrisa. and Roberts, Erica. 'Oral History Research', in Sandra B. Lewenson and Eleanor K. Herrman (eds) *Capturing Nursing History: a Guide to Historical Methods in Research* (New York, 2007), p. 127.

Bourke, Joanna. 'Disciplining The Emotions: Fear, Psychiatry and the Second World War', in Roger Cooter, Mark Harrison and Steve Sturdy (eds), *War, Medicine & Modernity* (Stroud, 1998), p. 231.

Bourne, Harold. 'The Insulin Myth', *Lancet* ii (1953), p. 964.

Brandt, Allan M. 'Racism and Research: The Case of the Tuskegee Syphilis Experiment', in Susan M. Reverby (ed.), *Tuskegee's Truths: Rethinking the Tuskegee Syphilis Study* (London, 2000), p. 15.

Braslow, Joel. *Mental Ills and Bodily Cures* (London, 1997).

Brickell, Chris. *Mates & Lovers* (Auckland, 2008), p. 93.

Brooker, Charlie. 'Nurse Therapist Trainee Variability: The Implications for Selection and Training', *Journal of Advanced Nursing* 8 (1983), p. 322.

Brooks, Jane. 'The First Undergraduate Nursing Students: A Quantitative Historical Study of the Edinburgh Degrees, 1960-1985', *Nurse Education Today* 31 (2011), p. 634.

Brown, George. 'The Mental Hospital as an Institution', *Social Science and Medicine* 7 (1973), p. 409.

Brown, June. 'Editorial – Ethical Considerations in Historical Research', *American Association for the History of Nursing Bulletin* 38 (1993), p. 1-2.

Busfield, Joan. *Managing Madness: Changing Ideas and Practice* (London, 1986).

Busfield, Joan. 'Restructuring Mental Health Services', in Marijke Gijswijt-Hofstra and Roy Porter (eds), *Cultures of Psychiatric and Mental Health Care in Post-War Britain and the Netherlands* (Amsterdam, 1998), p. 16.

Butler, Tom. *Mental Health, Social Policy and the Law* (Basingstoke, 1985).

Butt, Gavin, *Between You and Me: Queer Discourses in the New York Art World, 1948-1963* (Durham, 2005).

Cameron, John L. and Laing, Robert D. 'Effects of Environmental Change in the Care of Chronic Schizophrenics', *The Lancet* (1955), pp. 1384-1386.

Cant, Bob. *Footsteps and Witnesses: Lesbian and Gay Life Stories from Scotland* (Edinburgh, 1993).

Carpenter, Mick. *They Still Go Marching On* (London, 1985).

Chatterton, Claire. "'Caught in the Middle"? Mental Nurse Training in England 1919–51', *Journal of Psychiatric and Mental Health Nursing* 11 (2004), p. 32.

Chatterton, Claire. "'A Thorn in its Flesh?" Maud Wiese and the General Nursing Council', *The Bulletin of the UK Association for the History of Nursing* 1 (1) (2012), p. 41.

Chatterton, Claire. "'An Unsuitable Job for a Woman?": Gender and Mental Health Nursing', *The Bulletin of the UK Association for the History of Nursing* 2 (2013), pp. 4–49.

Church, Oscar M. and Johnson, Michael L. 'Worth Remembering: the Process and Products of Oral History', *International History of Nursing Journal* 1 (1) (1995), p. 22.

Clarke, Daniel F. 'Fetishism Treated by Negative Conditioning', *British Journal of Psychiatry* 109 (1963), pp. 404–408.

Clark Hine, Darlene. 'Reflections on Nurse Rivers', in Susan M. Reverby (ed.), *Tuskegee's Truths: Rethinking the Tuskegee Syphilis Study* (London. 2000), pp. 386–398.

Clarke, Basil. *Mental Disorder in Early Britain* (Cardiff, 1975).

Clendinen, Dudley and Nagourney, Adam. *Out for Good: The Struggle to Build a Gay Rights Movement in America* (New York, 1999).

Cocks, Harry. 'Review: The Growing Pains of the History of Sexuality', *Journal of Contemporary History* 39 (4) (2004), p. 665.

Cocks, Harry. 'Secrets, Crimes and Diseases, 1800–1914', in Matt Cook (ed.) *A Gay History of Britain, Love and Sex Between Men Since the Middle Ages* (Oxford, 2007), p. 110.

Cocks, Harry. *Nameless Offences: Homosexual Desire in the 19th Century* (London, 2010), p. 17.

Connerton, Paul. *How Societies Remember* (Cambridge, 1989).

Conrad, Peter and Schneider, Joseph W. *Deviance and Medicalization: From Badness to Sickness* (Philadelphia, 1980).

Cook, Matt. *London and the Culture of Homosexuality, 1885–1914* (Cambridge, 2003).

Cook, Matt. "'A New City of Friends": London and Homosexuality in the 1890s', *History Workshop Journal* 56 (2003), pp. 33–58.

Cook, Matt. *A Gay History of Britain: Love and Sex between Men since the Middle Ages* (Oxford, 2007).

Cook, Matt, "'Gay Times": Identity, Locality, Memory, and the Brixton Squats in 1970s London', *Twentieth Century History* 9 (2011), pp. 1–26.

Coon, Diane and Mitterer, Jane O. *Introduction to Psychology: Gateways to Mind and Behaviour* (New York, 2009).

Cooper, Angus J. 'A Case of Fetishism and Impotence Treated by Behaviour Therapy', *British Journal of Psychiatry* 109 (1963), pp. 649–653.

Cooper, David. *Psychiatry and Anti-Psychiatry* (London, 1967).

Cooper, Michael., Cooper, Christine and Thompson, Margaret. *Child and Adolescent Mental Health Nursing Theory and Practice* (Oxford, 2005).

Coppen, Allen. 'Body-Build of Male Homosexuals', *British Medical Journal* 26 (1939), pp. 1443–1445.

Costello, John. *Love, Sex & War: Changing Values, 1939–45* (London, 1985).

Crisp, Quentin. *The Naked Civil Servant* (London, 1968).

Crompton, Louis. *Byron and Greek Love: Homophobia in Nineteenth-Century England* (Berkeley, 1985), pp. 158–171.

Crossley, David. 'The Introduction of Leucotomy: A British Case History', *History of Psychiatry* iv (1993), p. 557.

Crossley, Nick. 'R. D. Laing and The British Anti-Psychiatry Movement: a Socio-Historical Analysis', *Social Science Medical* 47 (7), p. 878.

Crown, Sidney. 'Aversion Therapy for Homosexuality', *British Medical Journal* 31 (1962), p. 943.

Crozier, Ivan. 'Philosophy in the English Boudoir: Havelock Ellis, Love and Pain, and Sexological Discourses on Algophilia', *Journal of the History of Sexuality* 13 (2004), pp. 275–305.

Curran, David and Parr, Daniel. 'Homosexuality: An Analysis of 100 Male Cases seen in Private', *British Medical Journal* 1 (1957), pp. 797–801.

Dale, Pamela and Melling, Joseph. *Mental Illness and Learning Disability Since 1850: Finding a Place from Mental Disorder in the United Kingdom* (London, 2006).

Davidson, Roger. *And Thus will I freely Sing: An Analogy of Gay and Lesbian Writings from Scotland* (Edinburgh, 1989).

Davidson, Roger. 'Law, Medicine and the Treatment of Homosexual Offenders in Scotland, 1950–1980', in Ingrid Goold and Charles Kelly (eds), *Lawyers' Medicine: The Legislature, the Courts & Medical Practice, 1760 – 2000* (Oxford, 2009), p. 129.

Davies, Kerry. 'Silent and Censured Travellers? Narratives and Patients Voices: Perspectives on the History of Mental Health since 1948', *Social History of Medicine* 14 (2) (2001), p. 271.

D'Emilio, John. *Sexual Politics, Sexual Communities* (Chicago, 1998).

D'Emilio, John. 'Afterword: "If I knew then . . .", in Nan A. Boyd and Horacio N. Roque Ramirez (eds), *Bodies of Evidence The Practice of Queer Oral History* (Oxford, 2012), p. 269.

Dennis, Peter. *Daring Hearts: Lesbian and Gay Lives in 50s and 60s Brighton* (Brighton, 1992).

Dickinson, Tommy and Wright, Karen M. 'Stress and Burnout in Forensic Mental Health Nursing: A Review of the Literature', *British Journal of Nursing* 17 (2) (2008), p. 85.

Dickinson, Tommy, 'Nursing History: Aversion Therapy', *Mental Health Practice* 13 (5) (2010), p. 13.

Dickinson, Tommy, Cook, Matt, Playle, John and Hallett, Christine. '"Queer" Treatments: Giving a Voice to Former Patients who Received Treatments for their "Sexual Deviations"', *Journal of Clinical Nursing* 21 (9) (2012), pp. 1345–1354.

Digby, Anne. *Madness, Morality and Medicine: A Study of the York Retreat, 1796–1914* (Cambridge, 1985).

Dimond, Bridget. *Legal Aspects of Nursing* (London, 2004).

Dingwall, Robert., Rafferty, Anne Marie and Webster, Charles. *An Introduction to the Social History of Nursing* (London, 1988).

Doan, Laura and Waters, Chris. 'Homosexuality', in Lucy Bland and Laura Doan (eds) *Sexology Uncensored: The Documents of Sexual Science* (Cambridge, 1998), p. 176.

Dock, Sarah. 'The Relation of the Nurse to the Doctor and the Doctor to the Nurse', *American Journal of Nursing* 17 (1917), p. 394.

Doidge, William T. and Holtzman, Wayne H. 'Implications of Homosexuality Among Air Force Trainees', *Journal of Consulting Psychology* 24 (1) (1960), p. 10.

Drescher, Jack and Merlino, Joseph P. *American Psychiatry and Homosexuality: An Oral History* (New York, 2007).

Drucker, Donna J. 'Male sexuality and Alfred Kinsey's 0–6 scale: Toward "a Sound Understanding of the Realities of Sex"', *Journal of Homosexuality* 57 (2010), pp. 1105–1123.

Drucker, Donna J. *The Machines of Sex Research* (Amsterdam, 2014), p. 30.

Dwyer, Ellen. *Homes for the Mad: Life Inside Two Nineteenth-Century Asylums* (New Brunswick, 1987).

Dyer, Richard. *The Culture of Queers* (London, 2002).

Eisenbach, David. *Gay Power: An American Revolution* (New York, 2006).

Ellis, Havelock and Addington Symonds, John. *Studies in the Psychology of Sex, Vol. 1: Sexual Inversion* (London, 1897).

Ellis, Alan. 'The Effectiveness of Psychotherapy with Individuals who have Severe Homosexual Problems', *Journal of Consulting Psychology* 20 (1956), pp. 58–60.

Erickson, Stacy. *Field Notebook For Oral History*, 2nd edn (Boise, 1993).

Evans, Mary. *Missing Persons: The Impossibility of Auto/Biography* (London, 1998).

Evans, Richard. *In Defence of History* (London, 2001).

Faderman, Lillian. *Surpassing the Love of Man: Romantic Friendship and Love Between Women from Renaissance to the Present* (London, 1985).

Feidson, Eliot. *Profession of Medicine: A Study of the Sociology of Applied Knowledge* (Chicago, 1970), p. 54.

Flemming, Gerald W. T. H., Golla, Fredrick L. and Walter, William. 'Electric-convulsion Therapy of Schizophrenia', *Lancet* II (1939), pp. 1353–1355.

Fogerty, James E. 'Oral History and Archives: Documenting Context', in Thomas L. Charlton, Lois E. Myers and Rebecca Sharpless (eds), *History Of Oral History: Foundations And Methodology* (Lanham, 2007), p. 208.

Foot, Michael. *Aneurin Bevan, 1945–1960* (St Albans, 1975).

Foucault, Michel. *The History of Sexuality, Vol. 1: An Introduction* (Oxford, 1990).

Frankfort-Nachmias, Chava and Nachmias, David. *Research Methods in the Social Sciences.* (London, 1996).

Freeman, Walter and Watts, James. *Psychosurgery: Intelligence, Emotion and Social Behaviour Following Prefrontal Lobotomy for Mental Disorders* (Illinois, 1942).

Freud, Sigmund. *Three Essays on the Theory of Sexuality* (Vienna, 1905).

Freud, Sigmund. 'Some Neurotic Mechanisms in Jealously, Paranoia, and Homosexuality', *The International Journal of Psycho-analysis* (London, 1923), pp. 145–172.

Freud, Sigmund. 'Anonymous (letter to an American Mother)', reprinted in *The Letters of Sigmund Freud* (New York, 1935).

Freund, Kevin. 'Some Problems in the Treatment of Homosexuality', in Henry J. Eysenck (ed.), *Experiments in Behaviour Therapy* (London, 1960), p. 79.

Friedlander, Henry. *The Origins of Nazi Genocide: From Euthanasia to Final Solution* (Chapel Hill, 1995).

Frielander, Peter. 'Theory, Method and Oral History', in Robert Perks and Alistair Thomson *The Oral History Reader* (London, 1998), p. 314.

Gaarder, Jostein. *Sophie's World: A Novel about the History of Philosophy* (London, 1995).

Garber, Marjorie. *Vested Interests Cross-Dressing and Cultural Anxiety* (London, 1992).

Gillon, Raanan. *Philosophical Medical Ethics* (London, 1986).

Giorno, John. *You Got to Burn to Shine: New Selected Writings* (London, 1974).

Giosca, Nicolai. 'The Gag Reflex and Fellatio', *American Journal of Psychiatry* 107 (1950), p. 380.

Ginzburg, Carlo., Tedeschi, John and Tedeschi, Anne C. 'Microhistory: Two or Three Things That I Know about It', *Critical Inquiry* 20 (1993), pp. 10–35.

Gittins, Diana. *Madness in its Place: Narratives of Severalls Hospital, 1913–1997* (London, 1997).

Gluck, Sherna B. and Patai, Daphne. *Women's Words* (New York, 1991).

Gluck, Sherna B. 'What's So Special About Women?: Women's Oral History', in Susan Hodge Armitage, Patricia Hart and Karen Weathermon (eds), *Women's Oral History: The Frontiers Reader* (Lincoln, 2002), p. 7.

Goffman, Erving. *Asylums* (New York, 1961).

Goffman, Erving. *Stigma: Notes on the Management of Spoiled Identity* (Harmondsworth, 1963).

Goldhagen, Daniel J. *Hitler's Willing Executioners: Ordinary Germans and the Holocaust* (London, 1996).

Golla, Francis and Sessions-Hodge, Robert. 'Hormone Treatment of the Sexual Offender', *The Lancet* 11 (1949), pp. 1006–1007.

Gould, Debby. 'Professional Dominance and Subversion in Maternity Services', *British Journal of Midwifery* 16 (2008), p. 4.

Green, Anna. '"Unpacking" the Stories', in Anna Green and Megan Hutching (eds), *Remembering: Writing Oral History* (Auckland, 2004), p. 11.

Grele, Ronald K. *International Annual of Oral History, 1990: Subjectivity and Multiculturalism in Oral History* (New York, 1992).

Griffiths, Olive, Reid, Norman and Scott, Margaret. 'Reconstruction Scheme for Mental Nursing', *Nursing Mirror* (27 October 1945), pp. 46–47.

Hall Carpenter Archives Gay Men's Oral History Group, *Walking After Midnight: Gay Men's Life Stories* (London, 1989).

Hall, Lesley. *Sex Gender and Social Change Since 1880* (Basingstoke, 2000).

Hallett, Christine. 'The 'Manchester scheme': A Study of the Diploma in Community Nursing, The First Pre-Registration Nursing Programme in a British University', *Nursing Inquiry* 12 (4) (2005), p. 292.

Hallett, Christine. 'Colin Fraser Brockington (1903–2004) and the Revolution in Nurse-Education', *Journal of Medical Biography* 16 (2008), p. 89.

Hammonds, Evelyn M. 'Your Silence Will Not Protect You: Nurse Rivers and the Tuskegee Syphilis Study', in Susan M. Reverby (ed.), *Tuskegee's Truths: Rethinking the Tuskegee Syphilis Study* (London. 2000), pp. 340–347.

Haravan, Tamara. 'From Amoskeag to Nishijin: Reflections on Life History Interviewing in Two Cultures', in Ronald K Grele (ed.), *International Annual of Oral History, 1990: Subjectivity and Multiculturalism in Oral History* (New York, 1992), pp. 9–42.

Hegarty, Peter. *Gentlemen's Disagreement: Alfred Kinsey, Lewis Terman, and the Sexual Politics of Smart Men* (Chicago, 2013).

Heger, Heinz. *The Men with the Pink Triangle* (Boston, 1980).

Henry, George. 'Psychogenic Factors in Overt Homosexuality', *American Journal of Psychiatry* xiii (1940), p. 57.

Higgins, Patrick, *Heterosexual Dictatorship: Male Homosexuality in Postwar Britain* (London, 1996).

Hirschfeld, Magnus. *Transvestites: The Erotic Drive to Cross Dress* (London, 1991).

Hooker, Evelyn. 'Male Homosexuality in the Rorschach', *Journal of Projective Techniques* 21 (1957), pp. 18–31.

Holloway, Immy. *Qualitative Research in Health Care* (New York, 2005).

Hopkins, Harry. *The New Look* (London, 1963).

Hopton, John. 'Daily Life in a 20th Century Psychiatric Hospital: An Oral History of Prestwich Hospital', *International History of Nursing Journal* 2 (3) (1997), p. 33.

Hopton, John. 'Prestwich Hospital in the Twentieth Century: A Case Study of Slow and Uneven Progress in the Development of Psychiatric Care', *History of Psychiatry* (1999), p. 351.

Houlbrook, Matt. *Queer London: Perils and Pleasures in the Sexual Metropolis, 1918–1957* (Chicago, 2005).

Houlbrook, Matt and Waters, Chris. 'The Heart in Exile: Detachment and Desire in 1950s London', *History Workshop Journal* 62 (2006), p. 145.

Howard, Joanne and Brooking, Julia I. 'The Career Paths of Nursing Graduates from Chelsea College, University of London', *International Journal of Nursing Studies* 24 (3) (1987), p. 183.

Hughes, Everett C. 'Work and the Self', in John H. Rohrer and Muzafer Sherif (eds), *Social Psychology at the Crossroads* (New York, 1951), pp. 313–323.

Hughes, Everett C. *Men and their Work* (Glencoe, 1958).

Hunter, Richard. 'The Rise and Fall of Mental Nursing', *The Lancet* 1 (1956), p. 3.

Hutchinson, Sally. 'Responsible Subversion: A Study of Rule-Bending Among Nurses', *Scholarly Inquiry for Nursing Practice: An International Journal* 4 (1990), pp. 3–17.

Hutchinson, Sally. 'Nurses and Bending the Rules', *Creative Nursing* 4 (2004), pp. 4–8.

Hutton, Emanon L. and Fox, Gerald W. T. H. 'Early Results Of Prefrontal Leucotomy', *The Lancet* ccxli (1941), pp. 3–7.

Hyde, Montgommery. *The Other Love: An Historical and Contemporary Survey of Homosexuality in Britain* (London, 1970).

Illich, Ivan. Medical Nemesis: The Expropriation of Health (London, 1976).

Irwin, Barbara J. and Burckhardt, Judith A. *NCLEX-RN Strategies for the Registered Nursing Licensing Exam* (New York, 2008).

Jackson, Paul. *One of the Boys Homosexuality in the Military during World War II* (Montreal, 2010).

James, Basil. 'Case of Homosexuality Treated by Aversion Therapy', *British Medical Journal*, 17 (1962), p. 768.

James, Basil and Early, Donal F. 'Aversion Therapy for Homosexuality', *British Medical Journal* 23 (1963), p. 538.

James, Francis E. 'Insulin Treatment in Psychiatry', *History of Psychiatry* iii (1992), p. 221.

Jeffery-Poulter, Stephen. *Peers, Queers & Commons. The Struggle for Gay Law Reform from 1950 to the Present* (London, 1991), pp. 169–172.

Jenkins, Keith and Munslow, Alan. *Re-Thinking History* (London, 2003).

Jenkins, Keith. *Why History? Ethics and Postmodernity* (London, 1999).

Jivani, Alkarim. *It's Not Unusual: A History of Lesbian and gay Britain in the Twentieth Century* (London, 1997).

Jones, Ernest. *The Life and Work of Sigmund Freud* (London, 1964).

Jones, James H. *Bad Blood: the Tuskegee Syphilis Experiment* (New York, 1981).

Jones, Karen. 'The Culture of the Mental Hospital', in German E. Berrios and Hugh Freeman (eds) *150 Years of British Psychiatry 1841–1991* (London, 1991), p. 124.

Jones, Kathleen. *Mental Health & Social Policy, 1845–1959* (London, 1960).

Jones, Kathleen. *A History of Mental Health Services* (London, 1972).

Jones, Maxwell. *Social Psychiatry in Practice: The Idea of a Therapeutic Community* (Harmondsworth, 1968).

Jones, Paul. *Tales from Out in the City* (Manchester, 2009).

Jones, Wilfred L. *Ministering to Minds Diseased: A History of Psychiatric Treatment* (London, 1983).

Jordanova, Ludmilla. *History in Practice* (London, 2000).

Kahn, Charles. *World Histories: Societies Of The Past*, 2nd edn (Winnipeg, 2005).

Kameny, Frank. 'Psychiatrists Re-evaluate: Aftermath of Gay Zapping', *Vector* 7 (1971), p. 21.

Kantrovich, Nvzia V. 'An Attempt at Associate Reflex Therapy in Alcoholism', *Psychology Abstracts* 4282 (1930), p. 26.

Kaplan, Morris B. *Sodom and the Thames. Sex, Love and Scandal in Wilde Times* (New York, 2005), p. 23.

Kelley, Donald and Sacks, David. *The Historical Imagination in Early Modern Britain* (Cambridge, 1997).

Kelman, Herbert C. and Hamilton, Lee. *Crimes of Obedience: Toward a Social Psychology of Authority and Responsibility* (New Haven, 1989).

Kennedy, Elizabeth Lapovsky. 'Telling Tales: Oral History and the Construction of Pre-Stonewall Lesbian History', in Robert Perks and Alistair Thomson (eds), *The Oral History Reader*, 2nd edn (Oxon, 2006), p. 281.

Khulman, Thomas L. 'Gallows Humour for a Scaffold Setting: Managing Aggressive Patients on a Maximum Security Forensic Ward', *Hospital and Community Psychiatry* 39 (10) (1988), p. 1085.

King, Michael and Bartlett, Annie. 'British Psychiatry and Homosexuality', *British Journal of Psychiatry* 175 (1999), pp. 106–113.

King, Michael. *Wrestling with the Angel: A Life of Janet Frame* (Auckland, 2000).

King, Michael. 'Dropping the Diagnosis of Homosexuality: Did it Change the Lot of Gays and Lesbians in Britain?', *Australian and New Zealand Journal of Psychiatry* 37 (6) (2003), pp. 684–688.

King, Michael, Smith, Glenn and Bartlett, Annie. 'Treatments of Homosexuality in Britain since the 1950s – An Oral History: the Experience of Professionals', *British Medical Journal* 1136 (2004), pp. 187–201.

Kinsey, Alfred, Pomeroy, Warren and Martin, Clyde. *Sexual Behaviour in the Human Male* (Philadelphia, 1948).

Kirby, Stephanie. 'The Resurgence of Oral History and the New Issues it Raises', *Nurse Researcher* 5 (1997), p. 47.

Korman, Nancy and Glennerster, Howard. *Hospital Closure* (Milton Keynes, 1990).

Koven, Seth. *Slumming, Sexual and Social Politics in Victorian London* (Princetown, 2004).

Kraft-Ebing, Richard von. *Psychopathia Sexualis* (Philadelphia, 1892).

Kragh, Jesper Vaczy, 'Shock Therapy in Danish Psychiatry', *Medical History* 54 (2010), pp. 341–364.

Laing, Ronald David. *Sanity, Madness and the Family* (London, 1964).

Lindley, Peter. 'Sexual Deviation in a Young Man', *Nursing Mirror* 8 (1977), p. 63.

Lomax, Montagu. *The Experiences of an Asylum Doctor* (London, 1921).

Longhran, Tracey. 'Hysteria and Neurasthenia in pre-1914 British Medical Discourse and in Histories of Shell-Shock', *History of Psychiatry* 19 (2008), pp. 25–46.

Luker, Karen A. 'Reading Nursing: The Burden of Being Different', *International Journal of Nursing Studies* 21 (1984), pp. 1–17.

Macnicol, John. 'Eugenics and the Campaign for Voluntary Sterilization in Britain Between the Wars', *The Society for the History of Medicine* (1989), pp. 147–169.

March, Sue. *Gay Liberation* (New York, 1974).

Marwick, Arthur. *New Nature of History* (Chicago, 2001).

Max, Louis W. M. 'Breaking up a Homosexual Fixation by the Conditional Reaction Technique: A Case Study', *Psychological Bulletin* 32 (1935), p. 734.

McConaghy, Neil. 'Is Homosexual Orientation Irreversible?', *British Journal of Psychiatry* 129 (1976), pp. 356–563.

McCulloch, Michael J. and Feldman, Michael P. 'Aversion Therapy in Management of 43 Homosexuals', *British Medical Journal* 4 (1967), pp. 595–597.

McFarland-Icke, Bronwyn Rebekah. *Nurses in Nazi Germany: A Moral Choice in History* (Princeton, 1999).

McGuire, Robert J. and Vallance, Michael. 'Aversion Therapy by Electric Shock: a Simple Technique', *British Medical Journal* 1 (1964), pp. 151–153.

McKenna, Neil. *Fanny and Stella: The Young Men Who Shocked Victorian England* (London, 2013).

McKie, Andrew. '"The Demolition of a Man": Lessons Learnt from Holocaust Literature for the Teaching of Nursing Ethics', *Nursing Ethics* 11 (2004), p. 141.

McLaren, Angus. *The Trials of Masculinity: Policing Sexual Boundaries, 1870–1930* (Chicago, 1997).

Medico-Psychological Association, *The Handbook for the Instruction of Attendants on the Insane* (London, 1885).

Milgram, Stanley. *Obedience to Authority: An Experimental View* (New York, 1969).

Minister, Kristina. 'A Feminist Frame for the Oral History Interview', in Sherna Gluck and Daphne Patai (eds), *Women's Words* (New York, 1991), pp. 111–119.

Minton Henry, L. 'Community Empowerment and the Medicalization of Homosexuality: constructing sexual identities in the 1930s', *Journal of the History of Sexuality* 6 (1996), pp. 435–458.

Minton, Henry. *Departing from Deviance* (Chicago, 2002).

Moran, Carmen. and Massam, Margaret. 'An Evaluation of Humour in Emergency Work', *The Australian Journal of Disaster and Trauma Studies* 3 (1997), pp. 176–179.

Mort, Frank. *Capital Affairs: London and the Making of the Permissive Society* (New Haven, 2010).

Moss, Winnifred W. *Oral History Programme Manual* (New York, 1974).

Munhall, Patricia. 'Moral Reasoning Levels in Nursing Students and Faculty in a Baccalaureate Nursing Programme', *Image* 12 (1980), pp. 57–61.

Neushul, Peter. 'Fighting Research: Army Participation in the Clinical Testing and Mass Production of Penicillin During The Second World War', in Roger Cooter, Mark Harrison and Steve Sturdy (eds), *War, Medicine & Modernity* (Stroud, 1998), pp. 203–224.

Newburn, Tim. *Permission and Regulation: Law and Morals in Post-war Britain* (London, 1992).

Nolan, Peter. 'Mental Nurse Training in the 1920s', *History of Nursing Group of the Royal College of Nursing* 10 (1986), p. 18.

Nolan, Peter. 'Jack's Story', *Royal College of Nursing The History of Nursing Group* 2 (2) (1987), pp. 22–28.

Nolan, Peter. 'Attendant Dangers', *Nursing Times* 85 (12) (1989), pp. 56–59.

Nolan, Peter. 'A History of the Training of Asylum Nurses', *Journal of Advanced Nursing*, 18 (1993), p. 1197.

Nolan, Peter. *A History of Mental Health Nursing* (London, 1993).

Nolan, Peter. 'Reflections of a Mental Nurse in the 1950s', *Royal College of Nursing History of Nursing Journal* 5 (1994), pp. 150–156.

Nolan, Peter. 'Mental Health Nursing – Origins and Developments', in Monica E. Baly (ed), *Nursing & Social Change* (New York, 1995), p. 254.

Nolan, Peter. 'The Development of Mental Health Nursing', in Jerome Carson, Leonard Fagin and Susan A. Ritter (eds), *Stress and Coping in Mental Health Nursing* (London, 1995), p. 13.

Nolan, Peter. 'Swing and Roundabouts: Mental Health Nursing and the Birth of the NHS', *Mental Health Care* 1 (1998), pp. 371–374.

Nolan, Peter and Chung, Cheung. 'Science and Early Development of Mental Health Nursing', *Nursing Standard* 10 (48) (1996), pp. 157–161.

Nolan Peter and Hopper, Barone. 'Mental Health Nursing in the 1950s and 1960s Revisited', *Journal of Psychiatric and Mental Health Nursing* 4 (1997), p. 334.

Norton, Rictor. *Mother Clap's Molly House: The Gay Subculture in England, 1700–1830* (London, 1992).

Nursing Times, 'Friends of Menston Hospital', *Nursing Times* (28 November 1953), pp. 1215–1216.

Nye, Robert. *Sexuality* (Oxford, 2000).

Oswald, Isaac. 'Induction of Illusory and Hallucinatory Voices with Consideration of Behaviour Therapy', *Journal of Mental Science* 108 (1962), pp. 196–212.

Palmer, Michelle, Esolen, Marianne, Rose, Susan, Fishman, Andrea and Bartoli, Jill. "'I Haven't Anything to Say": Reflections of Self and Community in Collecting Oral Histories', in Ronald K. Grele (ed.), *International Annual of Oral History, 1990: Subjectivity and Multiculturalism in Oral History* (New York, 1992), pp. 9–42.

Parahoo, Kadar. *Nursing Research: Principles, Process and Issues* (London, 1997).

Partridge, Eric. *Dictionary of the Underworld* (Wordsworth, 1995).

Pattinson, Juliette. *Behind Enemy Lines: gender, passing and the special operations executive in the Second World War* (Manchester, 2007).

Patton, Michael. *Qualitative Research and Evaluation Methods* (Oxford, 2002).

Penn, Donna. 'Queer: Theorising Politics and History', *Radical History Review* 63 (1995), p. 30–31.

Perks, Robert and Thomson, Alistair. *The Oral History Reader* (London, 1998).

Perks, Robert and Thomson, Alistair. *The Oral History Reader*, 2nd edn (Oxon, 2006).

Peters, Jess J., Olansky, Sidney, Cutler, John C. and Gleeson, Geraldine. 'Untreated Syphilis in the Male Negro: Pathologic Findings in Syphilitic and Nonsyphilitic Patients', *Journal of Chronic Disease* 1 (1955), pp. 127–148.

Phelan, Jo C., Link, Bruce G., Pescosolido, Ann and Stueve, Bernice A. 'Public Conceptions of Mental Illness in 1950: What is Mental Illness and is it to be Feared?', *Journal of Health and Social Behaviour* 41 (2) (2000), p. 188.

Plant, Richard. *The Pink Triangle* (New York, 1986).

Plummer, Ken. *Telling Sexual Stories: Power, Change and Social World* (London, 1995).

Portelli, Alessandro, 'What Makes Oral History Different?', in Robert Perks and Alistair Thompson (eds), *The Oral History Reader*, 2nd edn (London, 1998), pp. 32–42.

Porter, Roy. 'The Patients View: Doing History from Below', *Theory and Society* 14 (2) (1985), pp. 175–198.

Porter, Kevin and Weeks, Jeffery. *Between the Acts: Lives of Homosexual Men, 1885–1967* (London, 1991).

Porter, Roy. *Madness: A Brief History* (Oxford, 2002).

Povinelli Elizabeth A. and Chauncey, George. 'Thinking Sexually Transitionally: An Introduction', *Journal of Lesbian and Gay Studies* 5 (1999), pp. 439–449.

Power, Lisa, *No Bath But Plenty of Bubbles: stories from the London Gay Liberation Front, 1970–73* (London, 1995).

Pressman, Jack D. *Last Resort: Psychosurgery and the Limits of Medicine* (Cambridge, 1998).

Rachman, Stanley. 'Aversion Therapy: Chemical or Electrical?', *Behaviour Research and Therapy* 2 (1965), p. 289.

Raymond, Michael. 'Case of Fetishism Treated by Aversion Therapy', *British Medical Journal* 2 (1956), pp. 854–846.

Rijlaarsdam, Gert., Van den Bergh, Huub and Couzijn, Michel. *Effective Learning and Teaching of Writing: a Handbook of Writing in Education* (New York, 2005).

Ritchie, Donald A. *Doing Oral History: A Practical Guide* (New York, 2003).

Rees, Percy T. 'Symposium on Prefrontal Leucotomy', *Journal of Mental Science* xc (1943), p. 161.

Rees, Tudor and Usill, Harley. *They Stand Apart: a Critical Survey of the Problem of Homosexuality* (London, 1955).

Reverby, Susan M. 'Rethinking the Tuskegee Syphilis Study: Nurse Rivers, Silence, and the Meaning of Treatment', in Susan M. Reverby (ed.), *Tuskegee's Truths: rethinking the Tuskegee Syphilis Study* (London. 2000), pp. 365–387.

Robb, Barbara. *Sans Everything: a Case to Answer* (London, 1967).

Rogers, Carl. *Becoming a Person: a Therapist's View on Psychotherapy* (New York, 1995).

Rollin, Henry R. 'The Red Handbook: an Historic Centenary', *Bulletin of the Royal College of Psychiatrists*, 10 (1986), pp. 65–81.

Roseman, Mark. 'Surviving Memory', in Robert Perks and Alistair Thompson (eds) *The Oral History Reader*, 2nd edn (Oxon, 2006) p. 242.

Rosen, Ismond. *Sexual Deviation* (Oxford, 1979).

Royal Medico-Psychological Association, *Handbook for Mental Nurses* (London, 1923/1939).

Rubenstein, Charlie R. 'Psychotherapeutic Aspects of Male Homosexuality', *British Journal of Medical Psychology* 31 (1958), pp. 14–18.

Rumbold, Graham. *Ethics in Nursing Practice* (Edinburgh, 1999).

Russell, Geoff F. M. *Policy for Action* (London, 1973).

Safier, Gina. 'What is Nursing History? What are the Advantages and Disadvantages of Oral History? How can it be used in Nursing History?', *Nurse Researcher* 25 (5) (1976), p. 384.

Sandbrook, Dominic. *White Heat: A History of Britain in the Swinging Sixties* (London, 2006).

Sandelowski, Marguerite. 'Focus on Qualitative Methods: Sample Size in Qualitative Research', *Nursing and Health* 18 (1999), pp. 179–183.

Schacter, Daniel. *Searching for Memory: The Brain, the Mind, and the Past* (New York, 1996).

Scott, Joan W. 'The Evidence of Experience', *Critical Inquiry* 17 (4) (1991), p. 776.

Scott, Paul D. *Definition, Classification, Prognosis and Treatment of Sexual Deviation* (London, 1964).

Scull, Andrew. 'Desperate Remedies: a Gothic Tale of Madness and Modern Medicine', *Psychological Medicine* 17 (1987), p. 562.

Scull, Andrew. *The Most Solitary of Afflictions: Madness and Society in Britain, 1700-1900* (New Haven, 1993).

Seager, Charles P. 'Aversion Therapy in Psychiatry', *Nursing Times* 26 (1965), pp. 421–424.

Sears, James. *Lonely Hunters: An Oral History of Lesbian and Gay Southern Life, 1948–1968* (Boulder, 1997).

Sears, James T. *Edwin and John: A Personal History of the American South* (New York, 2009).

Sedgwick, Eve K. *Epistemology of the Closet* (London, 1990).

Seel, Pierre. *I, Pierre Seel, Deported Homosexual* (New York, 1994).

Seldon, Anthony and Pappworth, Joanna. *By Word Of Mouth: 'Elite' Oral History* (New York, 1983).

Shorter, Edward. *History of Psychiatry: From the Era of Asylum to the Age of Prozac* (New York, 1997).

Silverstein, Christine M. 'From the Front Lines to the Home Front: A History of the Development of Psychiatric Nursing in the U.S. During the World War II Era', *Issues in Mental Health Nursing* 29 (2008), pp. 719–737.

Sinfield, Alan. *Out on Stage: Lesbian and Gay Theatre in the Twentieth Century* (New Heaven, 1999).

Skeggs, Beverley. *Formations of Class and Gender: Becoming Respectable* (London, 1997).

Skinner, Robert B. *Science and the Human Behaviour* (New York, 1953), pp. 34–37.

Smith, Glenn., King, Michael and Bartlett, Annie. 'Treatments of Homosexuality in Britain since the 1950s – An Oral History: the Experience of Patients', *British Medical Journal*, 1136 (2004).

Smith, Susan L. 'Neither Victim nor Villain: Eunice Rivers and Public Health Work', in Susan M. Reverby (ed.), *Tuskegee's Truths: Rethinking the Tuskegee Syphilis Study* (London. 2000), pp. 348–364.

Stacey, Judith. 'Can There Be a Feminist Ethnography?', in Sherna Gluck and Daphne Patai (eds) *Women's Words* (New York, 1991), pp. 111–119.

Stanley, Liz. *Sex Surveyed 1949–1994: from Mass Observations: "Little Kinsey" to the National Surveys and Hite Report* (London, 1995).

Starns, Penny. 'Fighting Militarism? British Nursing During The Second World War', in Roger Cooter, Mark Harrison and Steve Sturdy (eds), *War, Medicine & Modernity* (Stroud, 1998), p. 192.

Steppe, Hilde. *Krankenpflege im Nationalsozialismus* (Frankfurt, 1989).

Steppe, Hilde. 'Nursing in Nazi Germany', *Western Journal of Nursing Research* 14 (1991), p. 745.

Stolorow, Robert D. and Atwood, George E. *Context of Being: The Intersubjective Foundations of Psychological Life* (Hillsdale, 1992).

Strom-Olsen, Roger. 'Results of Prefrontal Leucotomy', *Journal of Mental Science* lxxxix (1943), p. 491.

Sugden, John, Bessant, Andrew, Eastland, Mike and Field, Ray. *A Handbook for Psychiatric Nurses* (London, 1986), pp. 219–220.

Sulloway, Frank J. *Freud Biologist of the Mind* (London, 1979), p. 297.

Summerfield, Penny. '*Reconstructing Women's Wartime Lives*' (Manchester, 1998).

Summerfield, Penny. 'Culture and Composure: Creating Narratives of the Gendered Self in Oral History Interviews', *Cultural and Social History* 1 (2004), p. 69.

Szasz, Thomas S. *The Myth of Mental Illness: Foundations of Theory and Personal Conduct* (New York, 1961).

Szreter, Simon and Fisher, Kate. *Sex Before the Sexual Revolution: Intimate Life in England, 1918–1963* (Cambridge, 2010), p. 6.

Taylor, Barbara. 'The Demise of the Asylum in Late Twentieth-Century Britain: A Personal History', *Transactions of the Royal Historical Society* XXI (2011), pp. 193–216.

Terry Jennifer, 'Lesbians under the Medical Gaze: Scientists Search for Remarkable Differences', *The Journal of Sex Research* 27 (1990), pp. 317–339.

Thomas, Philip and Bracken, Patrick. 'Critical Psychiatry in Practice', *Advances in Psychiatric Treatment* 10 (2004), p. 366.

Thomson, Alistair. 'Fifty Years On: An International Perspective on Oral History', *The Journal of American History* September (1998), pp. 584–588.

Thomson, Matthew. 'Sterilization, Segregation and Community Care: Ideology and Solutions to the Problem of Mental Deficiency in Inter-War Britain', *History of Psychiatry* 3 (1992), pp. 473–498.

Thompson, Paul. *The Voice of the Past: Oral History* (Oxford, 2000).

Thorpe, John G., Schmidt, Edward and Castell, David. 'Comparison of Positive and Negative (Aversive) Conditioning in the Treatment of Homosexuality', *Behaviour Research and Therapy* 1 (1963), pp. 357–362.

Tinker, Dorris E. and Ramer, Jeanette C. 'Anorexia Nervosa: Staff Subversion of Therapy', *Journal of Adolescent Health Care* 4 (1983), pp. 35–39.

Tomes, Nancy. *A Generous Confidence: Thomas Story Kirkbride and the Art of Asylum-Keeping, 1840–1883* (Cambridge, 1984).

Tosh, John and Lang, Sean. *The Pursuit of History* (London, 2006).

Towell, David. *Understanding Psychiatric Nursing* (London, 1975).

Trumbach, Randolph. 'London's Sodomites: Homosexual Behaviour and Western Culture in the Eighteenth Century', *Journal of Social History* 11 (1977), pp. 4–5.

Trumbach, Randolph. 'Renaissance Sodomy, 1500–1700', in Matt Cook (ed.), *A Gay History of Britain: Love and Sex Between Men Since the Middle Ages* (Oxford, 2007), pp. 49–50.

Upchurch, Charles. 'Forgetting the Unthinkable: Cross-Dressers and British Society in the Case of the *Queen* vs. *Boulton and Others*', *Gender and History* 12 (2000), p. 127–157.

Uphurch, Charles. 'Politics and the Reporting of Sex Between Men in the 1820s', in Brian Lewis (ed.), *British Queer History: New Approaches and Perspectives* (Manchester, 2013), pp. 17–38.

Vickers, Emma. *Queen and Country: Same-Sex Desires in the British Armed Forces, 1939–1945* (Manchester, 2013).

Vincent, John. *An Intelligent Person's Guide to History* (London, 2005).

Wagner, Philip S. 'Psychiatric Activities During the Normandy Offensive', *Psychiatry* 9 (1946), pp. 348 and 356.

Walk, Alexander. 'The History of Mental Nursing', *The Journal of Mental Science* 107 (1961), p. 10.

Walkowitz, Judith. *Prostitution and Victorian Society: Women, Class and the State* (Cambridge, 1980).

Warren, Carol A. B. *Identity and Community in the Gay World* (New York, 1974).

Waters, Chris. 'Havelock Ellis, Sigmund Freud and the State: Discourses of Homosexual Identity in Interwar Britain', in Lucy Bland and Laura Doan (eds) *Sexology in Culture Labelling Bodies and Desires* (Cambridge, 1998), p. 276.

Waters, Chris. 'Disorders of the Mind, Disorders of the Body Social: Peter Wildeblood and the Making of the Modern Homosexual', in Becky Conekin, Frank Mort and Chris Waters (eds), *Moments of Modernity Reconstructing Britain 1945–1964*. (London, 1999), p. 135.

Watson, John and Rayner, Rosaline. 'Conditioned Emotional Reactions', *Journal of Experimental Psychology* 3 (1920), pp. 1–14.

Webb, Christine. *Communication Skills* (London, 1992).

Webster, Charles. 'Nursing and the Early Crisis of the National Health Service', *The History of Nursing group at the RCN Bulletin* 7 (1985), p. 12–24.

Weeks, Jeffery. *Coming Out: Homosexual Politics in Britain from the Nineteenth Century to Present* (London, 1990).

Weeks, Jeffery and Porter, Kevin. *Between the Acts: Lives of Homosexual Men 1885–1967* (London, 1998).

Weeks Jeffery, *The World We Have Won The Remaking of Erotic and Intimate Life* (London, 2007).

Westwood, Gordon. *Society and the Homosexual* (New York, 1952).

White, Rosemary. *The Effects of the NHS on the Nursing Profession* (London, 1985).

Wildeblood, Peter. *Against the Law: the classic account of a Homosexual in 1950s Britain* (London, 1955).

Wolpe, Joseph. *Psychotherapy by Reciprocal Inhibition* (Stanford, 1958).

Woodward, Mary. 'The Diagnosis and Treatment of Homosexual Offenders', *British Journal of Delinquency* 9 (1958), pp. 44–59.

World Health Organization. *The International Statistical Classification of Diseases, Injuries and Causes of Death* (Geneva, 1949).

World Health Organization. *The International Classification of Diseases version 10 Classification of Mental and Behavioural Disorders* (Geneva, 1992).

Wright, Maurice B. 'Psychological Emergencies in War Time', *British Medical Journal* 9 (1940), p. 576.

Index

Note: 'n' after a page reference indicates the number of a note on that page. Page numbers in *italic* refer to figures.

273

Index

Early, Donal F. 69
ECT *see* electroconvulsive therapy
Eisenbach, David 208, 210, 212, 213
electrical aversion therapy 3, 65, 66, 69, 73–76, *75*, 208, 217, 218–219
electroconvulsive therapy (ECT) 94, 98–100, 104
Ellis, Havelock 20–62
Ely Hospital (Cardiff) 214
emetics 65, 66, 67, 72
epilepsy 97
episiotomies 181
espionage 53
eugenics 45, 82n.45, 149–150
euthanasia 150, 152, 155, 235
exhibitionism 6
Eysenck, Professor Hans 211

family life 48, 49, 79, 231
fetishism 6, 66, 72
film 48, 57, 73, 83n.67–68, 187, 202
First Aid Nursing Yeomanry (FANY) 188, 198n.28
Fisher, Geoffrey, Archbishop of Canterbury 48–49
Fisher, Kate 13
Flemming, Gerald W. T. H. 98
Foucault, Michel 22
Fox, Colin 52
Frame, Janet 100
Frank, Hans 45
free will 5
Freeman, Walter 101, *101*
Freud, Sigmund 22, 23, 62, 63, 211
Freudenberg, Dr 95
Freund, Kevin 66–67
Fryer, Dr John 209–210
Fyfe, Sir David Maxwell 51, 57, 58

Garland, Rodney 56–57, 182
gas chambers 23, 150
'gay', use of term x, 204–205
Gay Activist Alliance (GAA) 210, 211
Gay Community News 212
Gay Liberation Front (GLF) 200, 204, 208, 209, 210

gay liberation movement x, 29, 45, 47, 123, 200, 203–206, 208, 220, 222, 223, 241
Gay News 210
Gay Pride 204
gay rights movement 213
Gay Times 205
gender, and rule-bending behaviour 179, 190, 191, 196–197
Gender Dysphoria 220
gender reassignment surgery (GRS) xi, 9, 237
gender roles 47, 48
General Nursing Council (GNC) 26, 105, 106, 124–126, 164
genocide 150
geriatric patients 213–214
German Criminal Code 45
Gestapo 1, 46, 70, 149, 151
Giosca, Nicolai 42
Gittings, Barbara 209
Gittins, Diana 118
Glaister, John 58–59
Glasgow Daily Record 220
Glasgow Herald 61
Glasgow Royal Mental Hospital 114
Glenside Hospital (Bristol) *68*
Glover, Dr Edward 62
Gluck, Sherna 12
Goffman, Erving 206–207
Gold, Greta 52, 54, 74, 75, 76, 219, 248
Gold, Ron 211, 212
Goldhagen, Daniel 170
Golla, Frederick L. 98
Gould, Debby 180–181
GPs (general practitioners), referral by 77
Granger, Elizabeth 56, 183–184, 185, 186, 187, 188, 189, 190, 192–193, 194, 195, 196, 236, 244–245
Greenwood, James 17
Grele, Ronald K. 11
Griffin, Maude 72, 116, 247–248
Guardian 61, 78, 205

habit training 103, 188
Hallett, Christine 192
Hamilton, Lee 170, 239
Hammonds, Evelyn 154
Harrington, Valerie 93, 125, 129